AF737839

PARTNERSHIPS IN RESEARCH, CLINICAL, AND EDUCATIONAL SETTINGS

Advances in Applied Developmental Psychology

Irving E. Sigel, Series Editor

Vol. 1, *Advances in Applied Developmental Psychology,*
edited by Irving E. Sigel, 1985

Vol. 2, *Continuity and Discontinuity of Experience in Child Care,*
edited by Donald Peters and Susan Kontos, 1987

Vol. 3, *Parent Education as Early Childhood Intervention: Emerging Directions in Theory, Research and Practice,*
edited by Douglas R. Powell, 1988

Vol. 4, *Ethics in Applied Developmental Psychology: Emerging Issues in an Emerging Field,*
edited by Celia B. Fisher and Warren W. Tryon, 1990

Vol. 5, *Parent–Child Socialization in Diverse Cultures,*
edited by Jaipaul L. Roopnarine and D. Bruce Carter, 1992

Vol. 6, *The Psychological Development of Low Birthweight Children,*
edited by Sarah L. Friedman and Marian D. Sigman, 1992

Vol. 7, *Coming Home to Preschool: The Sociocultural Context of Early Education,*
edited by Richard N. Roberts, 1993

Vol. 8, *Child Abuse, Child Development, and Social Policy,*
edited by Dante Cicchetti and Sheree L. Toth, 1993

Vol. 9, *Two-Generation Programs for Families in Poverty: A New Intervention Strategy,*
edited by Sheila Smith, 1995

Vol. 10, *Sibling Relationships: Their Causes and Consequences,*
edited by Gene H. Brody, 1996

Vol. 11, *Interacting with Video,*
edited by Patricia Greenfield and Rodney R. Cocking, 1996

Vol. 12, *Mastery Motivation: Origins, Conceptualizations, and Applications,*
edited by Robert H. MacTurk and George A. Morgan, 1995

Vol. 13, *Applied Developmental Science: Graduate Training for Diverse Disciplines and Educational Settings,*
edited by Celia B. Fisher, John P. Murray, and Irving E. Sigel, 1996

Vol. 14, *Caribbean Families: Diversity Among Ethnic Groups,*
edited by Jaipaul R. Roopnarine and Janet Brown, 1997

Vol. 15, *Verbal Interaction and Development in Families with Adolescents,*
edited by Manfred Hofer, James Youniss, and Peter Noack, 1998

Vol. 16, *Children of the Dispossessed: Far-West Preschoolers 30 Years On, Second Edition*,
by Barry Nurcombe, Philip DeLacey, and Susan-Lee Walker, 1999

Vol. 17, *Where Children Live: Solutions for Serving Young Children and Their Families*,
edited by Richard N. Roberts and Phyllis R. Magrab, 1999

Vol. 18, *Partnerships in Research, Clinical, and Educational Settings*,
edited by Roger Bibace, James J. Dillon, and Barbara Noel Dowds, 1999

Forthcoming:

Vol. 19, *Communication: An Arena of Development*,
edited by Nancy Budwig, Ina C. Uzgiris, and James V. Wertsch

Vol. 20, *The Guided Acquisition of First Language Skills*,
by Ernst L. Moerk

PARTNERSHIPS IN RESEARCH, CLINICAL, AND EDUCATIONAL SETTINGS

edited by
Roger Bibace
Clark University

James J. Dillon
State University of West Georgia

and Barbara Noel Dowds
Regis College

Ablex Publishing Corporation
Stamford, Connecticut

Copyright © 1999 by Ablex Publishing Corporation

All rights reserved. No part of this publication may be reproduced, stored in a retrieval system, or transmitted, in any form or by any means, electronic, mechanical, photocopying, microfilming, recording or otherwise, without permission of the publisher.

Printed in the United States of America

Library of Congress Cataloguing-in-Publication Data

Partnerships in research, clinical, and educational settings / edited by Roger Bibace, James J. Dillon, Barbara Noel Dowds.

p. cm. —(Advances in applied developmental psychology; v. 18)

Includes bibliographical references and index.

ISBN 1-56750-454-X (cloth)—ISBN 1-56750-455-8 (pbk.)

1. Interpersonal relations. 2. Research—Psychological aspects. 3. Research—Social aspects. 4. Teacher—student relationships. 5. Physician and patient. I. Bibace, Roger. II. Dillon, James J. III. Dowds, Barbara Noel. IV. Series: Advances in applied developmental psychology (1993); v. 18.

HM1106.P37 1999

302—dc21 99-26833

CIP

Ablex Publishing Corporation
100 Prospect Street
P.O. Box 811
Stamford, Connecticut 06904-0811

To Ruth, my partner-in-life who makes good things happen. To my daughters, Amy and Sandra, their husbands, Donald and Ronnie, and to my son Mark, all of whom educated me over the years. To my grandchildren, Zach, Haleigh, and Sam, who ask intriguing questions and give stimulating answers.

Roger Bibace

I dedicate this volume to Professor Ina C. Uzgiris who taught me not only what it means to think developmentally, but how to be in the world in an honest, scholarly, and graceful way.

James J. Dillon

To my children, Julie, Jonathan, and Benjamin, whose probing questions and creative ideas have helped me to see the wisdom of "novices" and the wonders of partnerships. Your enduring curiosity, lively humor, and clear sense of self have enriched my life immeasurably.

Barbara Noel Dowds

CONTENTS

CONTRIBUTORS

This volume contains a total of 21 contributors, only 3 of which are not directly related to Clark University in some way. Therefore, this volume is definitely within the "Clark family."

Dita G. Andersson, School of Education, Boston College, 140 Commonwealth Avenue, Chestnut Hill, MA 02467

Nicholas H. Apostoleris, Frances L. Hiatt School of Psychology, Clark University, 950 Main Street, Worcester, MA 01610

Roger Bibace, Frances L. Hiatt School of Psychology, Clark University, 950 Main Street, Worcester, MA 01610

Mary Davis, Frances L. Hiatt School of Psychology, Clark University, 950 Main Street, Worcester, MA 01610

James J. Dillon, Department of Psychology, State University of West Georgia, 1600 Maple Street, Carrollton, GA 30118

Barbara Noel Dowds, Regis College, 235 Wellesley Street, Weston, MA 02193

Monica H. Ferraro, Frances L. Hiatt School of Psychology, Clark University, 950 Main Street, Worcester, MA 01610

Marion Reynolds Guerra, Goddard School of Science and Technology, 13 Richards Street, Worcester, MA 01610

Christina Hatgis, Frances L. Hiatt School of Psychology, Clark University, 950 Main Street, Worcester, MA 01610

Leslie Rupert Herrenkohl, Educational Psychology, University of Washington, P.O. Box 353600, Seattle, WA 98195-3600

Laura Johnson, J. Fitzgerald Elementary School, 140 Beal Road, Waltham, MA 02453

James D. Laird, Frances L. Hiatt School of Psychology, Clark University, 950 Main Street, Worcester, MA 01610

Robert F. Leeman, Psychology Department, Brandeis University, Waltham, MA 02154

Joseph McInerney, McCarthy-Towne School, Charter Road, Acton, MA 01720

Patricia Quinn, School of Law, Northeastern University, 400 Huntington Avenue, Boston, MA 02115

Johanna Sagarin, Children's Hospital, Fegan 10, 300 Longwood Avenue, Boston, MA 02115

Ximena Soto, Clark University, 950 Main Street, Worcester, MA 01610

Jaan Valsiner, Frances L. Hiatt School of Psychology, Clark University, 950 Main Street, Worcester, MA 01610

Mary E. Walsh, School of Education, Boston College, 140 Commonwealth Avenue, Chestnut Hill, MA 02467

Angela Wiley, Children and Family Research Center, University of Illinois, 1207 W. Oregon Street, Urbana/Champagne, IL 61801

Stephen Dine Young, Department of Psychology, Hanover College, Hanover, IN 47243

FOREWORD

Irving E. Sigel

This volume, edited by Roger Bibace and his colleagues, offers a unique perspective on an oft advocated concept *partnership*. How the Bibace model and the various versions of partnerships presented by the diverse authors in this book differ from the conventional ones, are the frameworks they have developed for ways that individuals from different disciplines or professions can work together on practical problems of mutual concern. What is unique about the partnership constructs as presented in this volume, is that from the authors' point of view, partnership is not synonymous with collaboration or cooperation, but embraces these ideas in a profoundly different way.

In commercial ventures, the goal for partners is to work together in a symmetrical relationship to make the business profitable. The final outcome is materialistic. By contrast, in the professional settings addressed in this volume, partnerships are asymmetrical by convention and expertise, without a materialistic profit as the outcome, but rather some nonmaterial gains in knowledge to solve some human problem. The three settings selected for this volume include partnerships between physician–patient, teacher–student, and researcher–participant, each asymmetrical with one member an expert and the other a novice. The expert contributes to the novice's attainment of a greater degree of expertise by engaging in the partnership arrangement. To achieve a state in which the inequities in terms of status, power, and knowledge exist, a psychological reallocation is required of each member's perspective on the relationship. In the partnership concepts offered in this book, the expert has to relinquish power in the service of engaging the novice, has to accept counter-arguments and differences in viewpoint. The partnership, to be authentic, requires that each participant surrender not only power but also ego in the service of the emerging partnership. The hypothesis to be eventually tested is whether in the short and even the long run such partnership interactions will enhance the quality of the mutual effort. On reflection, the models of partnering the authors propose have a humanistic orientation in which successful partnering requires members to interact within a context of mutual respect, open-mindedness, and dialogue.

Lest these models appear unrealistic and idealized, let me present a hypothetical situation that is prototypic of the partnering concept developed by Bibace and his colleagues. I describe a situation in which an educational researcher wishes to engage a classroom teacher in a joint research project. The researcher, "Dr. R," is interested in studying learning styles in 6th grade children. Dr. R. is an expert in all the necessary bases for undertaking the study, that is, research design, knowing the literature, and so on, but is without firsthand knowledge of the nature of 6th graders. "Mr. T," the teacher, is an expert educator with years of experience in working with 6th grade students. Two experts are now involved, each with different and not necessarily overlapping expertise. The children's feedback regarding their preferred learning styles should also be sought.

The question is, what does it take to make this joint effort a productive partnership in which each of the professionals (and the children who are also participants in the project) will benefit? It requires the application of the principles that Bibace and his colleagues advocate. Dr. R will have to describe his project before finalizing it, thereby profiting from Mr. T's experience if he wants to engage Mr. T. as a true partner and not just as an expediter. It is clear that in order to do this, each partner will have to listen to the other as well as to the children, create shared meanings about the project and its goals, and share information and ideas about ways to proceed. Above all, they will have to work within an ethical framework each agrees on, especially related to the children's psychological welfare and educational experiences.

Reflecting on this situation, one can readily ascertain the need for mutual respect of the professionalism of the other, for sharing some common goals as far as understanding children's learning styles, and for respecting the time commitments of all concerned, that is, not taxing any of the participants beyond a reasonable limit agreed on by the partners. The relationship will continuously evolve from maximal asymmetry to a symmetrical one. Achieving such a working relationship is admittedly time-consuming, but presumed by Bibace and his colleagues to be eminently productive for all.

A number of lingering questions remain within this partnering framework, which are important for filling out the model. What are the responsibilities of each partner to each other and the children (prototypically speaking), after the research is completed? Did they or should they have had this issue attended to before the project began? How are the results to be reported? These are some of the questions to be discussed in this volume in various contexts along with some more basic, practical issues of how to initiate and follow through on partnerships. Are the partnering effort and the inevitable delays in working out the details worth it? Does it compromise or enhance the research? Or, are the usual, conventional procedures, in which investigators ask for permission to go into a classroom to gather the data they want and then disappear, preferable?

In conclusion, Bibace and his colleagues address these questions in their belief that partnering is advantageous in appropriate settings. However, true partnership requires subordination of ego, acceptance of limitation of power and control, listening to the opinions and judgments of others, and willingness to create consensual decisions. Following these principles, the processes of partnering will proceed. Increasingly symmetrical, complementary, and reciprocal dialoguing interactions are needed. Whether and how this ideal state of affairs can be realized is the subtext of the unique proposals and demonstrations described in this volume.

It is a welcome addition to the Advances in Applied Developmental Psychology series by offering another viewpoint in how research and practice in developmental psychology can enrich each other.

PREFACE

This monograph articulates diverse aspects of partnerships compared to traditional relationships between professionals and patients, students, and research participants. The reader should appreciate that neither the editors nor the various contributors subscribe to *one* interpretation of "partnerships." Rather, the editors subscribe to the assumption that there are *multiple* interpretations of partnerships. These differences among editors and contributors are based on many factors. A professional's primary identity as clinician, teacher, and researcher certainly contributes to such different perspectives on partnerships. Or, such differences are correlated with the diverse, sometimes divergent, everyday practices of the contributors. Such practices are influenced by individual value orientations and the institutions in which the contributors work. The hope is that the reader will empathize, resonate, and be stimulated by at least *some* of the possibilities for enacting partnership relationships in their own settings.

Roger Bibace
James J. Dillon
Barbara Noel Dowds

INTRODUCTION: PARTNERSHIP IN THE SOCIAL WORLD: OPPORTUNITIES FOR SCIENCE AND PRACTICE

Jaan Valsiner
Clark University

Human beings are socially interdependent on one another. Yet they simultaneously create social distinctions among themselves that are the basis of creating new relations across these distinctions. Individuals join various kinds of joint efforts toward shared goals, and become partners to one another.

The present volume is a good example of partnership in action. The reader enters into the world of the reality of the "doing" of science in psychology, and into the practical contexts of education and medicine. These contexts often involve human relations of an impersonal kind: a doctor treats "the illness" (which is located in the life-world of the sick person), or a teacher brings the curriculum materials to the classroom and gets angry at children who fall asleep in class. The children's life-worlds may have entailed spending the night before helping their parents with their subsistence work, or sneaking out of home and parents' control to enjoy the forbidden pleasures of the nighttime. Yet the teacher does not know—or would not like to know—of either of these personal realities. In a similar vein, a research psychologist may confidently march into a real-life context in the expectation that most people are eager to take part in her or his study. Such self-assured feeling dies quickly, and the researcher is left begging, bribing, or giving "extra credit" to the few individuals who happen to be persuaded to devote their time to the glory of science.

The reality of researchers establishing and maintaining contact with fellow human beings who might allow them access to their personal worlds is usually overlooked in published research reports, and is only rarely brought out to the focus of researchers (Günther, 1998; Hong, 1998; Kojima, 1998). This is the "messy" part of research in which researchers are faced with the reality that their research goals are necessarily hostage to the generosity of the human beings whom the researchers have labeled "research participants." The label matters less than the social role assignment it denotes.

ILLUSION OF POWER AND CONTROL OF PSYCHOLOGISTS' ROLES

What is at stake here is the relinquishing (by researchers) of the "control"—or the illusion of control—over the course of the research process, and the arrival at the understanding that "the social other" is the actual joint constructor of the empirical evidence. Like in any social system, the question of power is crucial in human encounters as they become established in some formal system of social role relationship. That power can be negotiated between the role carriers in different ways—ranging from aggressive to affiliative—yet the issue of control remains central.

Different social systems may have developed different ways of negotiating and renegotiating power. Some persuade the populace to vote one or another party in and out of government, others send tanks to take over the parliament. Similar variability of power negotiations is seen in interpersonal relations. Some people turn to divorce court to bargain about child custody, others tolerantly accept the power games of the marital partner for the sake of a continuing relationship that would provide the children with "full" home environments.

In the middle of the many societal and interpersonal power negotiations stands psychology—science and practice—as a bastion of hope for the otherwise unruly humankind that creates its own suffering of the soul. In some ways, such a role would be a utopian example for any social science, which is the benefactor of the realities of human societies, rather than a creator of the social world. Thus, psychology's role in any society is inherently ambiguous. Borrowing from the practices of shamans and fortune-tellers on its practical side, and natural sciences on its research side, psychology is a discipline in identity crisis over most of its independent history. That ambiguity leads to tensions between the humanistic goals and institutional interests of application.

WANDERINGS OF PSYCHOLOGY IN ITS SOCIAL CONTEXTS

Psychology moves around in circles. The centrality of the research participant was crucial within the traditions of psychology of perception and reasoning, and within the introspectionist approach in general. Research participants were not called "subjects," but "observers"—they were to observe carefully either external stimuli (in perception research) of their intrapsychological processes (in case of introspectionist research), and (hopefully) accurately report their observations to the researcher. The latter had no control, other than that of external set-up of the experiment scene, over the psychological phenomena under study. The partnership of the introspecting research participant was even acknowledged in the form of the ownership marking of the data—often it was the participant, and not the researcher, who authored the published reports. The researcher got a footnote of thanks for setting up the experiment (Danziger, 1985). The social role relations of the researchers and the researchees have undergone major changes over the past century. Presently, the equal role of the persons who are studied with those who study them has become (again) recognized. Would it be reversed? Would researchers begin to assume a subservient stance toward the people they study, perhaps relabeling them "executive officers of research" and paying them high salaries? If so, then professional research participants would not differ much from professional athletes.

Psychologists Becoming Leaders: Controlling Rats and Predicting People

Changes in psychologists' roles in a society are linked with their becoming established as "experts" of their know-how, in their particular societies. In the 20th century, psychologists became important and took leadership roles in real societies. This entailed becoming socially accountable in terms of the society in which they worked, whether it was democratic (Danziger, 1990), simply socialist (Valsiner, 1988), or national socialist (Geuter, 1984). The major users of psychologists' know-how—aside of private patients in clinical psychology—became social institutions.

This appropriation of psychology by institutions meant a move away from previously preferred partners in research—usually one's own friends and colleagues—and their replacement by representative anonymous masses of subjects. A discipline can't be socially credible by the study of the next-door neighbor, but if the discipline briefly tests a million army recruits, its power acquires a kind of social prestige. This happened in psychology during World War I, and its boost to psychology's role in the texture of social institutions after that has remained profound.

Yet it was not only masses of humans who became studied. Aside from the large samples of soldiers, psychology turned to the study of individuals of a special kind: white rats. Of course, when psychology stopped the study of mental processes of higher kind and concentrated on controllable new equivalents for human beings—white rats—the use of the language of treating research participants as "observers" became obsolete. The rats were not reporting any observations; they ran around in cages, and—especially when hungry—began to push levers to earn rewards of food. Psychologists who "ran" the rats in mazes claimed to extract universal principles of management of the behavior of the other—the subordinate worker—in many other contexts. Other psychologists who studied samples of humans attempted to devise methods for the selection of potential employees, out of masses of candidates. Selection and training have been in the background of psychology in the U.S. as a social demand. This demand has led to proliferation of practical applications of psychology. It has also guided the research questions psychologists have asked. So it is not surprising that the same socioinstitutional demand has also framed the social role relations between the "experts" and the "consumers" of the expertise.

The white rat was indeed a good equivalent for the subordinate workers in a hierarchical corporation, and the researcher—who might have proudly boasted about "running subjects"— could feel important as a chief executive officer of a large corporation. Surely s/he had full control over the fate of the workers (rats in cages). The benefit of the psychologist was the impossibility of the laboratory rats to form trade unions—a tendency widely fought, at times unsuccessfully, by real leaders of business corporations.

Psychology in different societies, East or West, became socially appropriated. This meant that the social institutions who had made psychologists' work socially valuable—and economically supported—gained the control over what issues, on whom, and how, the discipline was to study. As individuals, human beings are of limited social importance, unless they happen to be designated by some label of their outstanding nature, be it genius, crazy, revolutionary, or criminal. The interest of social institutions has been on the prediction and control over the conduct of subgroups of human beings—usually those of inferior social status to the predictors and controllers. Such interest has been free of taking the perspective of the subordinates: human beings within the crowd. Instead, the interest has been in dividing the crowd (by testing and placement of individuals into socially appropriate classes) in ways that fit the interests of the social institutions to control the crowd.

By introducing new class distinctions of psychological kind into societies that were overcoming other distinctions, the crowd would be given new means of making intergroup distinctions, and creating prejudices. Yet here is an essential paradox: psychologists' ideals of improving the lives of other human beings can easily become used for the exploitation, or selective use, of some of the human beings in ways not most beneficial for them. The partnership ideal that unites this book is in effect work against that latter use of psychology. Psychology's moral imperative is to consider their subjects (research participants) as equal human beings, rather than merely "objects of investigation." It is from this humanistic perspective—human beings must not be used as tools for others' gain—that the dominant theme of the present volume emerges.

PARTNERSHIP IN FOCUS

In this book, a constructive effort is made to restore the role of psychologists' partners in their work—research participants, or patients in medical settings—into their deserving social roles as joint constructors of knowledge and practical results. This is done here without utopian efforts to overthrow the hierarchical power establishment of human society. The realities of power asymmetries are not denied, but are circumvented. The differences between "experts" and "nonexperts" in a given area of knowledge—like medicine—are presented as inevitable and beneficial if the partnership ideal is implemented. Two mutually intertwined notions—*equality* of human beings *as human beings* (the moral imperative) and *differences between* human beings in their interindividual variability of world views, skills, and expertise—are brought together into one general scheme. The researcher and the research participant (or doctor and patient, or teacher and student) are equal, yet different. The difference is not evaluative, with suppression of the subordinate (e.g., "the subject need not know what is happening" or "the patients do not know"), but rather a positive enhancement of the accomplishment by the expert through being informed by the partner. The expert may know what the client does not, but the client is the only person who knows his/her personal world. Any application of generalized expertise to individual cases requires collaboration by the person who participates in such application. The expert needs to understand his/her dependency on that collaboration, and the client needs to know how to ask questions about the general knowledge from the other person who—for the given knowledge domain—*happens to be in the role* of the "expert." Today, a car mechanic goes to a doctor with his or her health problem; tomorrow the roles are reversed, when the doctor takes his or her misbehaving car to the same car mechanic. Both would benefit from mutual cooperation, in both role relations.

Partnership as it emerges in this volume is based on the coconstructionist general notion of psychological phenomena (for an overview, see Valsiner, 1994), and on bidirectional notions of cultural communication. Human beings construct new knowledge, as well as social relationships, in the course of irreversible time and with the assistance of one another. In a way, partnership—when viewed as the necessary interdependence between human beings—is the very essence of human psychological functioning. Thus, it is curious that psychology needs to be reminded of its own axiomatic cornerstone.

PSYCHOLOGY IN PRACTICE: ACKNOWLEDGING THE OTHER

If our contemporary societies turn increasingly toward specialized (expert) knowledge in most areas of practical activities, then the issue of partnership as described in this volume has a wider relevance than the restoration of cooperative relationships in research, medicine, and education. By definition, the emergence of expert roles in a domain means the delegation of the vast majority of other human beings into the role of nonexperts. This practically means that, in sum total, human beings in contemporary society become increasingly ignorant of —and dependent on—the experts' know-how. The latter may have economic interests in the differentiation of the knowers and not-knowers. A century ago, no young parent of a child would think of paying his/her grandmother for advice on how to take care of children, but today we look for expert advice in this area by subscribing to "how to parent" kinds of journals, buy books on the topic, and go to pertinent workshops organized by parents. With this economically promoted expert/nonexpert role differentiation, it becomes all the more important for the clients—paying customers—to know how to ask relevant questions, and indeed to ask them. Asking questions and deciding on one's own life is a crucial counterweight to the totalitarianism of many uses of the expert roles, and to the rosy future for persons in consumerist societies in which purchasing new things and services is suggested as a solution to all problems.

Psychology may be the single discipline among the social sciences that can highlight the centrality of partnership in human societies. Its simultaneous focus on the person and the social context of the person allows for such openness of the approach. The message emerging from this volume is loud and profound—without implementing the partnership principles in our daily practice, the humanity of human beings can disappear. Surely we as readers do not want to lose that—yet it remains our joint effort with the authors of this volume to become partners—partners for the sake of our own lives, as well as those of others.

REFERENCES

Danziger, K. (1985). The methodological imperative in psychology. *Philosophy of the Social Sciences, 15,* 1–13.

Danziger, K. (1990). *Constructing the subject.* Cambridge: Cambridge University Press.

Geuter, U. (1984). *Die Professionalisierung der deutschen Psychologie im Nazionalsozialismus.* Frankfurt: Suhrkamp.

Günther, I. (1998). Contacting subjects: The untold story. *Culture & Psychology, 4*(1), 65–74.

Hong, G-Y. (1998). Logistics and researchers as legitimate tools for 'doing' intercultural research. *Culture & Psychology, 4*(1), 81–90.

Kojima, H. (1998). Researcher's story told and participants' story still untold. *Culture & Psychology, 4*(1), 75-80.

Valsiner, J. (1988). *Developmental psychology in the Soviet Union.* Bloomington, IN: Indiana University Press.

Valsiner, J. (1994). Culture and human development: A co-constructionist perspective. In P. van Geert, L. P. Mos, & W. J. Baker (Eds.), *Annals of theoretical psychology* (Vol. 10, pp. 247–298). New York: Plenum.

part I

The Partnership Approach in Research Settings

1

AN INTRODUCTION TO PARTNERSHIP IN RESEARCH: CHANGING THE RESEARCHER–PARTICIPANT RELATIONSHIP

Roger Bibace
Clark University and
University of Massachusetts Medical School

Stephen Dine Young
Hanover College

Leslie Rupert Herrenkohl
University of Washington

Angela Wiley
University of Illinois, Urbana/Champagne

ABSTRACT

Suggestions for partnerships in research include: 1) attitudinal shift to research participant as actors rather than as acted on; 2) avoiding jargon that serves to separate "experts" from "lay people" or the audience in general by making discussion and understanding unnecessarily difficult; 3) increasing the availability of entire sets of data to readers; 4) beginning research with participant-generated questions; and 5) instituting a feedback procedure whereby the participant has an opportunity to comment on the researcher's interpretations.

Disciplines socialize experts pervasively. Furthermore, the zeitgeist cuts across disciplines so that within a given historical era, they take on what Foucault (1971) termed the same basic "episteme." Under the broad and sometimes confusing umbrella of "post-modernism," it is relatively clear that the episteme of the current historical era is in a state of transition. One of the consequences of this epistemological shift within the social sciences has been a basic reconsideration of the nature of the subject matter to be studied—human beings and human society. More concretely, we argue that the fields of study of the authors (developmental, clinical, health, and educational psychology), as well as a host of closely related disciplines (anthropology, sociology, education, and medicine), are presently experiencing currents of dissatisfaction with regard to how people called "subjects" are thought of and treated in empirical research.

The most recent *Publication Manual of the American Psychological Association* (1994) substantiates the current transition. The manual recognizes a premise we share: "Appropriate identification of research participants and clientele is critical to the science and practice of psychology" (p. 13). As a substitute for the traditional term "subject," this prominent national organization now suggests that its members should "write about the people in your study in a way that acknowledges their participation. Replace the impersonal terms *subjects* with a more descriptive term when possible—*participants, individuals, college students, children, or respondents* for example." "Subject" is now considered to be appropriate only when discussing statistics (p.49).

While this shift in terminology as important, it should signify more than merely the substitution of one term for another. Rather it is the assumptions being made about people, as well as the methods and procedures being espoused, that we claim are in need of reconceptualization.

How individuals should be construed in psychology has been a persistent controversy. The current emphasis on "participants" as *actors* rather than as *acted on* would not have been acceptable to behaviorists such as Watson in the 1920s or indeed B.F. Skinner in the 1950s through the 1980s. And of course, the controversy extends beyond psychology. An entire recent issue of the *American Behavioral Scientist* (Ashmore, Wooffit, & Harding, 1994) is devoted to "one of the most fundamental and long-running debates in and on the social and behavioral sciences. The debate concerns the question of how the very entities that social scientists investigate—humans and their interactions—are to be conceptualized in the first place" (p. 733).

This chapter contributes to the further development of this crucial debate in several ways. First it extends the issue to include what we call the "research triangle," not just the researcher–participant dyad. We suggest that relevant audi-

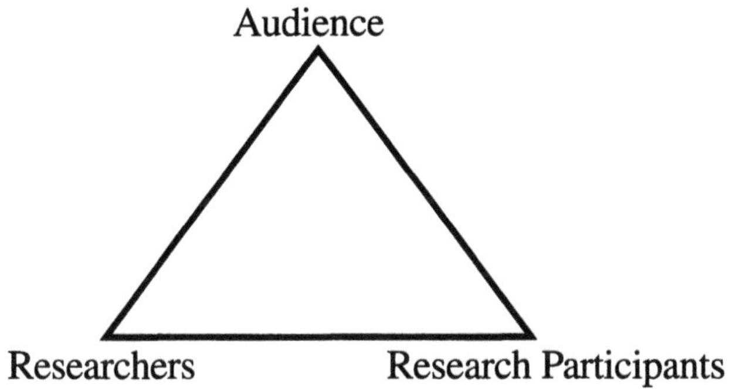

FIGURE 1.1. Three consituencies involved in research.

ences, the "generalized others" to which scientific works are directed, should also be part of the concepts and values that guide research with human participants. We take the position that research should be construed as an ongoing dialogical process that has no definite end point. This dialogical (or, perhaps, "trialogical") process minimally includes three constituencies: the researchers, the participants in the research, and the audience (other experts as well as so-called ordinary people) who read, react to, and potentially become part of *searching* and *re-searching* questions of widespread concern.

In addition to emphasizing the role of the audience in research, we also contribute by offering some suggestions for specific methodological changes that will mitigate the current dissatisfaction with the treatment of "subjects." Since we conceive of research as a dialogical process, this assumption requires that a set of procedures be established in order to ensure that the collaboration of the participant and readers is "substantial." The methodological changes we suggest work to open up what has been a rather constricted and well-dammed flow of information among the three points of the research triangle. While some of these suggestions are more relevant to studies that employ qualitative or interpretive methods, others are equally relevant to quantitative studies.

Our suggestions include:

1. changing terminology from "subject" to "participant,"
2. avoiding jargon that serves to separate "experts" from "lay people" by making discussion and understanding unnecessarily difficult,
3. increasing the availability of entire sets of data to readers,
4. beginning research with participant-generated questions, and
5. instituting a feedback procedure whereby the participant has an opportunity to comment on the researcher's interpretations.

Finally, we discuss how our suggestions move toward the possibility of truly "collaborative" and more "comprehensive" research in the social sciences.

SOME METHODOLOGICAL CHANGES

Eliminating the Term "Subject"

As a first step, we support the *APA Manual*'s (1994) recommendation that the term "participant" be used instead of "subject" when referring to human beings engaged in psychological research. As Danziger (1990) has aptly demonstrated, "subject" historically has been an unfortunate choice for psychology. On one hand, the term is inaccurate in that "subjects," traditionally, often have been treated more like "objects" without subjectivity. On the other hand, even in the sense that "subject" is accurate (research participants are "subjected to" various procedures), it reinforces the passivity of participants. For these reasons, it would be beneficial if all social science disciplines followed this suggestion.

The strength of the term "participant" is that it emphasizes the active nature of an individual's involvement in the research. Clearly a child being interviewed about his experience of his parents' divorce or a woman telling her story about her psychiatric admission are both playing a crucial role in the construction of knowledge and the advancement of the social sciences. Their contribution has often been unrecognized, and the term "subject" calls attention only to the degree to which they were passively involved in the scientific process. A change to "participant" in and of itself begins to move toward their recognition as contributors. The term will become even more apt as some of the other suggestions that follow are put into practice.

It should be noted that other terms are possible, some of which might imply even more activity than "participant" does. For example, "collaborator" or "coresearcher" are other terms that could be used. While the ideal of "participants" as "coresearchers" is admirable, we do not believe that it accurately describes the current state of research (or even research that applies some of the suggestions in this paper). Except in the most unusual cases (see the conclusion below), academic researchers will continue to take primary responsibility for developing projects and theories, seeking grants, recording findings, and preparing documents for widespread distribution. These functions place researchers in unique roles they will likely remain in, regardless of the important steps taken to give attention to the perspectives, experiences, and interpretations of the participants. A term such as "coresearcher" blurs this real and important distinction and thereby becomes inaccurate and disingenuous.

Mary Catherine Bateson (1989) in her book *Composing a Life* encounters the dilemma of using our current language to describe the researcher–participant relationship as she writes about the lives of five influential women, including herself:

> When I search for a word for my relationship with the women described in this book, I feel a need for a term that would assert both collegiality and the fact that the process is made possible by our differences. The thesaurus betrays me, denying me a term

> that affirms both symmetry and complementarity. The gap in the language parallels a gap in the culture. We are rich in words that describe symmetrical relationships, from buddy to rival to colleague. We are also rich in words that describe strongly asymmetrical relationships, many of which imply hierarchy and have curious undertones of exploitation and dominance. (p.102)

Bateson eloquently describes the difficulty she has faced in trying to characterize her relationship to the "subjects" of her book. She raises a crucial point regarding what the English language offers to characterize relationships in general. It is not surprising, therefore, that many researchers who have reflected on these issues have been unable to transform the deeply entrenched beliefs and assumptions reached by reliance on the term "subject." We hope this chapter is one attempt among many toward devising new ways of "speaking" and "thinking" regarding how we engage others who are involved in research activities. We will argue that, without denying the importance of differences in roles, a change in the way participants are thought of by researchers allows for more effective and informative investigations.

Avoiding Jargon

Technical language or "jargon" develops as a discipline becomes more established and specialized. Commonly understood phenomena are now referred to in ways that ordinary people cannot understand. "New" ideas surface couched in new terminology—"Old wine in new bottles."

While some specialized language is necessary in any scholarly undertaking, the overuse of jargon in speaking and writing is an obstacle in communication. Jargon keeps researchers separated not only from the participants in their study but from much of their potential audience as well. While other researchers have called for limiting the use of jargon (e.g., Bem, 1987), few individuals who have ever read a social science journal would argue that the amount of jargon found therein is essential for the communication of ideas.

Often, the reason for the unnecessary proliferation of technical language is simply a lack of immediate awareness by researchers of the specialized nature of their language and its obtuseness to "everyday" people or even to other scholars in different disciplines. Sometimes however, there is a more conscious attempt to separate the discipline from everyday activities and create a like-minded, isolated community of specialists. While a justification for this elitism is questionable in the area of molecular chemistry, it is less defensible when the topic of study becomes depression, drug use, poverty, or other widely experienced human phenomena.

Our basic recommendation then is to eliminate jargon wherever possible and to aim toward a language that can be understood by participants and by as large an audience as possible. Often this is not exceptionally difficult as a close examination of social science writings indicates that commonly understood words can be substituted for more technical terms. When greater precision is required and specialized language is necessary, then definitions and examples are helpful. An argument could be made that repeated definitions of widely used and understood terms within a given area would be unnecessary and cumbersome. However, we point out that it is often these "understood" terms that have entered what Bruno Latour (1987) calls the "black box"; they are no longer open to question or examination. If researchers were more often forced to explicate the technical terms they use so as to communicate better, it is possible that less of this "black boxing" phenomenon would occur.

Increasing the Availability of Data

Increasing the availability of data is a change that would have the greatest effect on the "audience" point of the research triangle. Easier access to data challenges the univocality of the researcher's interpretation. Since it is unrealistic that any researcher would have the last word on any psychological or social phenomenon, the audience should have the opportunity to participate in actively interpreting results. Science progresses as alternative interpretations (some contradictory, some complimentary) come together in dialogue and mutually inform one another.

While this is the ideal, often in interview-based and other forms of qualitative research, the text that is being interpreted is unavailable to all but the researchers. At best, a few pages of a transcribed interview are included in papers reporting on such investigations. A situation is created in which the primary researchers have access to more data and therefore have an interpretive advantage over readers who might want to generate alternative readings. An even more lopsided presentation of data usually exists in regard to quantitative data. Whatever advantages statistical methods have for summarizing and manipulating data, they also have the disadvantage of further separating the original phenomenon of interest and interpretations of it.

To counter this tendency with both qualitative and quantitative data, we suggest that researchers make their data as readily available to as large an audience as possible. While transcripts and similar data require a great deal of written space, the widespread availability of the Internet and computer databases has made the distribution of such material much more feasible. In addition, books are a traditional publishing form that are amenable to widespread disbursement of such data. Authors could present their own interpretations of the data, which could also be available in an appendix so that readers could draw their own conclusions.

For some forms of presenting research, there are, of course, practical limitations to this suggestion. A 20-page journal article reporting on research generated from a dozen two-hour interviews could hardly contain much in the way of raw data. However, such data could easily be accessed. While scientific ethics have long called for researchers to be able to present their data if called upon to do so, such sharing of knowledge in the area of qualitative research is relatively uncommon. If, however, the sharing of data as a means toward multiple interpretations were encouraged, efficient systems of distribution could be instituted. To begin with, having copies of data readily available that easily and quickly could be mailed or e-mailed would be helpful. Some grant monies could be dedicated to this endeavor, eliminating financial limitations as a possible discouragement toward all interested parties obtaining data.

Confidentiality is a major issue that must be addressed. As always, care should be taken to protect the identity of participants, especially in sensitive areas related to personal or clinical issues. In addition, participants need to be made aware that other individuals will have access to their stories; informed consent is essential.

Researchers should recognize that confidentiality and the desire to present as complete a data set as possible often conflict. Since transcription systems themselves are guided by researchers' theories about how oral language should be organized, coded, and presented in written form (Ochs, 1979), transcripts are, from this perspective, a step removed from videotapes or audiotapes. Researchers' transcription systems reflect their interests and the issues that they themselves are pursuing. Thus, if a reader has a slightly different interest in language data, it may not be reflected clearly in the transcript that the researcher provides.

Ideally, therefore, having audiotapes or videotapes widely available would be the best solution to this dilemma. Unfortunately, such mediums are often impossible to make confidential adequately. Although there may be certain situations in which participants might choose to waive confidentiality, those situations in which a waiver is not possible or desirable are much more common. In these instances, it is incumbent upon researchers to clarify the theories that guided their transcription system. Again, the overarching question guiding such disbursement decisions would be "How can I maintain confidentiality while simultaneously making accessible as much relevant information as possible?"

Participant-Generated Questions

Within psychology, the impetus for much of the qualitative and interpretive research has been the observation that psychology is a science that investigates how human beings construct their world with complex symbol systems such as language (Gergen, 1985; Kaplan, 1983; Mishler, 1986). Therefore, if researchers want to understand human beings, they must encounter the complexities of human language, either in spoken or written form. Thus, researchers have become interested in peoples' narrative accounts of their experience. Both open-ended and semistructured questionnaires and interviews allow participants to tell their stories. Careful thought is given to the questions that are asked so as to promote rich narratives. The same thoughtfulness is applied to many quantifiable questionnaires as well, even though the range of responses is more limited.

In an attempt to encourage participants to communicate their perspectives and opinions on a topic as clearly and fully as possible, the above scenario actually overlooks an important obstacle to that goal. While the questions are intended to allow for honest expression on the part of the participants, the fact that they are generated by the researchers prior to data gathering establishes a hierarchy of power. The researcher often stipulates both what issues are important and the sequence of questions to be investigated. Participants may be given some space to "roam," but the overall field of inquiry is dictated by the researchers.

The alternative is to allow the participants themselves to generate the relevant questions and thereby guide the research process. Focus groups are one type of procedure that have been used within the social sciences as a preliminary means of gathering information about the important questions when embarking on a new area of research (Morgan, 1988).

Other methods that focus on individuals instead of groups are also possible. In a study of substance abusers within our research group, we began our interview with the question, "What questions do you think are important to ask in order to understand substance use and abuse?" This one question allowed the participants to structure the interview around the issues they considered most important. When the participants were done responding spontaneously to this question, we presented them with a list of questions that we had compiled from a review of the professional literature on substance abuse. We marked those issues that had been brought up by the participants and asked if they thought that any of the other questions were especially relevant to the experience of substance use.

This procedure was designed to remove some of the traditional authority granted to the "expert" to decide what the important questions are. Engaging participants to generate their own questions concretely communicates the researcher's attitude. This attitude empowers the participants and indicates that the researcher will be a respectful listener.

One other related procedure that can help participants gain some measure of control over the research situation is to ask them what pseudonym, if any, they prefer to use in writings that emerge from the research process. While this procedure might seem minor, it has proven to be an effective tool in bridging the expert-novice gap. Clearly, a personal name does more than neutrally denote an individual. Names have a variety of connotations—consider the difference in associations to the names "Johnny" and "Jonathan." In addition, the stories participants tell regarding the reason for the name they have chosen are often illuminating. Asking the participants to name themselves further empowers them to define themselves and characterize their own accounts.

Participant Feedback Procedure

The most significant change to the methodological procedures of standard social science research that we will introduce is the implementation of a feedback mechanism in which participants comment on the interpretations made by researchers. Normally, the researchers' interpretations are the ending point; they would be written up and presented solely to a scholarly and professional audience.

Our suggestion is that, prior to the publication of interpretations, the interpretations should be presented to the participants who generated the data in the first place. While making results available to participants has generally been a part of responsible research, we are calling for researchers to go a step further. The reactions of the participants to the researchers' interpretations should also be recorded and included as part of the final product.

This feedback loop does not preclude researchers from making interpretations that participants do not agree with. However, researchers would be compelled to include these disagreements in their work. If nothing else, this dialogical procedure is more legitimate and true to the spirit of intellectual discussion than the standard procedure in which participants are represented by the researchers and are never given an opportunity to challenge that representation.

There are some precedents in which the subtle one-sided power of the researcher to represent events has been challenged by participants. One prominent example was a response by research participants to a *New York Times Magazine* article (Prose, 1990) about Carol Gilligan's research with teenage girls (Gilligan, Lyons, & Hammer, 1990). These participants were upset by the way they had been portrayed by Gilligan, and they questioned the researchers account of their experience. Such disagreements occurred despite the fact that many feminist social scientists, including Gilligan (1982), are explicitly concerned about the role of participants in social science research.

In addition to being respectful to participants, the inclusion of their disagreements and opinions would be provocative and informative to readers. Readers would have an opportunity to observe at what points the interpretations of the participants themselves and the interpretations of experts diverge and at what points they converge. While this procedure may add some effort to the conduct of research, these added dimensions of understanding would, in many cases, justify the effort.

This suggestion may sound radical in the domain of research. However, such dialogue is commonplace and central in the helping professions. Specialists, be they teachers, physicians or clinicians, must learn to speak to two audiences: specialists like themselves and ordinary people whom they call students, patients, or clients (Bibace & Walsh, 1982; Heymann, 1995a). Furthermore, Heymann (1995b) has asserted that a similar reflexive relationship should exist in medical research. Our suggestion is to further expand the practice to include social science research participants as well.

The participant feedback procedure extends to participants what is already an established practice between researchers and their audience. Many of the most exciting areas in the social sciences are those in which public commentary, criticism, and rebuttals are present either in written or oral form. In a sense then, the feedback procedure is simply an attempt to further balance the research triangle. However, in addition to giving participants a greater voice in social science research, our highlighting of this procedure should also call attention to the public, dialogical nature of scholarly dialogue in general and lead to a reconsideration of those arenas in which it is not practiced as much as it might be.

CONCLUSION: TOWARD "COLLABORATIVE" AND "COMPREHENSIVE" RESEARCH

We have been trying to envision an orientation toward research in which the methods employed work to decrease the distance between researcher and participant. Inherent in this goal is a desire to disturb the unquestioned role "experts" often have in social science research.

At the same time, we have continued to maintain a distinction between researchers and participants. In our proposed research process, investigators and participants each bring equal but different domains of expertise to the research—the investigators bring generalized training in theory and method while the participants bring the lived experience of the phenomenon being studied. Knowledge is formed out of a collaboration of these distinct orientations. This movement toward a differentiated egalitarianism is further elaborated in our emphasis on the active reader engaging in dialogue with the researchers and participants, thereby completing the research triangle.

There are possibilities for collaborative research beyond what we have been suggesting, however. Such an approach might feature researchers and participants starting at the same point, sitting down together and deciding on the very object of study. The research would proceed from there with all those involved participating similarly. In such a situation, the researcher/participant distinction changes altogether. Indeed, such research is not without precedent. For example, Freire (1988) has advocated a similar approach to education in Brazil. In the U.S. in the area of teacher-researcher partnerships, this form of research has been successful (Guerra & Smith, 1992; Jacobs, McCrohon, Reddy, & Rupert, 1993).

For social scientists with egalitarian tendencies who are interested in making immediate social changes, such a method might be more appropriate than the less radical methods we have been suggesting. We will leave those farther-reaching changes for others to discuss.

All of the suggestions that have been made are open to further refinement. They are intended to be starting points for future inquiry. Clearly, some of them are more or less appropriate for different types of research. In addition, other changes which would also work toward a restructuring of the researcher-participant relationship are certainly possible. As some of these suggestions are implemented and further thought is given to other changes, then our methods as social scientists will become more refined and better serve the goal of bringing researchers, participants, and readers closer together.

While our thinking is based, at least in part, on a desire to promote social equality, we also have a less ideological motivation as well. We believe that research in the social sciences that facilitates a complex, active role for the humans being studied is "better science." It deserves this characterization because it is more "comprehensive," the standard that Pepper (1970) and others have advocated as the primary criteria for judging science. We hope that the results of such investigations will be more developed, insightful, and in the end, useful.

REFERENCES

Ashmore, M., Wooffit, R., & Harding, S. (Eds.). (1994). Humans and others: The concept of agency and its attributions [Special issue]*American Behavioral Scientist, 37*(6).

Bateson, M. C. (1989). *Composing a life.* New York: Atlantic Monthly Press.

Bem, D. (1987). Writing the empirical journal article. In M. P. Zann & J. M. Darley (Eds.), *The compleat academic: A practical guide for the beginning social scientist* (pp.171–201). New York: Random House.

Bibace, R., & Walsh, M. E. (1982). Conflict of roles: On the difficulties of being both a scientist and practitioner in one life. *Professional Psychology, 13*(3), 389–396.

Danziger, K. (1990). *Constructing the subject: Historical origins of psychological research.* Cambridge: Cambridge University Press.

Foucault, M. (1971). *The order of things: An archeology for the human sciences.* New York: Pantheon Books.

Freire, P. (1988). *Pedagogy of the oppressed.* New York: Continuum.

Gergen, K. J. (1985). The social-constructionist movement in modern psychology.*American Psychologist, 40*(3), 266–275.

Gilligan, C. (1982). *In a different voice.* Cambridge: Harvard University Press.

Gilligan, C., Lyons, N. P., & Hammer, T. J. (1990). *Making connections: The relational worlds of adolescent girls at Emma Willard School.* Cambridge: Harvard University Press.

Guerra, M. R., & Smith, M. (1992). *'Science is wonderful': Evolving scientific discourse in a primary resource room.* Unpublished manuscript.

Heymann, S. J. (1995a). *Equal partners: A physician's call for a new spirit in medicine.* Boston: Little Brown.

Heymann, S. J. (1995b). Patients in research: Not just subjects, but partners. *Science, 269,* 797–798.

Jacobs, P., McCrohon, C., Reddy, M., & Rupert, L. (1993, November). *Seeing with new eyes: Becoming a teacher/researcher team.* Paper presented at the American Anthropological Association Annual Meeting, Philadelphia.

Kaplan, B. (1983). Genetic-dramatism: Old wine in new bottles. In S. Wapner & B. Kaplan (Eds.), *Toward a holistic developmental psychology* (pp. 53–74). Hillsdale, NJ: Lawrence Erlbaum.

Latour, B. (1987). *Science in action.* Cambridge: Harvard University Press.

Mishler, E. G. (1986). *Research interviewing.* Cambridge: Harvard University Press.

Morgan, D. L. (1988). *Focus groups as qualitative research.* Newbury Park, CA: Sage.

Ochs, E. (1979). Transcription as theory. In E. Ochs & B. Schieffelin (Eds.),*Developmental pragmatics* (pp. 43–72). New York: Academic Press.

Pepper, S. C. (1970). *World hypotheses: A study in evidence.* Berkeley: University of California Press.

Prose, F. (1990, January 7). Confident at eleven; confused at sixteen. *New York Times Magazine,* pp. 22–46.

Publication manual of the American Psychological Association (4th ed.). (1994). Washington, DC: American Psychological Association.

2

PSYCHOLOGY'S SUBJECT(S): MOVING TOWARD THE PARTNERSHIP MODEL

Christina Hatgis
Clark University

James J. Dillon
State University of West Georgia

Roger Bibace
Clark University and
University of Massachusetts Medical School

ABSTRACT

In this chapter, we examine various conceptions of psychological research participants. We consider some of the historical, intellectual, and social influences on these conceptions, as well as their implications for the types of knowledge investigators produce. A researcher's view of the investigatory process and its knowledge products is affected by whether s/he conceptualizes research participants as members of an aggregate subgroup of a population, individuals with measurable behavior, thoughts, and perceptions; or as people who cooperate to construct their own subjectivity in relation to others in social contexts, such as the experimental situation. With the latter notion of research participants, scientific investigation is seen as a relational process involving, at least, the scientific community, investigators, and research participants. By examining the implications of these different perspectives on the subject, we preview some of the thinking upon which fellow authors in this book have built innovative approaches to research and to the idea of the subject. Through changes in theory, practice, and reporting conventions, these researchers strive to position the research participant as more of a partner in the process of psychological investigation.

In this chapter, we consider some of the historical, intellectual, and social contexts within which psychologists have adopted the conception of the human person as a "subject." We attempt to elucidate the implications of different conceptions of the subject for the types of knowledge psychological investigators, educators, and clinicians produce. Through the discussion of changes in conceptions of the subject that have held sway within psychology, we trace the shifting emphases and elisions that accompany these conceptions. In doing so, we describe the context within which the partnership model of psychological practice now emerges.

As the field of modern psychology evolved, it borrowed some of its methods, values, and theoretical orientations from the more abstract or mathematical sciences, such as physics, biology, and chemistry. Over time this identification led to the trend in psychology in which the subject of study increasingly became conceptualized as a "dehumanized other." The partnership model emerges now as a corrective to the problematic implications of this trend in psychology; it is an attempt to re-situate psychology among the human sciences, to reinstate "the person" as the appropriate level of analysis for this field, and to specify the "person-in-partnership" as the primary context in which psychological investigation takes place.

THE EMERGENCE OF THE SUBJECT

Over the course of the last century, psychologists have moved through many different perspectives toward the subject of their investigations. Kurt Danziger's (1990) history of the conceptions of the research subject in psychology describes how early psychologists, such as the members of Wilhelm Wundt's laboratory, began by studying individual perceptual processes, using themselves as subjects, and using introspection as their prime method of observation. From information they gathered about themselves, these psychologists made inferences about perceptual processes that were believed to be common to all humans. Over time, other research models, such as the clinical experiment, emerged that involved different views of research participants. Instead of studying themselves as prototypic or exemplary humans, researchers focused attention on the psychologically deviant or mentally ill. The clinical experiment took on a form that was more similar to the physician–patient relationship in that the purpose was to diagnose and possibly cure the illness. In these relations, the division between the investigator and the object of investigation was clear: the "subject" was undoubtedly the "other." One of the important social conditions and defining aspects of this approach to research was the subordination and dependency that characterized the relationship of the patient to the investigator.

Yet another type of psychological investigation was promoted by Frances Galton, who, in the role of expert investigator, collected data from many subjects and ranked them on a scale of intellectual ability based upon the data he gathered (Danziger, 1990). An assumption of this approach to investigation was that individuals' abilities were attributable to stable, innate, or biological factors that could be measured and were substantively unaffected by social factors. Psychologists needed quantitative methods to handle the type of data this approach generated, since the information was statistical in nature. The proliferation of quantitative methods added another ingredient to the context within which psychologists determined what were the relevant, important, and interesting questions to ask.

Clinical and Galtonian research gave rise to a subsequent development in psychology which Danziger terms the "triumph of the aggregate" (1990, p. 68). This describes the predominance of a methodology that involved drawing comparisons between different groups. Such comparisons entailed attributing psychological characteristics to groups, rather than to individuals. Ultimately, definitions of collective subjects were not confined to those preexisting categories found in the sociocultural environment (e.g., gender, age, etc.), but they came to include the kinds of experimental groups that got created in the two kinds of investigative situations: experimental and correlational designs. In this manner, Danziger notes, psychology became a science that constructs its own categories. Danziger argues that these categories are artificial for two reasons. First, these groups do not correspond to preexisting social categories, but are explicitly created in the process of research. Second, they are artificial because of an idealization that is involved in their conceptualizations. In the case of experimental designs, the groups are idealized in the sense that they are regarded as a collective, characterized primarily by modifiability. Correlational design involves the opposite idealization; subject groups are conceptualized as an agglomeration of stable traits. The ways in which aggregate subjects became idealized—as mainly possessing relevant characteristics of malleability or stability—are important because they highlight aspects of the process of category construction that are generally obscured in prevailing views of scientific research.

This argument, however, fails to encompass another level of critique: the categories created in the research situation (whether by experimental conditions or correlational methods) are no more or less artificial than those created outside the experimental situation. Descriptive categories, even ones that are often taken for granted (such as gender and age), do not inhere as entities to be discovered within people; rather they are created in relation to specific goals. We are not saying that there is no such thing as age or gender; rather our intention is to emphasize that critical aspects of what defines these and other social categories are also constructed. These categories do not preexist historical, social, and cultural contexts. An example of this is the division of the human life span into stages—that is, infancy, toddlerhood, childhood, adolescence, adulthood, middle age, and old age. When these stages begin and end, what differentiates them, and in fact their very existence, are products of particular social, cultural, and historic conditions (such as public education, child labor laws, and the legal age of majority) and prevailing values and perspectives (e.g., whether sexuality begins in adolescence or childhood). So, this shift enables us to regard all three sources of categorization and the idealization of categories—experimental conditions, correlational methods, and sociocultural norms—as constructions. This recognition strengthens the force of the idea that subjects are produced through scientific and social practices.

If we take seriously the perspective that investigative categories are constructed through social practices, both scientific and otherwise, this moves us far from the idea that we, as scientists, are engaged in a process of merely observing, recording, and attempting to understand what is already there in the world. Instead, it brings us to an understanding of our work as a coconstructive relationship in which the investigator participates in the creation of the subject of investigation. In turn, the investigative process and the kind of knowledge it generates are shaped by the investigator's, or the social matrix's, conception of the subject. Finally, our roles as scientists and practitioners are defined and shaped by the practices we undertake in research, or in education and clinical work, in which our methods, our conceptions of the subject, and the knowledge we produce are interwoven. Thus we have a rich interdependency of practice, theory, and social roles, in which the scientist, the research subject, the methods, the knowledge generated, and the frame within which these elements come together, all exist in a nexus of mutually defining relations.

By the mid-20th century, psychology came to a point at which the prevailing notion of the subject had moved from the self as exemplary of others, to the other as different or deviant, and, finally, to the aggregate other. In this final form, nonexperimental variance, both within groups and within individuals, was taken as error; group means were the central concern. Whereas psychologists had once used data gathered from an individual to predict performance of other group members, they then came to use data gathered from the group to predict individual performance. This shift carried with it both a methodological and a conceptual disregard for the individual persons who were research subjects. If the view of research subjects as "participants" goes part of the way toward rectifying this omission, the "partnership model" goes further. Before discussing the partnership model in greater detail, we will touch upon some of the intellectual and social contexts and conflicts within which it has emerged.

THE PARTNERSHIP CONCEPTION OF KNOWLEDGE: AN ACT OF COLLABORATIVE CONSTRUCTION

The view of the experimental relationship as a constructive process in which both subject position and knowledge are created is a departure from the principles that guided early psychological investigators. Early experimental psychologists, like other scientists of their day, and like many psychologists of today, viewed their work as a process of discovering generalizable knowledge about human thought and behavior, or as unveiling hidden but universal processes. Today, there is widespread acceptance of the notion that science is produced among a community of investigators who share conceptions of legitimate data, methods, and reporting conventions. This view of science, as characterized by Kuhn (1970), holds that the conventions of scientific communities come into conflict with one another, and are subject to radical transformations that give rise to entirely new versions of what counts as evidence for claims of truth. Progression within a field from one paradigm to another may take the form of a dialectic rather than a clear-cut transition. Thus, coexistence of conflicting views may characterize the terrain at any given point in time. This appears to be the case in contemporary psychology.

Kimble (1984) articulates the tension between two coexisting but contrary paradigms in psychology along a dimension that is anchored by the "idiographic" perspective on one end and the "nomothetic" on the other. Kimble characterizes these two perspectives as broadly corresponding with qualitative versus quantitative approaches to psychological research and knowledge. Another way to describe the distinction he makes is the contrast between attention to particular cases versus general categories or groups. Although the distinction between these points of emphasis is problematic, it serves as a way of mapping the terrain of "two cultures" within psychology, which are often perceived as being in conflict. This conflict is one of the tensions the partnership model strives to reconcile. By foregrounding the cooperative, negotiated quality of the relationship between researcher and participant, the partnership model reminds research practitioners that they cannot merely study patterns and group tendencies. Rather, they must interact with individuals and, over many such interactions, researchers may thus perceive and understand patterns.

By foregrounding the relationship between investigators and participants in research practice, the proponents of the partnership model are aligned with social constructionists who regard knowledge as a social act involving the shared construction of meaning (Gergen, 1985, 1991, 1994). Although there are differences between these two approaches, there are points of intersection that may be helpful in elucidating the partnership model of psychological practice.

First, "subject" and "investigator," like other categories, are constructed and they exist in the particular context of the investigative situation. Second, the investigative situation is a relational process that sometimes involves shared goals and agreed-upon parameters. Finally, the categories of subject and investigator are negotiated in the playing out of their respective roles; that is to say, neither is fixed, and both contribute to the definition of the other. The role of the investigator is not separate from, but is shaped and contextualized by, the concomitant role of the subject or research partner.

In a discussion of the changing conceptions of illness and medical work in western Europe during the turn of the 19th century, Jewson (1976) describes a similar interdependence of the roles of "sick-man" and "medical-man." As the prevailing view of a patient's pathology shifted from a disorder of the whole person, to a dysfunction of a particular organic system, and finally to an abnormality of a cell complex, so, too, did the routine practices that characterized the doctor–patient relationship, as well as the salient features of the doctor's role. Such a dialectic in definitions of the key components of investigation is especially operative in the social sciences where our studies are about human beings, and therefore, about ourselves.

Thus, knowledge can be seen not as "something individuals *possess*, but rather, something they *do*" (Gergen, 1985, p. 10, emphasis in original). This perspective on knowledge seems especially useful as a framework for thinking about the importance of the processes of coconstructing questions, method, and feedback that occur in the interaction between investigator and subject-as-partner, that characterizes the partnership model of psychological practice (Bibace, in this volume; Bibace, Young, Herrenkohl, & Wiley, in this volume).

SOCIAL CONTEXTS FOR THE PARTICIPATORY RESEARCH SUBJECT

Particular social and political movements prepared the ground for a shift within psychology toward a more participatory model of the subject; in fact, they drove and required such a move. Although it is difficult to isolate such strands, and in doing so we risk inappropriately elevating the importance of some over others, we focus on only a few. Our purpose is merely to suggest some of the ways these movements created the circumstances for deep shifts in views and practices relating to research participants within psychology. Some of the many prevalent forces of the past 50 years, as conceptions of the psychological subject began to shift, include post-holocaust reconsiderations of the ethics and accountability of scientific practice, the civil rights movement, and the rising influence of feminism.

The role of scientists in the holocaust (Proctor, 1988) and in the Tuskegee syphilis study (Jones, 1993) called for a new level of self-awareness and accountability among researchers, and a new conceptualization of the research subject. It was no longer morally or politically tenable to make someone a martyr for science (Engel, 1977). This revised stance took the form of patients' and subjects' rights to informed consent to participate in psychological and medical research and treatment. Institutionalized insistence on these rights ensured a shift in practice and fueled a shift in attitudes toward subjects as participants.

The mid-20th century rise of feminism also shaped changes in prevailing conceptions of what psychologists and other scientists study and in their methods. For our present purposes, one important shift that can be traced to the influence of feminism is the shift in the researcher's perspective from objective observer to engaged participant. In a series of essays on the relationship between gender and science, Evelyn Fox Keller (1985) shows how the geneticist Barbara McClintock's seminal work in discovering genetic transposition was made possible by McClintock's reconceptualization of the perspective of researcher. Keller further argues that this reconceptualization is gendered. According to Keller, McClintock adopted a role as researcher that subverted the dichotomies of "subject–object, mind–matter," (for our purposes, such a role also subverts the researcher–subject dichotomy) that "are directed toward a cosmic unity typically excluding or devouring one of the pair" (p. 163). Instead, McClintock offers a paradigm of research that is motivated by a "respect for difference that remains content with multiplicity as an end in itself" (p. 163). Keller characterizes McClintock's view of the goals of science as distinct from prevailing scientific goals of prediction and control; for McClintock the goals of science involve "understanding and empowerment" (p.166). The stance necessary to achieve such goals is one of a relationship or connection between the researcher and the objects of investigation, rather than one that sharpens the division between these two perspectives.

The most important point for the present discussion is to see how, in her feminist and gendered analysis of scientific practice, Keller underlines the way that the stance one assumes in relation to the object of study affects "both the kinds of questions one asks and the explanations that one finds satisfying" (1985, p. 167). In this manner, her work exemplifies a trend in the philosophy of science that takes the relationship between scientists and their objects or subjects of study as a central concern and a definitive aspect of the whole enterprise of research.

Thus, we have seen, in several of the current social and theoretical shifts, a movement toward: (1) self-reflexivity on the part of investigators to understand and assume responsibility, insofar as they are able, for their role in shaping the products of their investigation, and (2) recognition of the people who are partners in the investigative process as such, with fuller elaboration of their roles as partners. Through these shifts a concept emerges of the relationship between participants as peers, but not equals; the relative contributions of each partner are of equal importance, but they are not the same.

THE PARTNERSHIP MODEL

In their work toward a more integrative and comprehensive approach to research in the social sciences, investigators have incorporated the active participation of subjects in a variety of ways. This is a fieldwide effort, as exemplified by the American Psychological Association guidelines for renaming and reconceptualizing the subject as a "participant" in psychological research. This shift within psychology mirrors a broader transformation as discussions of these efforts and their practical and theoretical implications appear in publications from various disciplines within the human sciences (see, for example, Bibace, Young, Herrenkohl, & Wiley, in this volume; Farrow, Moss, & Shaw, 1995; Fisher & Fyrberg, 1994; Gibson-Graham, 1994; Moss, 1995; Shaw, 1995). However, we argue that the participant model does not go far enough to reinstate the full person into the role of research subject. By adopting a conception of investigators and subjects as "research partners," we attempt to approximate a more complementary and mutually beneficial relationship between these parties.

In the following section we briefly discuss some of the problems the partnership model attempts to address, the conflicts it embraces, its central principles, and the kinds of practices involved in approximating these principles. These topics are elaborated more fully throughout this volume, as contributing authors describe various exemplifications of the kind of work we envision.

Problems and Conflicts

The central problem the partnership model addresses is one of incompleteness. Inherent in the relation of expert to novice is an assumption that the expert's vantage point is superior, and therefore more complete in terms of access to knowledge. We disagree. Rather, the vision of knowledge that guides our work is that knowledge is achieved through an interweaving of multiple perspectives; from each perspective there is a different kind of expertise. We do not imagine this perspective to redress fully the problem of incompleteness, because no matter how inclusive we are of multiple perspectives, we can never completely know our limitations. Rather, we believe this perspective represents movement toward a desired, though perhaps unattainable, goal.

A second problem our model attempts to address is that we recognize in our peers, our students, and ourselves a tendency to adopt methodologies and their inherent assumptions uncritically. In doing so, we risk losing sight of the implications of, and alternatives to, our perspectives. The partnership model guards against this by requiring us to:

1. be more self-reflexive of our own stance, methods, and assumptions;
2. hold ourselves to a higher standard of accountability to the individual participants of our research; and
3. reckon with the alternative interpretations that our participants and others offer about the information we gather.

An important element of the partnership model is the view of conflict as productive. Rather than seeking to resolve differences between various perspectives (for example, among investigators, or between investigators and research participants), we want to foreground the tensions and differences. We value, or more strongly, require the coexistence of differing points of view, and we recognize that part of the "mess" we invite is exactly what was efficient to exclude in traditional, more asymmetrical relations between scientists and subjects.

An assumption we hold is that all of our vantage points have limitations. It is only through elaboration of multiple vantage points that we can hope to comprehend more fully the phenomena we investigate. This view is similar to feminist philosopher of science Sandra Harding's idea of "strong objectivity" (1993). As Rachel Joffe Falmagne (1998) discusses, Harding values objectivity in science, but argues that "strong objectivity" can only be attained through a reciprocal process that incorporates multiple social standpoints, both dominant and marginalized. Thus, objectivity, for Harding, is not the view one has from an ideal or neutral standpoint; rather it is a dynamic composite of views from many standpoints.

Examining changes in conceptions of the research participant suggests new ways in which the concept of the subject becomes problematized in attempts to transform it. For example, as one envisions the shift of the relationship between researcher and participant toward a partnership model, the question arises of whether this is necessarily an egalitarian vision, or if it is a vision of complementary but nonequivalent partners. Currently, our conception is to regard researchers and participants as being engaged in an ongoing process of negotiating the balance of their interdependence. Chapter 1 refers to Mary Catherine Bateson in its discussion of the difficulty of conceiving of relationships that are neither symmetrical nor entirely asymmetrical. Bateson attributes this difficulty, in part, to the paucity of the English language to describe relations of interdependence which she terms symmetrical and complementary (Bibace, Young, Herrenkohl, & Wiley, in this volume). That is to say, there are relationships between how we talk, what we imagine is possible, and what we construct in our relationships with others. If we conceptualize relationships as either balanced or imbalanced with respect to the distribution of power, for example, this dualistic view constrains our notions of what we can possibly create. Alternatively, our relationships, complex as they are, will likely strain at the seams of such dualistic formulations. This dialectic tension is at work in the present dialogue about the investigator–participant relationship: Changes are occurring at the levels of talk, imaginings, and action.

Principles

Among the principles we strive for as we articulate the partnership model, one of the most important is the principle of symmetry and reciprocity in relationships between psychologists and research participants, students, or patients. In traditional conceptions of these relationships, the expert defines the important and interesting questions about a given domain of investigation and then elicits and evaluates the participant's responses to these questions. In the partnership model of the research relationship, there is reciprocity in that both parties generate questions, and both evaluate the other's responses or interpretations of responses to these questions. By advancing this kind of reciprocity in the researcher–participant relationship, the partnership model promotes mutual accountability and responsibility. This relationship entails negotiated agreements, and ongoing disagreements, about the research goals and the means to attain them. In order to negotiate, research partners must have dialogue. In order to have such dialogue, researchers must take account of participants' assumptions, values, and goals; without this step dialogue is seriously thwarted. For some research methodologies, the introduction of dialogue between researchers and their participants may be one of the more radical changes that the partnership model instigates.

Several questions arise at this point. For example: What forms will this dialogue take? Is it not disingenuous to equate the perspectives of participants who have never considered a particular problem, with those of experts who may have spent their careers striving to understand and articulate the same problem? How do we achieve relationship symmetry in such a circumstance? Some of the answers seem clearer if we consider the particular methods involved in partnership model research and practice, which is the subject of the following section. Others may remain open questions as we attempt to refine our approach and understand its implications and particular problems.

Practices

Bibace, Young, Herrenkohl, and Wiley (in this volume) offer several methodological revisions designed to move psychological research toward a partnership conception of the research enterprise. An organizing principle of these revisions is that research is a dialogic process of knowledge production. To further this notion, the authors argue for maximizing the inclusion of multiple perspectives, especially the perspectives of research participants, in the interpretation of research findings. They emphasize the negotiation process between researcher and participant, from the stage of identifying research questions, through interpreting data, and, finally, to reporting results.

Negotiation continues among investigators, the scientific community in which they are members, and research participants on the goals of research and the means toward achieving them. Perhaps in a less explicit sense, the values inherent in an investigation are also a point of negotiation. Through the steps of research investigation the investigator does more than obtain permission to conduct a study, recruit participants, and complete a protocol. In addition to these steps, the investigator also constitutes him or herself as a member of the scientific community, worthy to conduct the investigation and to publish the information it yields. Thus, these negotiations construct the subject positions of investigators as well as participants. As this process of examining views of the research subject unfolds, it becomes apparent that in transforming our conceptualization of research participants, we reconceptualize the roles of investigators and the interpretive community as well.

A final aspect of the partnership model that needs mention is the view that this approach offers a more comprehensive, and therefore a better, science (Bibace, Young, Herrenkohl, & Wiley, in this volume). The methodological changes suggested increase the opportunity for representation of multiple perspectives (i.e., eliciting participant feedback, increasing community access to data, incorporating participant-generated questions).

However, the knowledge produced by such methods is not comprehensive, only more comprehensive than before. One can never represent the view from a truly comprehensive vantage point. In addition, this multiperspectival work is more fully contextualized; that is, the partnership model exemplifies a move toward a more historically and socially grounded view of what scientists produce. By incorporating multiple perspectives, such as those of participants and audiences, we more comprehensively appreciate and delineate the situation, the community, and, ultimately, the limits within which our knowledge is produced. Thus, by following such an approach, we, as scientists, can become more specific, local, and less universalistic in our knowledge claims; more humble; and, therefore, self-reflexive, in our cognizance of the constraints within which we conduct our work. We argue that this move does not diminish the significance of our work; it enables us to be aware of the complexity of the circumstances that make our work possible at all.

REFERENCES

Danziger, K. (1990). *Constructing the subject: Historical origins of psychological research.* Cambridge: Cambridge University Press.

Engel, G. L. (1977). Physician-scientists and scientific physicians: Resolving the humanism-science dichotomy. *American Journal of Medicine, 81,* 107–111.

Falmagne, R. J. (1998). A time of epistemic transformation and responsibility: Essay review of "Ethnography and Human Development: Context and Meaning in Social Inquiry." *Human Development, 41,* 134–144.

Farrow, H., Moss, P., & Shaw, B. (1995). Symposium on feminist participatory research. *Antipode, 27,* 71–74.

Fisher, C. B., & Fyrberg, D. (1994). Participant partners: College students weigh the costs and benefits of deceptive research. *American Psychologist, 49,* 417–427.

Gergen, K. J. (1985). Social constructionist inquiry: Context and implications. In K. J. Gergen & K. E. Davis (Eds.), *The social construction of the person.* (pp. 3–18). New York: Springer-Verlag.

Gergen, K. J. (1991). *The saturated self: Dilemmas of identity in contemporary life.* New York: Basic Books.

Gergen, K. J. (1994). Exploring the postmodern: Perils or potentials? *American Psychologist, 49,* 412–416.

Gibson-Graham, J. K. (1994). 'Stuffed if I know!': Reflections on post-modern feminist social research. *Gender, Place and Culture, 1,* 205–224.

Harding, S. (1993). Rethinking standpoint epistemology: "What is strong objectivity?" In L. Alcoff & E. Potter (Eds.), *Feminist epistemologies* (pp. 49–82). London: Routledge.

Jewson, N. D. (1976). The disappearance of the sick-man from medical cosmology, 1770–1870. *Sociology, 10,* 225–244.

Jones, J. (1993). The Tuskegee syphilis experiment: "A moral astigmatism." In S. Harding (Ed.), *The "racial" economy of science: Toward a democratic future* (pp. 275–286). Bloomington: Indiana University Press.

Keller, E. F. (1985). *Reflections on gender and science.* New Haven, CT: Yale University Press.

Kimble, G. A. (1984). Psychology's two cultures. *American Psychologist, 39,* 833–839.

Kuhn, T. S. (1970). *The structure of scientific revolutions* (2nd ed.). Chicago: University of Chicago Press.

Moss, P. (1995). Reflections on the 'gap' as part of the politics of research design. *Antipode, 27,* 82–90.

Proctor, R. N. (1988). *Racial hygiene: Medicine under the Nazis.* Cambridge: Harvard University Press.

Shaw, B. (1995). Contradictions between action and theory: Feminist participatory research in Goa, India. *Antipode, 27,* 91–99.

3

TOWARD A COEXISTENCE CONCEPT OF CAUSAL REASONING ABOUT ILLNESS IN CHILDREN AND ADULTS

Roger Bibace
Clark University and
University of Massachusetts Medical School

James J. Dillon
State University of West Georgia

Johanna Sagarin
Children's Hospital, Boston

ABSTRACT

Recent research on conceptual development in children's reasoning about illness suggests the presence of specialized abilities not expected to occur within the Piagetian sequence until many years later. A case for the "hardwiring" of these abilities is often subsequently made. The following study attempts to examine whether these precocious responses are part of an overall concept of illness, or are a function of a specialized experimental task. Forty-one children between 7 and 12 years, and 38 college students between 18 and 22 years were interviewed about their conceptions of various illnesses. Participants were then given a series of cards each containing one of six developmental levels of reasoning about illness. Scores for initial interview responses were compared with choices of the "best" response on the card sort. Results suggest that when given an array of options, both children and adults will opt for highly developed forms of reasoning, but in the absence of the array, rely on less mature forms of reasoning. Implications for a "coexistence" concept of development are discussed.

Currently, somewhat of a controversy has developed between researchers operating from a cognitive-science perspective and those operating from a more traditional cognitive-developmental perspective. Specifically, recent research with infants and children (e.g., Baillargeon, Spelke, & Wasserman, 1985; Carey, 1985; Chi, 1978; Gelman & Baillargeon, 1983; Spelke, 1988; Wellman, 1990) indicates the presence, at very early ages, of highly specialized cognitive abilities not expected to occur within the Piagetian cognitive-developmental sequence until many years later. This controversy is also reflected in the domain of children's conceptions of illness. For example, Lyon, Kate, and Stoat (1995) have shown that both healthy and ill three- and four-year-olds correctly distinguish in various stories between children who are acting immorally and children who are sick or being treated. Kalish (1996) has suggested that four- and five-year-old children's ascriptions of illness generally match adults'. Schonfeld and colleagues (1995) have demonstrated gains after educational instruction of at least two years' growth in level of conceptual sophistication in children's understanding of the causality of AIDS. Sigelman and colleagues (1996) have pointed to similar gains concerning conceptual understanding of the causes of AIDS and flu, AIDS risk factors, and AIDS generally. These authors suggest that contrary to Piagetian formulations (e.g., Bibace & Walsh, 1980), young children can grasp scientific theories of disease, and may not necessarily grow through a series of developmental stages to come to reason in scientific, formal-logical ways about illness.

We suggest that some distance can be made toward sorting out this issue by focusing on the structure of the *experimental task* itself. That is, certain experimental tasks may induce developmentally extraordinary responses, which are not normally in evidence as part of the individual's cognitive repertoire. In this context, Fischer & Bidell (1991) suggest that we distinguish between a "precocious behavior" and a "skill." Precocious behaviors occur in highly specific contexts in response to remarkably simplified tasks that require the child to engage a limited number of components. A skill, on the other hand, is the capacity to engage in a given behavior across a *wide variety* of contexts in response to complex tasks in which the child must engage several components. In what they call the "argument from precocity," the researcher takes the presence of a precocious behavior (e.g., animate vs. inanimate or causality vs. immorality distinctions) as *prima facia* evidence that a sophisticated *concept* is present at a particular early age. They argue that it is misleading to find a precocious behavior through ingenious experimental methods and then to treat this finding as showing a stable capacity or concept that is seen to be independent of the special experimental context in which it occurred.

In an example of such an "ingenious" methodology, Kalish (1996), in his recent study on preschoolers' conceptions of illness, read the child a character description and presented pictures depicting the cause of the character's illness and his/her symptoms. Then he asked the child a series of "forced-choice" questions, such as: Is the individual "sick or not?" Does the individual "need a medicine from a doctor or not?" Similarly, Lyon, Kate, and Stoat (1995), in their study on preschoolers' ability to distinguish between illness and immorality, first told the child a story, and then said, "Sometimes these children did things that are naughty, sometimes they did things that are nice, and sometimes they did things that are just o.k. You can help me figure out which children did things that are naughty." Note that these experimental tasks involve putting the child in the position of an *evaluator.* Specifically, the child is invited to draw contrasts and to make comparisons among a range of presented options in order to choose the "best" one. Such tasks surely differ from traditional Initiation-Response-Evaluation (IRE) tasks (e.g., Mehan, 1979; Sinclair & Coulthard, 1976) in which the experimental task consists of questions posed by the researcher, spontaneous responses given by the participant, followed by an evaluation by the researcher.

An experimental task in which the child is put in the position to compare, contrast, and evaluate various presented options can be seen as among the highest level of "distancing strategies" in Sigel's (1970; 1993) Psychological Distancing model of conceptual development. Sigel has persuasively shown that performance is greatly enhanced as a function of the demand characteristics of the experimental task, specifically, the degree of "distance" that the child is prompted to take from the concrete experimental situation (e.g., asking the child to draw inferences, render cause-and-effect judgments, make plans, formulate hypotheses). The question is, however, whether children who demonstrate these precocious behaviors in experimental settings will exhibit the same precocious responses *outside* of these specialized, high-level-distancing contexts. The following study is designed to compare the direct responses of children and adults to questions about illness with their responses from among a "forced-choice" array of options.

METHOD AND PROCEDURE

Participants

The participants in this study included 38 college students (26 females and 12 males), 11 ten- to twelve-year-olds (4 males and 7 females), and 30 seven- to nine-year-olds (8 male and 22 female). The children were drawn from an elementary school that consisted of a 50% mixture of Hispanic and Caucasian students. The college students were drawn from a predominantly white university.

Procedure

In school, the children were given assent forms to sign and consent forms for their parents to sign. The children who finally participated in the study were those who returned both signed forms to their school. The college students were recruited in classes and given consent forms to sign at the time of the interviews.

Each interview lasted from approximately one half hour to one hour. The interviews consisted of the Bibace and Walsh (1980) conceptions of illness protocol which relies on Piaget's clinical interview method (see Appendix A) and a card sort task. With the conceptions of illness protocol, participants were asked questions relating to different illnesses: "sick," cold, headache, heart attack, cancer, and AIDS. For each illness, participants were asked what it was, how people got it, how one might prevent it, what some misconceptions about that illness are, and finally, should children with that illness go to school.

After participants gave their spontaneous responses during the interview, they were asked to perform a card sort task. For each of the aforementioned illnesses, participants were given six cards with "other kids' responses" on them and asked to put them in order from "best" to "worst." Each of the six cards was representative of one of the developmental stages elaborated in Appendix B.

Scoring

Each participant's spontaneous responses were scored according to the following three major categories, each with two subdivisions, as illustrated in Appendix B: phenomenism, contagion, contamination, internalization, physiological, and psychophysiological. Each participant was scored according to these six subcategories. Raters did not score their own interviews. Reliability, as assessed by Kappa (Cohen, 1968), was found to be .96.

RESULTS

Participants' scores for spontaneous responses were compared to their own choice of the "best" response during the card sort task. Wilcoxon signed rank tests (Siegel & Castellan, 1988) were used to compare the two measures for college students and seven- to nine-year-olds. Because of the small number of participants for the ten- to twelve-year-olds, sign tests were also used to compare the two responses for this age group. For the college students, the comparisons of their spontaneous responses on questions about AIDS with their card sort responses did show significant improvement:

$$z(N = 38) = -2.20, p \leq .05$$

For the ten- to twelve-year-olds, the comparison of their spontaneous responses on questions about colds with their card sort responses was significant:

$$p\ (N = 11) = .0195, p \leq .05$$

Comparisons of their spontaneous responses on questions about AIDS with card sort responses also showed significant improvement:

$$p\ (N = 11) = .0010, p \leq .01$$

For the seven- to nine-year-olds, comparisons of their spontaneous response on questions for colds with card sort responses also showed significant improvement

$$z(N = 30) = -2.52, p \leq .0059$$

Comparisons for AIDS for this same group was also significant:

$$z(N = 30) = -4.23, p \leq .00003$$

DISCUSSION

For both children and adults, the same individual, on the very same day, reasons about illness in qualitatively different ways. Different task demands appear to elicit different reasoning potentials within the individual. Research on children's and adults' reasoning about illness (e.g., Bibace & Walsh, 1980; Walsh & Bibace, 1991) in which participants are not given an array of options to choose from, but must spontaneously generate a response, suggests an asymmetrical relationship between children's and adults' causal reasoning about illness such that children *never* demonstrate the more abstract levels of thought. But as the present study indicates, children, under certain experimental conditions, will employ forms of causal reasoning about illness that are more developmentally advanced than the forms that they typically employ. Conversely, Bibace, Sagarin, and Dyl (in press) have shown that in college students there is a coexistence of magical and concrete forms of reasoning with formal and abstract forms. Thus, for both children and adults, there appears to be a great deal of intra-individual *variability* with respect to forms of reasoning about illness. This variability leads us to embrace an alternative theoretical model of development than currently exists in the field.

Siegler (1994) has argued that *variability* is, in fact, the "key" to understanding cognitive development generally. He characterizes the basic concepts of five extant theories of development as "steps" (p. 406). That is, most theories of development involve "replacement" concepts. With replacement concepts, development is seen to occur in a linear, stage-by-stage fashion; step three, for example, cannot coexist with step one. Siegler suggests "waves" as a preferred metaphor to "steps" (p. 410). This is seen as an improvement because we are enabled to account for the immense variability we see within and between various ages and stages of cognitive development. We would argue that as powerful as this wave metaphor is, it still lacks the possibility of coexistence of *all* stages together within a single individual. The results of this study support a coexistence concept of psychological development in that the *same participant*, on the *same day*, can perform at significantly different stages of cognitive development with respect to his or her reasoning about illness.

The theoretical model we suggest is based principally upon the work of the psychologist Heinz Werner (1948, 1955), and is amplified by such figures as Subbotsky (1993), and Siegler (1994). We contrast our "coexistence" concept of development with two principal conceptions of development: a continuity concept of development, and a replacement concept of development. With continuity concepts, development is seen to unfold "maturationally" in a continuous, linear sequence. With replacement concepts, development is seen to occur in a linear, stage-by-stage fashion. By contrast, with coexistence concepts, initial immature forms of thinking are not seen as supplanted with development, or as unfolding out of earlier forms, but come to *coexist* alongside later more mature forms. We argue that a coexistence concept of development is more comprehensive because it accounts for group differences related to age, and also encompasses individual and *intra-individual* differences, which we have observed in our study.

Under typical researcher–participant interactions (e.g., Bibace & Walsh, 1980), in which the researcher asks a question, the child answers the question, and the researcher evaluates the response, children and adults differ significantly with respect to the frequency and developmental sophistication of forms of reasoning about illness. Specifically, older children and adults rely on cognitive processes (abstract, formal, scientific) that young children *never* demonstrate. However, the novel feature of the coexistence concept of development can be demonstrated through the sorting task employed in the present study. If the child is encouraged to sort, to compare, and to rank order responses that exemplify all the categories relied upon by the *researcher*, then the young child's choices clearly indicate a preference for responses based on more mature cognitive processes compared to his or her own spontaneously generated answers. It is this "potential" or "latent" knowledge that can be mobilized by certain experimental conditions in contrast to the usual "interviewing" of the child. And, of course, the ingenious experimental conditions created by many cognitive scientists have repeatedly demonstrated the child's hitherto unsuspected knowledge.

Our claims for the coexistence concept of development are, in summary, that the coexistence concept has heuristic value and challenges developmental psychology to: 1) acknowledge the existence of less mature forms of thought in more cognitively mature individuals, and 2) recognize the educational implications stemming from the possibility that more mature forms of thought can be elicited even from young children by employing carefully constructed techniques. Traditional replacement concepts of development, continuity concepts of development, and the theoretical framework of cognitive science could perhaps profit from a reexamination in terms of the coexistence concept of development.

APPENDIX A: CONCEPTIONS OF ILLNESS PROTOCOL*

1. How do people get sick?
2. What is a cold?
   2a. How does a person get a cold?
   2b. Can people do something so they won't get a cold?
3. What is a headache?
   3a. How does a person get a headache?
   3b. Can people do something so they won't get a headache?
4. What is a heart attack?
   4a. How does a person get a heart attack?
   4b. Can people do something so they won't get a heart attack?
5. What is cancer?
   5a. How does a person get cancer?
   5b. Can people do something so they won't get cancer?
6. What is AIDS?
   Probe: What are the symptoms of AIDS? (For children: When a person has AIDS, what is the sickness like?)
   6a. How does a person get AIDS?
   Probe: How does (the cause) lead to (the symptoms)?
   6b. Is there anything people can do so they won't get AIDS? (How does ________ help them not to get AIDS?)
   6c. Sometimes people talk about the ways you don't get AIDS. Do you know any ways that you don't get AIDS?
   6d. Should kids with AIDS go to school? Why? Why not?

APPENDIX B: DEVELOPMENTAL LEVELS OF REASONING ABOUT ILLNESS**

Magical Level: Explanations Based on Association

Phenomenism. The child describes the illness in terms of any phenomenon he or she has experienced as associated with the illness without clear differentiation of cause and effect, for example, "A cold is from . . . it's when your nose runs."

Contagion. The child describes the illness in terms of body experiences or symptoms. He or she associates a specific external cause with the illness, but cannot explain how the cause leads to the effect, for example, "A cold is a runny nose and it's like from going outside in winter." (How?) "It's from being out in the winter."

---

*(Bibace & Walsh, 1980)

**(Bibace, Schmidt, & Walsh, 1994)

Concrete Level: Explanation Based on Sequence

Contamination. The child describes illness in terms of experienced symptoms and explains its cause as originating in external acts or situations. The child explains how a sequence of causal events leads to the illness by contacting or involving the body as a whole, for example, "A cold is from when you're swimming in cold water or out in the snow. It stays in your body . . . it goes up onto your chest."

Internalization. The child describes the illness and explains how a sequence of mechanical actions leads to changes in specific internal body parts, for example, "A cold is when your nose gets stuffed up and you can't breathe. It's from the germs getting into your nose and lungs and clogging them up so you can't breathe. You sneeze to get the germs out."

Abstract Level: Explanations Based on Interaction

Physiological. The older child or adult describes an entire internal disease process involving the interaction of multiple causes and effects on multiple body parts, for example, "A cold is a change within the body resulting in symptoms like coughing, sneezing, running nose, headaches, and stuffed-up sinuses. You catch the germs that are all around us. Coughing and running nose are the side effects of the body's fighting them off, it makes mucous to carry away the dead germs."

Psychophysiological. The older child or adult explains how multiple causes and effects interact by describing transformations at the cellular level, for example, "A cold is the collection of symptoms that define the immune system's response to an invading virus. The white blood cells . . . And this happens when the person is experiencing a lot of stress."

REFERENCES

Baillargeon, R., Spelke, E. S., & Wasserman, S. (1985). Object permanence in five month olds. *Cognition, 20*, 191–208.

Bibace, R., & Walsh, M. E. (1980). Development of children's concepts of illness. *Pediatrics, 66*(6), 912–917.

Bibace, R., Schmidt, L. R., & Walsh, M. E. (1994). Children's perceptions of illness. In G.N. Penny, P. Bennett, & M. Herbert (Eds.), *Health psychology: A lifespan perspective* (pp.13–30). Philadelphia: Harwood Academic.

Bibace, R., Sagarin, J., & Dyl, J. (1998). The heuristic value of Werner's co-existence concept of development. *Journal of Applied Developmental Psychology, 19*, 153–163.

Carey, S. (1985). *Conceptual change in childhood.* Cambridge: MIT Press.

Chi, M. T. H. (1978). Knowledge structure and memory development. In R. Siegler (Ed.), *Children's thinking: What develops?* (pp. 73–96). Hillsdale, NJ: Lawrence Erlbaum.

Cohen, J. (1968). Weighted kappa: Nominal scale agreement with provision for scaled disagreement or partial credit. *Psychological Bulletin, 70,* 213–220.

Fischer, K. W., & Bidell, T. R. (1991). Constraining nativist inferences about cognitive capacities. In S. Carey & R. Gelman (Eds.), *The epigenesis of mind: Essays on biology and knowledge* (pp. 199–235). Hillsdale, NJ: Lawrence Erlbaum.

Gelman, R., & Baillargeon, R. (1983). A review of some Piagetian concepts. In J. H. Flavell & E. M. Markman (Eds.), *Handbook of child psychology* (pp. 167–230). New York: John Wiley.

Kalish, C. (1996). Causes and symptoms in preschoolers' conceptions of illness. *Child Development, 67,* 1647–1670.

Lyon, T. D., Kate, P. M., & Stoat, R. (1995, March). *Sick vs. bad: Healthy and ill preschooler's ability to distinguish between illness and immorality.* Paper presented at the meeting of the Society for Research in Child Development, Indianapolis, Indiana.

Mehan, H. (1979). *Learning lessons.* Cambridge: Harvard University Press.

Schonfeld, D. J., O'Hare, L. L., Perrin, E. C., Quackenbrish, M., Showalter, D. R., & Cicchetti, D.V. (1995). A randomized, controlled trial of a school-based multifaceted AIDS education program in the elementary grades: The impact on comprehension, knowledge, and fear. *Pediatrics, 95*(4), 480-486.

Siegel, S., & Castellan, N. J. (1988). *Nonparametric statistics for the behavioral sciences.* New York: McGraw-Hill.

Siegler, R. S. (1994). Cognitive variability: A key to understanding cognitive development. *Current Directions in Psychological Science, 3*(1), 1–5.

Sigel, I. E. (1970). The distance hypothesis: A causal hypothesis for the acquisition of representational thought. In M. R. Jones (Ed.), *Miami Symposium on the Prediction of Behavior, 1968: Effect of early experience* (pp. 99–118). Coral Gables, FL: University of Miami Press.

Sigel, I. E. (1993). The centrality of a distancing model for the development of representational competence. In R. R. Cocking & A. Renninger (Eds.), *The development and meaning of psychological distance* (pp.141–158). Hillsdale, NJ: Lawrence Erlbaum.

Sigelman, C., Derenowski, E., Woods, T., Mukai, T., Alfeld-Liro, C., Durazo, O., & Maddock, A. (1996). Mexican-American and Anglo-American children's responsiveness to a theory-centered AIDS education program. *Child Development, 67,* 253–266.

Sinclair, J., & Coulthard, R. (1976). *Towards an analysis of discourse: The English used by teachers and pupils.* London: Oxford University Press.

Spelke, E. S. (1988). Where perceiving ends and thinking begins: The apprehension of objects in infancy. *Minnesota Symposium on Child Psychology, 20,* 197–234.

Subbotsky, E. V. (1993). *Foundations of the mind: Children's understanding of reality.* Cambridge: Harvard University Press.

Walsh, M. E., & Bibace, R. (1991). Children's conceptions of AIDS: A developmental analysis. *Pediatric Psychology, 16,* 273–285.

Wellman, H. M. (1990). *The child's theory of mind.* Cambridge: MIT Press.

Wellman, H. M., & Gelman, S. (1992). Cognitive development: Foundational theories of core domains. *Annual Review of Psychology, 43,* 337–375.

Werner, H. (1948). *Comparative psychology of mental development.* New York: International Universities Press.
Werner, H. (1955). Microgenesis and aphasia. *The Journal of Abnormal and Social Psychology, 7,* 347–353.

4

TOWARD A PARTNERSHIP WITH RESEARCH PARTICIPANTS

Barbara Noel Dowds
Regis College and University of Massachusetts Medical School

Monica H. Ferraro
Clark University

ABSTRACT

The structure of a traditional experimenter–subject interaction in psychology takes the role of scientist to be that of expert authority. While it is an approach that has contributed richly to psychology in America, it is also a limiting framework. Here we describe some of the limitations and explore some of the alternatives.

The structure of a traditional experimenter–subject interaction in psychology has, for many decades, reflected the value orientations implicit in psychology's "normal science" paradigm. The most recent edition of the *Publication Manual of the APA* (1994), while renaming "subjects" as "participants" (which we believe is an ethically and scientifically important change), selected as sample papers the reports of two studies (pp. 258–272) that utilized traditional experimenter–subject interactions. This view of experimenter–participant interactions, which is derived from the natural sciences and strives for "objectivity," takes the role of the scientist to be that of expert authority (see Chapter 2). It is an approach that has contributed richly to psychology in America and within which many psychologists and educators, including one of this chapter's authors, have worked for years (e.g., Dowds &

Fontana, 1977; Dowds & Marcel, 1998). It is also a limiting perspective. This chapter describes some of the limitations and explores some of the alternatives, while acknowledging the strengths and accomplishments of psychology's normal science paradigm.

Within the normal science paradigm, we adhere to "role-prescribed" behaviors as expert researchers. Experimenter–subject interactions are driven by the researcher's questions. Rarely do we as researchers seek to answer what others, particularly research participants, think are the important questions. Beutler, Williams, Wakefield, and Entwistle (1995) suggested that "scientists may be missing important avenues for identifying critical areas of research" (pp. 989–990) because researchers pay scant attention to clinicians' views and writings. We suggest that scientists "may be missing important avenues for identifying critical areas of research" because we pay little attention to or do not even consider the views, ideas, and questions of our research participants. This tendency is consistent with the longstanding tension between psychology's scientific and humanistic cultures (cf. Kimble, 1984). Scientists typically study behavior from a nomothetic perspective, utilizing experimental and quantitative research methodologies. Yet as scientists we could also conceptualize our research participants' views as idiographic findings, as worthwhile ideas for empirical confirmation or disconfirmation (Beutler, Williams, Wakefield, & Entwhistle, 1995). In order to do this, we must learn to listen to our research participants, to engage in dialogue with them, and to value their ideas and insights. Rather than the typical situation in which we as researchers determine the research topic and the hypotheses, we might work collaboratively with our research participants, including issues and questions they believe to be important in our investigations (cf. Chapter 1).

THE TRADITIONAL EXPERIMENTER–SUBJECT PARADIGM

In our traditional "role-prescribed" behaviors as expert researchers, we determine not only the broad "what" (topic and hypotheses) of the investigation but also the particular "hows" (the ways in which the topic is investigated) by choosing a methodology (e.g., experiment, survey, structured interview) and specific instruments to investigate the questions we have articulated. This traditional experimenter–subject relationship results in answers from research subjects that are *constrained*. The subjects' answers are constrained because they are framed and limited by the parameters of our questions, which, in turn, are framed and limited by the necessarily somewhat limited perspectives we hold. In addition, subjects' answers are constrained by the power structure of the relationship, in which the subjects' roles are so narrowly circumscribed, that besides answering our questions as we have framed them or participating in the experiments as we have designed them, the subjects' only other option is to withdraw from the study.

A concrete example of role constraints is evidenced in a recent research project in which one of the authors participated (Dowds, Quinn, & Apostoleris, 1996), in which we investigated psychosocial factors and pregnancy outcomes. We chose psychological variables that we believed were important, including locus of control. Then we chose a particular measure for each of the variables, and for measures like locus of control, we, like most researchers, chose an already established questionnaire. When we asked our subjects to complete the questionnaire, we interacted with them in as standardized a way as possible. If they had questions about a particular item, we tried not to follow up on the individualized meaning the question had for them. Instead we suggested that they just respond with the first answer that came to mind. It was our hope that, by having enough subjects complete the measure, whatever error was there would be evenly distributed, and we would be absolved from having to worry about individual idiosyncrasies. When all of the subjects completed the questionnaires, we scored them and then related the scores to the outcome measures, which were also chosen by us, the researchers. We were interested in group data and patterns, not individual responses. We wanted to see if there were statistically significant relationships between locus of control and the outcome measures. Specifically, we hypothesized that there would be a positive relationship between internal locus of control and avoidance of risky behaviors and that there would be a negative relationship between chance locus of control and avoidance of risky behaviors. We tested our hypotheses using partial correlations to control for differences in education. Alternatively, we might have subdivided the sample into groups, based either on already established norms or on the sample's median scores, to see if there were statistically significant differences between groups on the outcome measures. As scientists using either statistical approach, we are utilizing a nomothetic, quantitative approach. From within this perspective, our subjects have utilitarian value to us as researchers.

There are certain advantages to this approach. The traditional experimenter–subject approach is probably less time consuming than a partnership approach in which both the researchers' and the research participants' interests and ideas must be addressed. In addition, there is a certain comfort with well-established roles, including experimenter–subject roles, probably especially so for experimenters. This comfort with our roles as experimenters contrasts with the uncertainty of trying new approaches. Perhaps most importantly, much of what we psychologists know about human behavior is the result of "normal science" investigations. From experimental studies such as Milgram's (1963, 1965) classic work on obedience to questionnaire studies such as those employing Eysenck's inventory of personality traits (e.g., Barrett, Petrides, Eysenck, & Eysenck, 1998; Eysenck, 1964), we have learned a great deal from research within psychology's "normal science" paradigm, with its traditional experimenter–subject roles. Moreover, the knowledge that we have gained contributes to many areas of society, including the education of children, treatment of the ill, and improvements in the "fit" between employees and tasks. Thus, at least in some important ways, psychology's "normal science" does work.

CHANGING PARADIGMS

Just as our views of research "subjects" were derived from a particular time and place in history, our evolving ideas about research "participants" derive from our current context. Influences outside psychology, such as the civil rights movement and feminist and humanist studies on the role of power in the creation of knowledge, have led to a focus on empowerment or equity for all individuals regardless of race, gender, or class. This has resulted in an intellectual climate in which equity (or lack thereof) can be examined in socially prescribed roles such as physician–patient, teacher–student, and researcher–research participant. Further, it has contributed to some social/behavioral scientists trying to "lessen the psychological distance" between expert scientist and research subjects, or "building bridges between experts and novices." We believe this concern for the well-being of the other is an important gain for us as scientists, and for us as a society. (For further discussion of ethical considerations, see Chapter 10.)

Will we gain more than we may lose by adopting a different paradigm for research? After all, we as psychologists really do have some expertise. Do we want to trust the outcome of our research to our "subjects?" One analogy that comes readily to mind is that of traditional parent–child roles in which parents know best, set the parameters, and enforce the rules. The flow (of directions, knowledge, etc.) is from parent to child. The authoritarian parent role, like the traditional experimenter role, has its advantages. Yet in each case there is a richness of ideas and of interaction that is lost. And, as any of us who has been a parent knows, we do *not* always know best or come close to knowing it all. Our children, knowing our love for them, may feel free to tell us this, and help us learn with them about ideas and possibilities that either we or they alone would not have considered. However, our research participants are not likely to feel as free with us. Like the subjects in Milgram's experiments (1963, 1965), they are likely to do as they are told and not much else. They are not likely to challenge us, to expand our horizons, or to share with us their insider perspectives. We, as scientists, lose when we only engage in typical experimenter–subject interactions. That is, there are certain types of research projects, certain topics of investigation that are hampered from a scientific standpoint when we limit the participation of our subjects to doing only what they are told, to thinking only within our frames of reference. As individual investigators and as a science, we lose ideas and possibilities.

CONTRASTING PARADIGMS IN THE STUDY OF PSYCHOSOCIAL FACTORS AND PREGNANCY

Let us return to the example of psychosocial variables related to pregnancy outcome. As noted earlier, we had hypothesized that locus of control would be predictive of adherence to healthy behaviors during pregnancy. Locus of control has been used to predict a variety of health related behaviors (e.g., Strickland, 1978; Wallston & Wallston, 1978, 1982; Wilson et al., 1986). Several studies have examined locus of control in relation to pregnancy. Labs and Wurtele (1986), using the Fetal Health Locus of Control (FHLC) questionnaire, which reflects three dimensions of locus of control (Internal, Chance, and Powerful Others), each measured by a subscale of the FHLC, found that women high in an Internal locus of control were less likely to smoke or to drink caffeinated beverages than were women low in an Internal locus of control. Also using the FHLC scale, Tinsley, Trupin, Owens, and Boyum (1993) reported that a high Internal locus of control predicted lower usage of cigarettes, nonprescription drugs, and street drugs. Using the Multidimensional Health Locus of Control Scale, Kruse, Zweig, and LeFevre (1988) found that a high Powerful Others orientation was related to risk avoidant behaviors, including a lower probability of smoking and drinking during the pregnancy. We used this literature as the basis for our hypothesis that women high in an Internal locus of control orientation would be most likely to avoid behaviors during pregnancy that posed a risk to the baby, while women high in a Chance orientation would be least likely to avoid such behaviors. Women high in a Powerful Others orientation were expected either to be at an intermediate level of risk avoidant behaviors or to be similar to those with an Internal locus of control orientation because they would be likely to follow the recommendations of their health care providers, whom we conceptualized as Powerful Others to a pregnant woman.

As part of a study investigating a biopsychosocial approach to pregnancy and birth outcomes, 61 women receiving prenatal care gave informed consent. The sample included women from a range of socioeconomic backgrounds.

The women completed several measures including the FHLC scale (Labs & Wurtele, 1986) which measures locus of control with respect to maternal behaviors. According to Labs and Wurtele, the FHLC purpose is to facilitate the prediction of factors contributing to compliance with health-related recommendations during pregnancy.

The women also completed a self-report measure of risk avoidance behavior. This measure was a weighted composite of self-reported risky behaviors including smoking, alcohol consumption, illegal drug use, missing prenatal appointments, improper use of prescription medications, inconsistent use of prenatal vitamins, poor diet, lack of sleep, and lack of exercise.

Contrary to predictions, after controlling for education, FHLC scale scores were not significantly related to the self-reported measure of risk avoidance or to birth outcomes. That is, our results were inconsistent with our hypotheses. Had we these results in the past, we might simply have said, in effect, "O.K. that's the end of that idea. Either there are no group differences or our measure is inadequate." Yet because we were in a state of disequillibrium, not just because the data did not support our hypotheses, but also because we were not fully satisfied with our role as researchers, we did not just drop the idea. Many of us, in addition to being researchers, are clinicians and are interested in variability within an individual as well variability between groups. At an experiential level, we know firsthand the difficulties of being both scientist and practitioner (Bibace & Walsh, 1982). We were in the process of struggling with some of the underlying assumptions as researchers, not yet having articulated the partnership model, yet no longer satisfied with the traditional researcher–subject paradigm. For all these reasons, we decided to *talk with* some of the women in our study. In talking with them, we wanted to focus on their reality, their lived experiences, and their reflections as the core of the investigation.

Let us look at a subsample of nine women (or approximately 15 percent of the sample) who were interviewed. These women were selected on the basis of their responses to the FHLC Scale, with three women high on the Chance orientation, three women high on the Internal orientation, and three women high on the Powerful Others orientation. Each of the nine women had delivered a healthy baby by the time of the follow-up interview. The interviews were designed to provide qualitative information on the women's social learning histories. For example, a woman high on the chance locus of control was asked, "You indicated that you thought that chance played a role in the health of your baby; what are some of the experiences you've had that led to this belief?" A woman high on the internal locus of control was asked, "You indicated that you thought that what you did while you were pregnant was very important for the health of your baby; what are some of the experiences you've had that led to this belief?"

An analysis of the qualitative interviews suggests that women high in Chance orientation who tended to avoid risky behaviors had a history of a prior pregnancy with a poor outcome. That is, in terms of their learning history, these women had learned that even if they engage in all the recommended behaviors, they may still encounter health related complications (mother or baby) or even lose the baby. As one woman poignantly explained about her prior experiences, "My son developed pneumonia and died a few days after he was born. I've also had several miscarriages. I think I feel the way I do because I did everything I was supposed to do, I took care of myself but there were still problems. There were no explanations the doctors could give me for why my son died or for the miscarriages."

Another woman described her past experience as follows:

> I do feel there is a certain degree to which I play a part in the health of my baby, but there are some things I have no control over. For example, with my first pregnancy I went into early labor, and I started labor early this time too. . . . There is no reason, no answer as to why that happens to me. It just does. I have no control over it and it's not related to anything I do. It just happens for no reason, at least they (the doctors) can't give me one. . . . I did my part of the responsibility, I ate right and avoided things like alcohol. It makes me upset why I can't have a normal pregnancy while so many women can.

Another woman stated that,

> I think that a woman can have some control by taking care of herself the best she can for her baby's sake, but when it comes to some type of biological problem, it's out of her control, it's bad luck. . . . You know what, I just thought of something that never struck me before! All of my babies were born tongue tied—they all needed an operation. Just my children, not their cousins or anyone else in the family. Even though I never thought about it before, it is probably why I think about hereditary factors a lot. I guess the combination between my husband and myself causes this problem, Also (with this pregnancy) the baby's size was really small and the amniotic fluid was low. . . . I was doing everything I could, like eating as much as I could to help the baby's growth, but no matter how much I tried to eat my baby was not going to get big, genetically she was meant to be small . . . it was just meant to be that way.

Thus for some women with a chance locus of control, something beyond their control had determined the outcome of a prior pregnancy. So, although they engaged in healthy behaviors like women with an Internal locus of control, they knew from prior experience that this might not be enough to ensure the health of their baby. This learning history was reflected in their responses to the FHLC scale, in their endorsement of a Chance locus of control. Had we not spoken with them, we could not have known this. By listening to these women's stories we were able to understand why they believed that chance was important in determining the outcomes of their pregnancies, even though they believed that engaging in healthy behaviors during their pregnancies was also important. By listening to them, we learned from them. They were the experts.

THE PARTNERSHIP PARADIGM

By listening to our research participants, we also reduce the likelihood of misunderstanding. We are less likely to think we're getting at one thing, while they think we are getting at something else. For example, at a workshop on partnerships at the 1996 meeting of the Society for Research on Adolescents (Belfor et al., 1996), a researcher reported that, partway through a study with adolescents, she realized that the phrasing of the question, "Are you sexually active?" meant one thing to her as the researcher but something quite different to at least some of the participants. In response to this question, one adolescent replied, "No, I just lay there." While this example is humorous, it does highlight some of the problems with the traditional experimenter–subject relationship. The most likely way to maximize the possibility that we and our research participants get at the same thing is by working together in partnership. That is, when we learn some of their "language" and they learn some of ours, we increase the likelihood of mutual understanding. Moreover, when we learn what questions are important to them and when we address those questions in our research, we will no longer be in a one-way utilitarian relationship. We will also give to them. This permits more of a partnership relationship, one built on reciprocity, respect, and mutual accommodation.

It is important to note that reciprocity, respect, and mutuality do not imply equality. Researchers do have expertise. Participants do have an "inside" perspective. Each group complements the other; each can contribute to increasing our understanding of human behavior. This perspective allows for difference and even for greater expertise in one partner's repertoire (see the literature on mother–infant mutuality [Isabella & Belsky, 1991; Stern, 1985], or better yet, watch a mother and infant as they "dance" together). In addition to assimilating data that our research participants provide, can we also learn to accommodate our research participants? Can we learn to "dance" with them?

In some ways the current situation in psychological research seems similar to that in medicine. When medicine began to thrive as a science, it was able to cure many diseases. Patients came to doctors to be examined, diagnosed, and treated; the doctor was the expert who "took care of" the patient. While this sounds like a caricature, it could be said that the patient's task was to provide a diseased body, the rest was up to the physician. As the successes of modern medicine (and good sanitation) have begun to plateau, we have realized the limitations (as well as the strengths) of the biomedical model. We have broadened our perspectives. We now talk about the biopsychosocial model (Engel, 1980), about the importance of the patient's behaviors in preventing disease and in coping with chronic disease (e.g., McDaniel, Hepworth, & Doherty, 1992; Rolland, 1994; Taylor & Aspinwall, 1990), and about holistic medicine (e.g., Cohen, Tyrrell, & Smith, 1991; Greenfield, Kaplan, Ware, Yano, & Frank, 1988; Pelletier, 1992). Yet the physician still has expertise with respect to the medical literature and the prevention and treatment of disease. Similarly, the psychologist or educator, as researcher, still has expertise with respect to the literature, research design, and data analysis. But in both medical practice and psychological research we are beginning to appreciate the importance of the other (patient/research participant). Neither patient nor research subject is simply an entity that we, as experts, just treat or plug into an experimental design. Rather, patients and research participants are individuals with whom we can form partnerships that, in many cases, may lead to a more comprehensive treatment approach and a more comprehensive understanding of human behavior.

Considering our research participants' ideas is important because if we exclude any specific group, we lose "a segment of the scope of psychological ideas" (Bohan, 1995, p. 2), whether that group consists of scientists or research participants, males or females, empowered or disempowered members of our society. We have much to learn from each other. We need to learn how to learn from one another.

Research methods that might enable us to do this are not yet well articulated. Focus groups are one approach. But there are additional steps that could be taken. For example, after the focus group's discussion, the researchers typically abstract themes or summaries of information. Another step toward a partnership model could occur by then going back to the focus group and asking if the participants believe that these researcher-derived themes and summaries accurately and completely represent the participants' views. That is, do the research participants think the researchers have *heard* what they were saying? Another step, before conducting additional focus groups, would be to ask the current research participants what they believe are important questions for the next groups to consider. What do they, with their insider perspective, suggest are important issues or hypotheses to be explored? And, from an ethical perspective, would it not be important and just to know the ends that they seek, the means that they value? Research partnerships could be further enhanced (between researcher and participant and between researcher and research community) by incorporating research data, particularly qualitative data, into presentations and papers and by seeking out and incorporating alternative interpretations that participants or reviewers might have. Philosophically, we are attempting to circumvent, at least partially, the "egocentric predicament"; that is, the various selves we are stuck with: ourselves as socialized into a particular theoretical perspective, ourselves as committed to a particular hypothesis. In attempting to create partnerships with our research participants, we are consciously trying to circumscribe, or at least partially surmount, our diverse egocentricities. We are trying to build on our shared humanity, to listen to, respect, and learn from our research participants. We can help to build partnerships within the research community by making data available to others (within ethical limits that respect the confidentiality of participants) as occurs, for example, at the Henry A. Murray Research Center at Radcliffe College.

We may need to develop additional research methodologies in order to maximize the possibility of partnerships in research. It is important to give credence to differing methodologies because we lose valuable data if we exclude a particular methodology, whether that methodology be quantitative or qualitative. We argue that what is necessary is a differentiated approach. Researchers need to develop an appreciation that different methodologies may be appropriate in varying contexts, to answer different questions, and to achieve divergent ends.

Perhaps what is needed is the ongoing acknowledgment that psychology operates within multiple paradigms, each with its own strengths and weaknesses (White, 1977). An understanding of the history of psychology as derived from and enriched by both the natural sciences and philosophy (cf. Benjamin, 1992) might be useful in this regard. The tensions between basic and applied research, between laboratory and clinical investigations, are not new. The contrast between causal explanations derived from work in the lab and understanding derived from work in the field stem from fundamentally different world views (Pepper, 1942/1970) that are not easily, if at all, integrated. These disparate paradigms within psychology can be viewed as either a hindrance or a source of richness. If we, as scientists, develop an appreciation of many methodologies, if we develop an appreciation of the value of our research participants' perspectives, we have the opportunity to increase our scientific knowledge of human behavior and to increase the humaneness with which we live our lives.

REFERENCES

Barrett, P. T., Petrides, K. V., Eysenck, S. B. G., & Eysenck, H. J. (1998). The Eysenck Personality Questionnaire: An examination of the factorial similarity of P, E, N, and L across 34 countries. *Personality and Individual Differences, 25,* 805–819.

Belfor, N., Bibace, R., Davis, M. J., Delpappa, E., Young, S. D., Dowds, B. N., Ferraro, M. H., & McMenamy, J. (1996, March). *Adolescent research participants as partners not subjects: Values, concepts and methods.* Workshop at the meeting of the Society for Research on Adolescents, Boston, MA.

Benjamin, L. T. (Ed.). (1992). The history of psychology [Special issue]. *American Psychologist, 47*(2).

Beutler, L. E., Williams, R. E., Wakefield, P. J., & Entwistle, S. R. (1995). Bridging scientist and practitioner perspectives in clinical psychology. *American Psychologist, 50,* 984–994.

Bibace, R., & Walsh, M. E. (1982). Conflict of roles: On the difficulty of being both scientist and practitioner in one life. *Professional Psychology, 13,* 389–396.

Bohan, J. S. (1995). *Re-placing women in psychology* (2nd ed.). Dubuque, IA: Kendall/Hunt.

Cohen, S., Tyrrell, D. A. J., & Smith, A. P. (1991). Psychological stress and susceptibility to the common cold. *New England Journal of Medicine, 325,* 606–612.

Dowds, B. N., & Fontana, A. F. (1977). Patients' and therapists' expectations and evaluations of hospital treatment: Satisfactions and disappointments. *Comprehensive Psychiatry, 18,* 295–300.

Dowds, B. N., & Marcel, B. B. (1998). Students' philosophical assumptions and psychology in the classroom. *Journal of Nursing Education, 37,* 219–221.

Dowds, B. N., Quinn, P., & Apostoleris, N. H. (1996, March). *Locus of control and risk avoidance during pregnancy.* Poster session presented at the annual meeting of the Eastern Psychological Association, Philadelphia, PA.

Engel, G. L. (1980). The clinical application of the biopsychosocial model. *American Journal of Psychiatry, 137,* 535–544.

Eysenck, H. J. (1964). The measurement of personality: A new inventory. *Journal of the Indian Academy of Applied Psychology, 1,* 1–11.

Greenfield, S., Kaplan, S. H., Ware, J. E., Yano, E. M., & Frank, H. J. L. (1988). Patients' participation in medical care: Effects on blood sugar control. *Annuals of Internal Medicine, 3,* 448–457.

Isabella, R. A., & Belsky, J. (1991). Interactional synchrony and the origins of infant-mother attachment: A replication study. *Child Development, 62,* 373–384.

Kimble, G. A. (1984). Psychology's two cultures. *American Psychologist, 39,* 833–839.

Kruse, J., Zweig, S., & LeFevre, M. (1988). Health locus of control and behaviors related to pregnancy. *Family Medicine, 20,* 422–425.

Labs, S., & Wurtele, S. (1986). Fetal health locus of control scale: Development and validation. *Journal of Consulting and Clinical Psychology, 54,* 814–819.

McDaniel, S. H., Hepworth, J., & Doherty, W. J. (1992). *Medical family therapy.* New York: Basic Books.

Milgram, S. (1963). Behavioral study of obedience. *Journal of Abnormal and Social Psychology, 67,* 371–378.

Milgram, S. (1965). Some conditions of obedience and disobedience to authority. *Human Relations, 18,* 57–76.

Pelletier, K. R. (1992). Mind-body health: Research, clinical, and policy implications. *American Journal of Health Promotion, 6,* 345–358.

Pepper, S. C. (1970). *World hypotheses: A study of evidence.* Berkeley, CA: University of California Press. (Original work published 1942)

Publication Manual of the American Psychological Association (4th Ed.). (1994). Washington, DC: American Psychological Association.

Rolland, J. S. (1994). *Families, illness, and disability.* New York: Basic Books.

Strickland, B. (1978). Internal-external expectancies of health related behaviors. *Journal of Consulting and Clinical Psychology, 46,* 1192–1211.

Stern, D. N. (1985). *The interpersonal world of the infant.* New York: Basic Books.

Taylor, S. E., & Aspinwall, L. G. (1990). Psychosocial aspects of chronic illness. In P. T. Costa & G. R. VandenBos (Eds.), *Psychological aspects of serious illness: Chronic conditions, fatal diseases, and clinical care* (pp. 3–60). Washington, DC: American Psychological Association.

Tinsley, B., Trupin, S., Owens, L., & Boyum, L. (1993). The significance of women's pregnancy related locus of control beliefs for adherence to recommended prenatal health regimens and pregnancy outcomes. *Journal of Reproductive and Infant Psychology, 11,* 97–102.

Wallston, K., & Wallston, B. (1978). Development of the multidimensional health locus of control scales. *Health Education Monographs, 6,* 160–170.

Wallston, K., & Wallston, B. (1982). Who is responsible for your health: The construct of locus of control. In G. Sanders & J. Suls (Eds.), *Social psychology of health and illness* (pp. 65–88). Mahwah, NJ: Lawrence Erlbaum.

White, S. H. (1977). Social proof structures: The dialectic of method and theory in the work of psychology. In N. Datan & H. W. Reese (Eds.), *Life-span developmental psychology: Dialectical perspectives on experimental research* (pp. 59–92). San Diego, CA: Academic Press.

Wilson, W., Ary, D., Biglan, A., Glasgow, R., Toobert, D., & Campbell, D. (1986). Psychosocial predictors of self care behaviors (compliance) and glycemic control in non insulin dependent diabetes mellitus. *Diabetes Care, 9,* 614–621.

5

FOCUS GROUPS AS A MEANS FOR ELICITING THE EXPERTISE OF RESEARCH PARTICIPANTS*

Barbara Noel Dowds
Regis College and University of Massachusetts Medical School

Mary Davis
Clark University

Roger Bibace
Clark University and University of Massachusetts Medical School

ABSTRACT

Because of our increasing appreciation of the importance of listening to others' views, we conducted focus groups on unintended pregnancy with female adolescents, with male adolescents, and with clinical staff. These focus groups are

---

*Portions of this chapter are adapted from Davis, M., & Bibace R. (1996, March). *Unintended pregnancy: Teenagers, their beliefs, and reaction to those of experts.* Poster session presented at the annual meeting of the Eastern Psychological Assocation meetings, Philadelphia, PA.

The authors thank Melissa A. Smith for searching PsychLit for studies on unintended, unplanned, and unwanted pregnancies.

discussed from within the framework of a partnership model. We consider implications for both research and consultation.

Our work in the Department of Obstetrics and Gynecology at University of Massachusetts Medical School led to our interest in unintended pregnancy among adolescents. As we began to review the literature and discuss ideas, we realized how well we fit the stereotypes of academics in ivory towers, ready to investigate a topic based on a literature review and discussions with other colleagues, but having little "insider information." We knew we had a choice: we could pursue a more traditional study, in which we designed the questions (perhaps using the questionnaires of other researchers who had already developed reliable and valid measures), or we could use our emerging understanding of the potential for partnerships with research participants. We believed that the partnership model would provide us with more of an "insider's perspective." We also believed we could learn about the strengths and limitations of partnerships with research participants by trying to establish them rather than just thinking about them theoretically.

We decided to talk with three groups: a) adolescents who had or might become pregnant, b) adolescents who had or might impregnate someone, and c) those in our health care setting who work most consistently and directly with pregnant adolescents. In deciding to draw upon these groups' expertise as well as our own, we were explicit that we wanted to learn from them. We were not attempting to see if they knew what we knew, as is the case with some psychological research. Rather we were trying to learn what was important from their perspective. We believed that without including their perspectives, we might well miss important ideas.

Recall the poem of the six blind men and the elephant (Saxe, 1936), in which one man, feeling its side, thought the elephant was like a wall; another, feeling a tusk, described the elephant as being like a spear; a third, feeling the trunk, declared it like a snake; and so on. As this poem illustrates, partial pictures can be quite misleading. Thus we should be more able to "see" the whole picture if we acknowledge our limitations and seek additional knowledge from those who "see a different part of the elephant." We did not want to privilege our perspectives as researchers, or those of female adolescents, or male adolescents, or health care professionals. We wanted to be able to see each perspective.

In order to obtain these perspectives, we implemented focus groups because that methodology is consistent with the partnership model. Focus groups are not expert driven; participants express their views, questions, and concerns. Participants do not talk to the researcher; they discuss among themselves.

In this chapter, we present first the focus groups with adolescents, then the focus group with our health care providers who work with pregnant adolescents. Finally, we discuss how the focus groups have influenced our thinking about research and consultation.

FOCUS GROUPS WITH ADOLESCENTS

We approached teenagers as partners rather than subjects by inviting them to present their beliefs concerning the causes of unintended pregnancy, and then asked them to respond to experts' beliefs regarding this issue. We hoped that this approach would provide some answers, or some new perspectives, to the problem of unintended pregnancies. Data presented by the National Institute of Child Health and Human Development (1994) indicate that the unintended pregnancy and abortion rates in the United States are the highest in the industrialized world.

We included both males and females as participants because, although much of the research and prevention strategies are aimed at females, unintended pregnancy is not a phenomenon that is caused by women acting alone. It is important to note that expert-driven research has, however, focused primarily on females, *as if* unintended pregnancies are just a "woman's issue." A review of published articles investigating unintended, unplanned, or unwanted pregnancies and cited in PsychLit from 1974 to 1997 showed that fewer than 25 percent included males. In contrast, 98 percent included females. Although there has been a slight increase in the inclusion of males in recent years (looking at the studies since 1990, 26 percent included males), there is clearly a tendency to investigate this issue without including half the relevant population.

Participants were 34 teenagers (14 males and 20 females) recruited from two coed inner city youth centers of a western Massachusetts city. They ranged in age from 13 to 18 years, with a mean of 16 years ($SD = 1.41$). Five of the females were mothers and two of the males were fathers.

Facilitators were introduced to teenagers by youth workers employed by the city to staff the youth centers. All participants indicated their interest to the youth workers. Most expressed surprise that a group of researchers from a local university and medical school were highly interested in their opinions and beliefs. At both centers almost all of the "regulars" who were there on the same days as the researchers, wanted to participate. We had to hold a number of focus groups to accommodate the high level of interest. In terms of gender, both males and females were very willing to cooperate. Thus there was little self-selection within the adolescents who attended the youth centers. However, there are probably many differences between adolescents who choose to come to the centers and those who do not.

Despite the adolescents' willingness to participate, there was one observation that caused concern among the facilitators: fear expressed by the female adolescents that the males might overhear their discussions. We had to arrange to meet with the female participants in a private room at the center to allay their fears about possible violent consequences should their beliefs be overheard by certain males. There was no evidence of such fears on the part of the males adolescents, but male facilitators chose also to meet in private rooms.

In the focus groups, the teens tended to take turns speaking, and some expressed both nonverbal (nodding their heads) and verbal agreement with what their peers communicated. Although they were encouraged to express their views if they disagreed with a speaker, this was a rare occurrence, especially among the females who had largely similar views on the causes of unintended pregnancies. Another observation about the groups was that when they contained one or more mothers, there appeared to be a slightly lesser willingness among the non-mothers to express their beliefs about unintended pregnancy. Instead, the mothers in the group would mostly provide their views, and the non-mothers seemed to listen with respect to what they had to say. (We had, based on our clinical experience, chosen to conduct separate focus groups for males and females. We had not thought to conduct separate groups for those who were parents and those who were not.)

Data were collected by audiotaping seven single-sex focus groups (three male and four female) which were conducted for approximately 90 minutes. Each focus group consisted of four to five teenagers and one non-directive facilitator of the same gender. There was an unstructured and a structured segment. The unstructured portion began with the facilitator stating "Researchers have found that 50 percent of all pregnancies are unintended—that is, unwanted or mistimed. Why do you think this might be so?" While there was some hesitation about beginning, once someone spoke, the others were usually clamoring to talk. The facilitators remained nondirective, sometimes asking a question to clarify what had been said, sometimes asking whether others thought the same or differently about an issue just discussed. Individuals presented their own beliefs, and discussed the experiences of teenagers they knew. After approximately 40 minutes, or when it was clear that participants had presented their beliefs as comprehensively as possible, the structured segment was initiated. During this segment, facilitators asked participants to react to four research findings, presented as causes for unintended pregnancy among teenagers. All participants received a copy of the statements and were asked to indicate agreement or disagreement. They were then asked to elaborate on the reasons for their reaction, discussing each finding in turn. The four statements, preceded by "Some experts believe that," read as follows:

1. Girls give sex in order to get love, and boys give love in order to get sex.
2. Girls who are sexually active at early ages are likely to experience sex against their will.
3. A thirteen-year-old who has been taught about birth control is no more likely to use contraceptives than one who has not.
4. Boys are emotionally clogged, and are unable to express their feelings.

Using verbatim transcripts of focus group sessions, the beliefs of males and females concerning unintended pregnancies were extracted. Researchers focused on the content of the adolescents' statements and coded themes that were present across transcripts. Inter-rater reliability, assessed by a kappa coefficient, was .82.

The percentages of males and females citing various causal factors were calculated. These results are presented in Table 5.1.

Males and females were both quite likely to report that a cause of unintended pregnancies was not using contraception. They also reported contraceptive failure as a cause, though it was much less frequently mentioned by both males and females. However, here the similarities between the two groups dropped dramatically, and their differing perspectives on the causes of unintended pregnancies became apparent. Males were much more likely than females to see the female as at fault and to view her as wanting welfare benefits. Females were much more likely to mention the male's request for no contraception and their own fear that if they did ask for condom usage, the male might become violent.

Looking first at the adolescent male focus groups, one male, in describing how it is the female's fault, explained, "You know how in parties sometimes they get drunk and shit, they flirt around and pick you up." Another quickly agreed, "I think so, they get drunk, they do, they do sex, and then they act that 'Oh, it was your fault, I'm going to take you to court, cause you did that against my will.' That do happen. That happens a lot of times."

Males also expressed the view that welfare is part of the problem. One commented, "I think they should make it harder for girls. It's easy for a girl to get pregnant and get so much public assistance, so much benefits, and what not, that is what messes us all up." Another male agreed, asserting, "It should be harder cause girls nowadays, having a baby has turned into like, for some young girls, like a star and shit, like a star." Another blamed the

> agencies, AFDC and all that. They rely on that, you know what I am saying. Like I figure a girl, I seen this happen, a girl gets pregnant right, she gets AFDC, and she gets what, two checks a month, then she claims she has no place to live, and then she gets section. Once she gets section she get her own place, she's straight! See what I am saying, figure, she has a home now, she has a kid, she has, regardless, even though

TABLE 5.1.

Percentages of Males and Females Indicating Their Beliefs Regarding the Causes of Unintended Pregnancy

	Males	Females
Contraception is not used	64%	75%
Contraception fails	21%	35%
Female is at fault	71%	25%
Females receive welfare	64%	15%
Males request non-use of contraception	0%	50%
Females fear violent reaction of males if asked to use condoms	0%	35%

> she has a monthly income, a yearly income, it's not all that great, but still you know what I am saying. Just lay back and have another kid.

In marked contrast, females talked about the males' dislike of contraception, particularly condoms. In their view, the male may want a pregnancy to occur:

> If you get into a relationship with a guy, and if you are younger, I think that most young girls I know, most of my friends don't want a baby, but there are a lot of guys who will say that to a girl, like "Oh, I want you to have my baby, I want you to have my baby," and a lot of the girls get caught up in what the guy is saying so they do it. But I think that the girl doesn't want it herself.

Another said she "heard about guys who have put holes in condoms purposely to get their girlfriends pregnant." Many commented about how "the guy doesn't want to put on a condom." As one described it,

> The guy might complain "Oh come on, come on, you can't do this to me, you got me this excited." A lot of times, its like "you can't stop me now." They don't want to use a condom . . . it doesn't feel the same for them.

In talking about why girls have sex without using a condom, one female explained, "You don't know if he is gonna get mad and hit her." Another observed, "A lot of guys can either get silent or get mad, like if they are ready and the girl is like 'No, no' and pushes them away." Or the boyfriend might respond, "'What are you trying to say, that I got something?' and then I'm not gonna say it again, cause I'm going to make him mad." None seemed comfortable with making the guy angry.

The reactions of males and females to the experts' views were tallied from their written responses of agreement or disagreement to each of the four statements. We used a chi-square test to compare males' and females' responses. The results are presented in Table 5.2.

In the case of statement 1, most males and females (88 percent of the sample) agreed. Also no significant differences between males and females were found for statements 2 and 3. Specifically, a majority of males and females agreed with statement 2 (70 percent of the sample), and a majority disagreed with statement 3 (71 percent of the sample).

The chi-square values reported in Table 5.2 indicate that males and females differed significantly only in their responses to statement 4. The majority of males (71 percent) disagreed with the statement, while the majority of females (85 percent) agreed.

What are some of the implications from these focus groups? First, in light of findings illustrated in Table 5.1, it is noteworthy that males largely have been excluded from research investigating unintended pregnancy. It is disconcerting that 50 percent of females pointed to a male's request for noncontraceptive use, and 35 percent to fear of a male's violent reaction to a request for condom use as reasons for unintended pregnancies. The concern about violence from their partners if they

TABLE 5.2.
Comparing Male and Female Adolescents' Reactions to Expert Findings

	Chi-square value
1. Girls give sex in order to get love, and boys give love in order to get sex.	0.15
2. Girls who are sexually active at early ages are likely to experience sex against their will.	2.62
3. A thirteen year old who has been taught about birth control is no more likely to use contraceptives than one who has not.	2.62
4. Boys are emotionally clogged, and are unable to express their feelings.	11.10*

* $p < .001$

request condom usage is consistent with their fear of violent reactions if certain males overheard their discussions. We believe fear of violence must be addressed both in research studies and in intervention programs.

It is striking that none of the males mentioned either males' request for noncontraceptive use or females' fear of violence as a response to females' request for condom usage. Instead, 71 percent believed that the female is at fault, and 64 percent believed that pregnancy is a technique used by women to claim welfare benefits. Both males and females seem to agree that contraception is not being used, but the explanations for this differ between the sexes. In essence, the reactions of male participants point to a low level of responsibility for the male role in a pregnancy.

It is important to note that the female's fear of a violent response if she asks her partner to use a condom and the male's derogation and blaming of the female are not typically studied in research on unintended pregnancy. Most of that literature has focused on demographic variables, on attitudinal and personality variables, and on sex education. Very little work has focused on issues of power and respect (or lack thereof). That is, the results from the focus groups in this study suggest that expert-driven research is missing significant, and perhaps central, issues in the investigation of unintended pregnancy.

At a more general level, the findings of this study point to the usefulness of approaching research participants as partners, not merely subjects. Permitting participants to present their beliefs and experiences unconstrained by specific questions has value, in that it is possible to learn of participants' actual experiences. By describing the experiences they have encountered or observed, the participants provide researchers with directions on what to address in future investigations. Finally, these adolescents, by explicitly rejecting some expert views, indicated that they do not agree with all of the experts' assessment of them and their motivations.

This suggests, at a minimum, that experts have not yet been able to articulate, fully and accurately, the adolescents' self-perceptions and beliefs regarding unintended pregnancies.

In conclusion, while quantitative research has many merits, it is also clear that permitting participants to present their beliefs and experiences unconstrained by specific questions has value. The female participants highlighted the coercive nature of sexual relations with some males. In doing so, they articulated a dilemma they face: while they may support the use of contraceptives, they feel prevented from doing so by their partners. The importance of targeting males' refusals to use condoms is one implication suggested by these findings. Extending the participant pool of intervention programs to include both males and females, rather than a continuing emphasis on females seems critical.

FOCUS GROUP WITH CLINICAL STAFF

In addition to learning from adolescents themselves, we also realized we could learn from the staff in our clinic, many of whom have years of experience working with pregnant teenagers. They provide continuity of care in the clinic of our teaching hospital, sometimes caring for patients during more than one pregnancy, sometimes getting to know family members and friends of the patients. Professionally, the staff is from the Departments of Nursing and Social Work. Most of them work in the clinic; some work in the community. Most speak only English; some are bilingual, speaking Spanish or Vietnamese and also serving as translators in the clinic.

The staff knew one of the authors as a psychologist/behavioral scientist who worked a half day a week with the obstetrical/gynecological residents, providing feedback on doctor–patient interactions and addressing the psychosocial context of patients' lives. After talking with one of the nurse-midwives about a pilot study on unintended pregnancy, she realized what an important resource the staff could be in helping us think about unintended pregnancy among our clinic population. The staff was excited about contributing to the project, and we held a focus group over an extended lunch hour. When the facilitator arrived, the room was packed, and she was introduced to staff she had not previously met. Since the turnout was much larger than anticipated, taping was impractical, and the facilitator took notes. As with the adolescents, we approached the staff as partners by inviting them to present their beliefs concerning the causes of unintended pregnancy. Also, as with the adolescents, the role of the facilitator was nondirective. The focus group began with the question, "How do you understand why unintended teenage pregnancies occur?" Everyone in the room participated: some confidently presented clearly conceptualized reasons, some presented their ideas more tentatively, and some nodded their agreement. When someone nonverbally indicated disagreement, she was invited to express her thoughts about the idea or observation with which she disagreed. The discussion was lively, with many of the staff contributing, building on each other's comments, and extending them in new directions.

Like the adolescents, the staff saw lack of contraceptives as a major contributor. "They don't use birth control. They have information on it, but they don't make use of birth control." (Staff comments are presented in quotes; however, because the focus group was not taped, the quotes are meant to convey the ideas, but are the facilitator's construction into complete sentences from her notes on the staff's discussion, rather than a staff member's exact words.)

Unlike the adolescents, the staff did not raise the issue of contraceptive failure. This is somewhat surprising since from their clinical experience they know this does sometimes occur. Perhaps they do not see contraceptive failure as a major contributor.

Like the female adolescents, the staff addressed the issue of males' dislike of contraception, but they also included the females' inability, from a psychological perspective, to confront the male on this issue. As this was a major theme in the group's discussion, several of their comments are included. "Males often pressure their partners not to use birth control, and the young females don't have the communication skills to negotiate. They don't know how to talk with the males. They don't know how to protect themselves from STDs either." Another commented,

> As young females they don't think they can say no to sex with their partner. There's a lot of peer pressure to be sexually active. Many young females don't think they can delay becoming sexually active. They are lacking assertiveness. Lots of girls don't feel they have a choice, especially if the guy is older. Some may see sex as a way to get the partner more committed to the relationship.

(This last point was occasionally mentioned by the adolescents as well.) Although the staff was aware of some males' need to control, ("Sometimes there are blatant control issues by the male partner. Sometimes if the female is doing well, his self-esteem goes down, and he wants her pregnant"), none raised the issue of violence or the females' fear of getting their partner angry. However, staff did raise the issue of prior abuse. "Some of them have a 'heavy history of abuse, especially sexual abuse.' So they are involved in sex at an early age. They have a two-week 'good' relationship with somebody, and then they have sex." Staff members also commented on the importance of cultural differences. "There may be some cultural and language barriers. For example, many Puerto Rican males believe neither they nor their partners should use any birth control."

Like the male adolescents, the staff also raised the issue of alcohol, but without blaming the female. "Drugs and alcohol may lower inhibition about having sex."

Also like the male adolescents, the staff discussed the role of welfare. "Our society supports pregnant women—we give them medical care, housing, income.

Our clinic gives lots of social support to these women—they come back for more. We need to empower women, not just give, give, give." Or as another said,

> The welfare system hasn't helped people lead their lives differently. It is difficult to get a job without daycare. Some jobs have no benefits. Somebody who graduates from high school might get a lousy job, lose it, fall by the wayside, get pregnant, and then get money to go to school.

In contrast to these views, some of the staff mentioned structural issues that work against adolescent use of contraceptives. "For some it may be difficult to get transportation to the clinic. For some cost may be a factor; other countries have national health insurance and birth control pills are cheaper."

Some staff commented on the adolescents' lack of cognitive maturity. "They get into having sex without thinking it through. They don't have the maturity to step back and think about the situation." Or as another said, "Some want to experience having sex and think that pregnancy will not happen to them—the adolescent's sense of invulnerability. Some may be lacking in 'fertility awareness' in this regard and insist it can never happen to them." One vivid example of adolescents' unrealistic expectations is that "after a pregnancy scare or after giving birth, some will say they don't need birth control because they're 'never, ever ever' going to have sex again!"

Others commented on developmental, life stage issues. For example, adolescents are " in transition and have no life plan. They lack goals in life." Another staff member observed that "Some of what we call unintended pregnancies may be intended." Consistent with this were the observations that "Some adolescents see pregnancy and having a baby as a way 'to become an adult'—it's a rite of passage. Having a baby is a way to increase self-esteem" and that "having a baby gives her someone who will finally love her the way she wants to be loved."

The clinical staff also raised two other themes, the role of the family and the role of society. Let us look first at the family. Many of the staff comments are presented both because this issue was seldom raised by the adolescents and because the staff commented on several different patterns. Some thought that adolescents "don't want their mothers to know they are having sex. Some are 'in denial.' They don't want to be seen in a clinic or a pharmacy obtaining a prescription." Others felt that families probably don't talk to their kids about sex so it may be "hard for adolescents to talk to their mothers. They need a big sister." From a different perspective, some staff members observed that "many adolescents have mothers and some have sisters who have had babies at young ages. That is, they have important role models in this regard. And some have also had role models of multiple partners being involved with their mothers." By becoming adolescent parents they may be doing what is expected of them. "If the mother had an early pregnancy, she may think it's OK that her daughter do the same. The mom and daughter may have a tacit understanding." Yet for other adolescents, "there may a thrill in doing something that is disapproved of." In some families, becoming pregnant may fulfill the need of the adolescent's parent. For example, "Some mothers around menopause may want their daughters to have a baby and be willing to take care of the baby to avoid the empty nest syndrome." On the other hand, the pregnancy may seem to serve the adolescent's needs: "Many teenagers get pregnant as a way to get out of the house. For Hispanic patients whose parents are from the 'old country,' they want to escape the 'tight reins' of their parents and have freedom like other teenagers in this country."

With respect to society, one staff member observed that "There's less stigma in society toward early sex and pregnancy. Even schools are accepting of it and provide day care. It's more normalized now that it used to be." Another wondered, "Is our society more impulsive than others?" She commented on the prevalence of drive-through restaurants and cited an example of a teenager "who was bored so she had sex." Another observed that "Sex is casual in our society. It's offered freely, like sitting down and having a piece of apple pie with someone." One of her patients had told her about a boy who for "his 16th birthday supposedly had 16 partners." Someone related the pressures from society with the teenagers' developmental stage, noting that "Sex is so romanticized on TV. Yet adolescents are not mature enough to make these kinds of difficult decisions."

What are some of the conclusions we can draw? First many of the issues raised by the adolescents were also raised by the staff. Like the focus groups with the female adolescents, the focus group with the staff highlights the importance of male coercion, in whatever form, as an important issue in unintended pregnancies. Yet the staff was more likely to speak at an abstract level about "pressure from the male," while the female adolescents were more likely to equate pressure with the potential for violence. We believe listening to these young voices about the potential for violence is important. Another similarity the staff had, though here with the focus groups of male adolescents, was the role of welfare in adolescent pregnancy. We believe that in future focus groups with female adolescents it would be important to raise this issue so they could give "voice" to their views.

The staff also discussed the families of pregnant teenagers, presenting many possible ways the adolescent's family may influence the possibility of teenage pregnancy. In future research it would be valuable to have focus groups of families, perhaps mothers of adolescents in particular. Although the adolescents themselves did not tend to raise issues of family influence, it seems likely that the staff pointed to an important omission by the adolescents.

Finally, conducting a focus group with the staff led to some specific research questions and to enhanced collaborative relationships with the staff. With respect to the former, here is one question that was generated: How many of the young females actually enjoy having sex or just do it because they feel they have to (because of pressure from society with its continual glamorization of sex)? This and other questions might lead to new interventions. For example, if many girls reported that they did not enjoy sex and they were given permission and opportunities to discuss this with not yet sexually active girls, would there be a small increase in age of first sexual encounter?

With respect to enhanced collaboration with the staff, two members approached the facilitator after the meeting to express their interest in becoming involved in research. Other staff members approached the facilitator both that day and in the weeks to follow to thank her for the opportunity to share their views.

IMPLICATIONS FOR RESEARCH AND CONSULTATION

Focus groups with adolescents have highlighted the need for research on unintended pregnancies to include males as well as females, because, at least in our work, males and females have differing perceptions about "causes" and "blame." The participants raised a number of issues that need further study, most notably females' concerns about their sexual partner's response, including the possibility of violence, if they urge their partner to use condoms. The female adolescents' concern led us (Ferraro, Bibace, Belfor, Davis, Delpappa, & Dowds, 1996) to offer a cautionary note to Amaro's (1995) call for empowerment of women in negotiating the realities of HIV prevention. In addition, the derogation of female adolescents by the males in our study is another issue that deserves further study.

As noted earlier, we chose to have single-sex focus groups based on our experience as clinicians. We believed we would be able to elicit more forthright discussions. A next step might be to take the beliefs of the females and present them to the males for their response (just as we had asked the males to respond to the experts' beliefs) and take the beliefs of the males and present them to the females for their response. As we noted above, asking the females to address the males' views about the role of welfare would be one such issue. Others would be for males to address the females' views of male contraception refusal and their fear of male violence.

Another possible step in future focus groups would be to build in a second round of focus groups, in which we present the findings of the research group to the participants and ask for their feedback or evaluation. They could let us know if they thought we were successful in adequately representing their beliefs, or they could offer clarification or further comments.

The possibility of a second round of focus groups could also be implemented as a methodological solution to the observation, in the current research, that when teenage mothers were present in a group, their views tended to dominate. Thus we would suggest having single-sex groups of parents and non-parents. Then, after the major themes have been elicited, one could have a second round of focus groups, presenting themes from the first round to newly re-formed groups, some of which are homogeneous and some heterogeneous with respect to parenthood.

We believe the use of focus groups can be both informative and transformative. Rather than seeing ourselves as "experts," we have learned that we have much to learn from the research participants. They have knowledge to share with us if we are willing to provide an appropriate context for them to do so.

This realization shaped our response to a request from a clinical staff member about patients who are "frequent flyers" at the ER. We suggested a focus group with patients who are the most frequent users of the ER, observing that they were the "experts" about why they chose the ER rather than the clinic. The staff member thought about this suggestion and later said it had "totally changed" her view. She took the suggestion back to her hospital committee. She had joined us in the belief that by listening to patients, we could learn from them. If we are able to conduct the focus groups, we will do so with the belief that the patients do indeed have some expertise and will be able to help us understand their choices. We might also ask them to generate ideas about what they think would reduce their use of the ER. Or we might ask them to come for a second time, after we have had a chance to transcribe and consider the results of the initial focus groups. This might allow us to generate possible approaches to reducing ER usage that they could then evaluate in a second round of focus groups.

We are, in essence, urging the inclusion of community members in discussions designed to increase our understanding of what is important to them. We believe focus groups are an efficacious means toward understanding "the other's" perspectives on important health care issues. We think this understanding of the other has the potential to lead to fiscal savings. In an excellent article that discusses some of the practical issues involved in conducting focus groups, Loevy & O'Brien (1994) provide a succinct rationale for the economic value of focus groups:

> Managers frequently develop new health care services without any input from the intended program participants. Then, when client satisfaction or client participation levels are low, managers must backpedal to discover the errors in planning or implementation. Even when the mistakes are identified, the obstacles encountered in changing the program and remarketing it to a disenchanted or disinterested community may be insurmountable.
>
> Focus groups provide an effective means for including [the community] in program planning, thus avoiding the problem of installing the wrong set of services in the wrong place. Through focus groups, researchers and managers alike have the opportunity to present a program plan, often based on a series of demographically valid assumptions, and then adjust the plan to meet the specific local social, economic, or ethical needs expressed during the focus groups. (p. 102)

In this situation, incorporating the community as partner is important prior to implementation of services but after some initial planning and program design. In the context of our "frequent flyers" or other situations in which a problem arises, focus groups can be used to increase our understanding of the problem and to "try out" possible solutions. In a research context, one could involve the community as partners earlier in the process, when generating scientific hypotheses. In another research context, the American Psychological Association has recently utilized focus groups in its public opinion study and public education initiatives (Halgrimson & Herndon, 1998). In a consultation, one could meet with a group as a facilitator, as is planned for a staff in-service on ER usage. In the planning of the in-service, the clinical staff member and consultant have worked as partners, each respecting what the other brings, each seeking the questions and feedback of the other. In the in-service we will attempt to do the same with the staff members, actively recruiting their questions, their ideas, and their feedback.

We would like to end with a caution. To be effective and ethical, focus groups should be conducted in an atmosphere of mutual respect; ideally, from our viewpoint, from within a partnership framework. We do not believe focus groups would be either efficacious or ethical if used from within an authoritarian framework where the leader believes s/he possesses the "right" answers or where the leader has power to do harm to the participants for their expression of what s/he may perceive as "wrong" views.

REFERENCES

Amaro, H. (1995). Love, sex, and power: Considering women's realities in HIV prevention. *American Psychologist, 50,* 437–447.

Ferraro, M. H., Bibace, R., Belfor, M. N., Davis, M. J., Delpappa, E., & Dowds, B. N. (1996). Empowerment—an ideal long-term goal: But what about now? *American Psychologist, 51,* 655–656.

Halgrimson, S., & Herndon, P. (1998). Focus groups help shape APA campaign radio ad. *The American Psychological Association Monitor, 29,* 26.

Loevy, S. S., & O'Brien, M. U. (1994). Community-based research: The case for focus groups. In A. J. Dan (Ed.), *Reframing women's health* (pp. 102–110). Thousand Oaks, CA: Sage.

National Institute of Child Health and Human Development. (1994). Unintended pregnancy in the United States. *NIH Guide 23* (18). (RFA-HD-94-22).

Saxe, J. G. (1936). The blind men and the elephant. In H. Fellmen (Ed.). *The best loved poems of the American people.* New York: Doubleday.

6

WHAT CHILDREN WANT TO KNOW ABOUT MEDICINE

Roger Bibace
Clark University and
University of Massachusetts Medical School

James J. Dillon
State University of West Georgia

ABSTRACT

This chapter attempts to answer the question, "What do children want to know about medicine?" The concern is not with what children *do* know about medicine, but with what they *want to know*. Consistent with the guiding partnership approach presented in this volume, the focus group is offered as an alternative research methodology. The focus group avoids many of the pitfalls of the traditional experimental design. Important data were found that, the authors argue, would have been missed by traditional IRE experimental designs. Implications for research are discussed.

This chapter examines a question that, to our surprise, is rarely asked in health psychology research: What do children want to know about medicine? We are not concerned with what children, from an adult standpoint, *should* know about medicine, or, for the more developmentally oriented, what children of various ages *can* or *cannot* know about medicine. Rather, we are concerned with what the *children themselves* actually want to know about medicine. In keeping with the partnership ideal described in Chapter 21, this study attempts to allow *the child* to determine the relevant questions and topics of interest. From this perspective, we became aware that the usual methods and procedures relied upon to elicit responses from participants were inappropriate.

Ordinarily, even a very young child will *not* ask an adult researcher questions in a one-on-one interaction. Rather, the child will wait to be *asked questions* by the adult. Further, a child very rarely, if ever, *directly contradicts* or *derogates* the questions asked by an adult authority. Other methods are necessary if the spontaneous responses that occur in children's everyday lives are to be observed. Given this concern, we decided that the focus group, as opposed to the traditional experimental design, would be the best means of ascertaining what children want to know about medicine. In the pages that follow, we hope to persuade you that our decision was a good one.

We begin by exploring the nature of the focus group interview. As opposed to experimental settings, focus group settings are relaxed and comfortable. Participants either sit in a circle or around a table so each participant can view the others. Participants are usually thanked for their participation and are then instructed as to the purpose of the interview. In our case, participants are reassured that this is not a test situation, and that there are no "right" or "wrong" answers, and that everything said in the room will stay in the room. Participants are reminded that everything that they say is important. To create a sense of intimacy and community, facilitators are encouraged to use first names in addressing participants and to use the "we" pronoun as opposed to the "I" pronoun. An ambiguous question is usually presented to get a discussion going. When the discussion lags, facilitators have at their disposal various prompts:

a) "sophisticated naiveté," in which the "expert" acts as though this was the first time her or she was hearing about a particular topic, for example, "Oh I didn't know that, tell me more";
b) incomplete statements in which a question is partially asked, for example, "So if you stopped breathing you'd. . . .";
c) encouraging additional points of view, for example, "Does anyone see it differently?";
d) requests for more information, for example, "Could you explain that further?" or "Can you give me an example?"

After completing the focus group interview, participants are thanked again for their participation and asked if they have any additional questions that they want to ask.

We believe that focus groups are important because the spontaneous comments, questions, and reactions of participants are indicative of the *attention* that is evidenced by the topics and contexts that are the subjects of discussion. We subscribe to Freud's (1963) assumption that the *attention* is most broadly indicative of *value orientations*. Thus, Freud's notion of "cathexis" very broadly encompasses "what" is being discussed; what is being discussed subsumes *all kinds* of reactions to the subject under discussion. Focus groups are also in keeping with our partnership ideal in that they attempt to address the egocentric predicament of the researcher directly. In traditional research designs, the self-centeredness of the researcher is restricted to the domain under discussion. Usually, no avenue is available to the researcher to determine how the participant understands a particular term or question, what is on the participant's mind, what the participant is interested in, etc. Focus groups are an improved means of escaping this self-centered predicament.

We follow Kitzinger (1995) on the validity and necessity of the employment of focus groups to answer certain kinds of research questions. Focus groups are frequently employed in research for political and commercial advertising. Companies and political campaigns, the latter of which are typically not profligate spenders, will invest great sums of money to gather information from such interviews. We believe this is a testament to the focus group's power and validity. What are the strengths of focus groups? First, focus groups encourage communication among *participants* and not between researcher and participant. As such, participants are much more comfortable voicing their *own views* without needing to feel like they have to give the "right" or "expected" answer, or that they have to say what the *researcher* wants them to say. In a sense, participants are encouraged, in a serious way, to "be themselves." In a talk given at Clark University, Peter Tulviste gave a highly illustrative example from a child in an experiment. The child answered the researcher's question by asking, "Do you want me to tell you what I would say in school, or what kids say when they are playing together?" We believe that this is really an extraordinary example because it highlights what children very rarely do: *to answer a question with a question.* In doing this, the child violates the traditional Initiation-Response-Evaluation (IRE) experimental sequence. Both children and adults typically answer as best they can the questions being asked by a doctor, teacher, or researcher. Further, the child indicates that responses given in experimental settings are *context dependent.* This child is aware that teachers in a school setting "require" or "approve of" one type of answer which is quite different from the "answers" that they give to one another when an authority figure is not present.

The second strength of the focus group is that it encourages participants to explore issues that are important to them in their own words, often generating their own questions. Third, researchers can tap into the different forms of communication that people use in their day-to-day interactions with each other. Fourth, participants can explore and clarify their own views in ways that are less accessible in a single, structured interview. They can modify their initial response, they can respond to feedback from others, disagree with others, etc. Fifth, participants in a focus group can move toward more symmetrical sequences of interaction characterized by reciprocity and complementarity occasioned by the dialogue between all parties. Specifically, participants can modify their initial responses in the light of feedback, mental elaboration, etc. We have found in many of our studies that the first answer that a participant gives (and which is typically taken as "the" answer in traditional protocols) is rarely his or her definitive answer. The participant is often prone to reconsider and further articulate his or her answer as time and the discussion goes on.

Surely the focus group has its weaknesses. For example, it is extremely difficult to test causal claims. As such, the focus group is surely not an *experimental* design. Further, as Kitzinger (1995) notes, group dynamics may often silence shy and reserved individuals, despite special attention paid by facilitators. Lastly, the focus group is a nonstandardized testing procedure. As such it is similar to the semi-structured interview. With such methods, comparisons between groups are conceptually difficult. Nevertheless, we believe that for certain questions and research purposes, the focus group's strengths far outweigh its weaknesses.

Focus groups for the following study were the outgrowth of the USP Committee on Children and Medicine (Bibace, 1996). This was a multidisciplinary committee composed of medical anthropologists, pediatricians, health educators, psychologists, and pharmacists. The interviews were conducted in Baltimore by Fay Menacker, Robert Smith, and April Stubbs, in New York City by Pilar Aramburuzabala and Nadia Minian, and in Worcester by Patricia Quinn, Joe McNeil, and Dan Green. Participants were 44 children attending a public school in Baltimore (more than 86 percent of the participants were African American), 26 children attending a public school in New York City (100 percent Hispanic), and 30 children attending a public school in Worcester (53 percent Hispanic and 47 percent Caucasian).

Focus groups were carried out with two to nine participants in each group following general guidelines for focus groups described above and further in Kitzinger (1995). Each focus group lasted approximately one hour. The group discussions were audiotaped and transcribed. What did we find?

Children's statements were organized into two groups: *personal* questions that children ask about medicine and *impersonal* questions that children ask. We added a third category that pertained to *what the children did not say,* questions which children do not ask. Personal questions revolve around the child as an individual or are specific questions with personal consequences, such as:

1. Is this medicine for me or someone else?
2. How come this medicine makes me feel bad?
3. Is this medicine for *this* illness or a different illness?
4. Is this a medicine or a drug?

The most common *impersonal* questions children in these groups asked were:

1. Is this medicine for a child or an adult?
2. Does it come in a pill or a liquid?
3. Where does the medicine come from?
4. How is the medicine made?

Lastly, there are a number of questions children do not ask, which include gender and ethnicity as related to medicine. Children also do not ask *why* people use illicit drugs.

In a general way, what children want to know about medicine is consistent with their everyday, personal experiences. Very frequently, children say medicines are "good" because they "make you feel better." And medicines are "good" *because* "Mom" gives them to you. Children also voice a variety of concerns and fears about medicine. Very often, these feelings are ambivalent. For example, especially for children, the very stuff that makes you feel better—"medicine"—could also kill you. Many children in our study explicitly asked whether medicine has "poison" in it. The danger implied in taking someone else's medicine was also clearly stated by a second grader who interrupted another child to say that "if you take someone else's medicine you get what they have." This last statement is consistent with a cardinal principle of cognitive-developmental psychology, namely: the lack of differentiation between the self and the other (Werner & Kaplan, 1963). Applied here, this principle lends coherence to the idea that if you take the other person's medicine then "you get what they have." Advertisers understand this principle very well: eat Wheaties and you too can become an Olympic athlete. It is not only children who have such "beliefs" or who are "persuaded" by such advertisements.

Children often confuse what we would call the effects of the disease with the side effects of the medicine. In a dialogue between two first graders in Baltimore, one child said that "cancer *medicine* made the hair fall out." Whereas another child disagreed saying it was the "*cancer* that made the hair fall out."

Although the basic assumption that children make is that medicines make you feel better, several children in Baltimore, New York, and Worcester expressed skepticism, saying "medicines do not cure" the illness. For example, a second grader reported feeling worse after using ear drops for an infection; another child reported throwing up after drinking Pepto Bismol; and a seventh grader mentioned that medicines "make one drowsy." Even children as young as kindergartners mentioned what we would call an incongruity between the side effects of the medicine and the belief that it should make you better. Many of us, not only children, think absolutistically. So it should not be surprising that children are puzzled: how come something that should make you feel good makes you feel bad? Perhaps health professionals should provide explanations that balance the need for understanding possible side effects with the benefits of taking the medicine in the first place.

In addition to the concerns about taking the wrong medicine for an illness, taking someone else's medicine, and how medicines sometimes make you feel worse is *the confusion between medicines and drugs*. The following is an exchange among second graders in New York City:

Child: I heard of this medicine that teenagers take it and they get violent.
Interviewer: Are these medicines like these ones? (Pointing to medicines on the table.)
All the children: No.
Interviewer: What medicines are you talking about?
Child: Drugs.
Interviewer: Are these drugs?
Most of the children: No.
One child says: Yes, they are good drugs.

Excerpts like this were common with the New York and Worcester focus groups. Many participants knew that medicines were "good drugs" and that there were "bad drugs," but they were reluctant at times to call medicines "drugs." One way older children (fifth graders onward) differentiate between "good drugs" and "bad drugs" is the place where they are bought, for example, "Bad drugs are sold on the corner of streets"; or by their appearance, for example, "Bad drugs come in a powder."

A further confusion that leads to the child's tendency to confuse drugs and medicine is due to a phenomenon that Werner & Kaplan (1963) call "word realism." With word realism, there is very little differentiation between a word and the thing to which the word refers. In the present case, since one can still buy medicine from a "drugstore," there is a tendency to assume that what is purchased at such stores must be a drug. When a child relies on "word realism" the "drugstore" as a place where medicine is sold does not help in understanding.

The problem is more complicated because most of the children are trying to differentiate between drugs and medicines as if it were solely a class inclusion problem involving the question of which is the broader, more inclusive class: medicines or drugs? Initially, only medicines are mentioned. When "drugs" as a word and referent become part of the child's world, they are juxtaposed as "bad" to medicine as "good." Educational programs in schools, such as DARE in Worcester, contribute to such a dichotomy.

Finally, based on what children wanted to know, we derived a set of questions that are often pertinent to adults, but which the children themselves did *not* ask. Not a *single* child in any of the three sites, from kindergarten to sixth grade, ever raised the question regarding *why people took what we call illicit drugs*! Further, the purpose the substance could be used for (medicinal or recreational) was never mentioned by any of the children in the present study. In the everyday world of the child there is an experiential incongruity between medicines that should make you feel good and its bad side effects. But there is no comparable incongruity regarding drugs. The child wants to know: if drugs are so bad for you, then why do people take them?

There were a number of additional questions that children never asked. We know that children can be sexist. Some boys, for instance, call girls "icky." But children never said that there are medicines for girls and not for boys. This observation is surprising since children see boys and girls as so qualitatively different. One would expect that children would transfer this difference into the belief that each would require different medicines. Most of the children believed that if you took someone else's medicine it was not good for you. But the "someone else" was never specified by either gender or race. The only connection to ethnicity occurred with Hispanic children in New York who *linked good medicine with location*, that is, where the medicine came from. That is, if the medicine was made in a *familiar* geographic location, such as Santo Domingo, then the medicine was good. In contrast, for many Hispanic children in New York, medicines made in the United States "didn't work."

The materials we collected, especially a dissertation by James Dillon (1998), shed some light on the source of these questions raised by children. This issue pertains to the child's understanding of how the body works. To simplify, the body for these children is a container. Dillon's data with some 100 children show, for instance, that children do not have an understanding of distinctly biological principles such as digestion, circulation, inheritance, etc. The clearest connection between medicines and the body as a container is seen in children's concerns regarding the question: Is the medicine for a child or for an adult? Children as young as kindergartners said there was a difference between medicines *for children* and medicines *for adults*. For example, a kindergartner said, "If you take medicine and it is not for kids, then the kids die." This idea was mentioned in most other groups. In only one case, a third grader in New York believed that medicines for kids and for adults were "exactly the same thing," while another participant in this group believed that it was dangerous for children to take adults' medicines. In all other groups, all participants acknowledged the danger of children taking medicines for adults. When we examined *why* there was a difference between medicines for adults and for children, the near universal finding was that the body of a child was not seen as being large enough to hold the "big" adult medicine. For example, a second grader responded, "The body is not big enough to hold a lot of germs in a little body so you only need a little medicine."

Further, children do not know about the relationship between dosage and weight regarding medicine. They acknowledge the child/adult difference *through the size of the container*. Large bodies are seen to have many germs, so strong medicine that is kept in a large container is needed. Small bodies, which are seen to contain fewer germs, require weaker medicine that comes in smaller containers. It follows that from a child's perspective, a mismatch of medicine and body size leads to problems.

In the pages that follow, we make a few methodological and theoretical suggestions based on our experiences conducting this study. The first suggestion involves the viability of the focus group as a research tool. We strongly believe that the dialogue inherent in the focus group process highlights an extremely important feature; namely, how developmental change comes about. Children, just like scientists, are continuously comparing, labeling, evaluating, contrasting, choosing.

It is just such cognitive activities that have been systematically studied and ordered by Sigel (1993) as the psychological "distancing activities" that bring about change. For example, relying on Sigel we have conducted two studies (Bibace, Dillon, & Sagarin, 1996; Bibace, Sagarin, & Dyl, 1998) that show that asking children, at various ages, to compare and evaluate by sorting and rank ordering the responses of *other* children results in dramatic increases in cognitive maturity, as compared to the child's own responses in the very same session and in the same domain of illness. Similarly, Dillon's (1998) dissertation demonstrates the impressive changes in a child's depiction of the inside of their bodies, in the very same session and as a result of only two levels of Sigel's psychological distancing activities, High and Analogy. These distancing strategies are discussed in detail in Dillon's chapter on ethics, Chapter 10.

We also received an unexpected benefit from the focus groups. In Baltimore, in New York, and initially in Worcester, we showed children various common medicines. The idea was to help children to talk about their experiences. This worked very well. From the standpoint of an experimental design, it worked too well. Because the visual perception of these familiar medicines captured the attention of the children, they were often so distracted that they were unable to offer *their own* insights and ideas. This observation leads us to make a suggestion that addresses children's concerns and fears when a child takes an adult's medicine. Prescription medicines are mostly packaged in brown plastic containers with a white cap. The suggestion is that children's medicines could be identified by a different colored container with a contrasting colored cap. That is, using perception for a constructive child-centered end.

There are a number of perceptual features regarding the medicine container and its cap that could reassure children that the medicine is for children and not for adults. Color is one perceptual feature, size is another. What existing evidence is there for such a suggestion? Some evidence can be marshaled from biological and sociocultural perspectives. We should choose a color that emphasizes *brightness and contrast.* Specifically, we suggest a contrast between a yellow cap and a blue container. The contrast between the *yellow cap* and the *blue container* is heightened because we know that contrast is sharpened when there is no space between the two contrasting regions.

These psychological features of perception have been grounded recently in the primary visual cortex (Rossi, Rittenhouse, & Paradiso, 1996). Most of us were taught the distinction between sensations and perceptions. That is, the traditional understanding is that we first experience sensations that then give rise to perceptions. But Rossi and colleagues have a different view. They write:

> The primary visual cortex is often described as an initial processing stage that sends information to higher cortical areas where *perception* of brightness, color, and form occurs. However, a significant percentage of neurons in primary visual cortex were shown to respond in a manner correlated with *perceived brightness*, rather than

responding strictly to the light level in the receptive fields of the cells. This finding suggests that even at the first stage of visual cortical processing, spatial integration of information yields perceptual qualities that are only indirectly related to the pattern of illumination of the retina.

Why this excursion into neuroscience? One reason is of the "wouldn't it be lovely" variety. We think it would be great if it were possible to have brightness and color contrasts in medicine *caps* and *containers* that would be child-centered and reassure children that it is for children not adults. Certainly, we should empirically investigate children's ability to discriminate the differences between a child and an adult's medicine in this way and to determine whether it is reassuring. But suppose it is too bureaucratically difficult to get manufacturers to change. Then we can use stickers to get the message across. Or a mother could involve the child by having the child paint the white cap their favorite color, using non-toxic paints of course.

Crossculturally, Adams and Osgood (1973) have found similarities in feelings about colors among 23 cultural groups. Blue was a universal favorite. Another study by Saito (1992) determined that with 400 individuals in nine ethnic groups living in the U.S., there was only one color that was preferred by all groups: vivid blue. Birren (1950) claimed that blue is a universal favorite. Of course there are cross-cultural differences, for example, the Japanese preference for white. Twenty-five percent of Japanese participants selected white as their first, second, or third choice. However, these researchers were studying color *preferences.* Following Rossi and colleagues (1996), I assume that ability to *discriminate,* to *immediately perceive* brightness and color contrasts is more basic. The question is whether such immediately perceived discriminations will be consistent across cultures.

Children's concerns with both the *personal* (Is this my medicine?) and the *impersonal* (Is this medicine for a child or for an adult?) parallels two basic and qualitatively different questions in clinical medicine: the *personal* (What is the best treatment for this *person* who has this disease?) and the *impersonal* (What is the best treatment for this disease?). The medical history of *this patient* and his/her personal lifestyle has to be considered in addition to the recommended treatment for a *disease* based on the evidence gathered from randomized controlled studies. The bridge between the personal and the impersonal is the clinician's judgement arrived at in the negotiation between health professionals and patients. As will be elaborated in Chapter 21, this linkage between the personal and the impersonal is important because it bridges the distance between the "generalizations" relied on by professionals and the particular person with whom the clinician, pharmacist, or parent is interacting. When dealing with particular children as individuals, the professional or parent should, from our partnership perspective, *ask and not assume* what color the child thinks the tops of medicine containers should be. The normative data regarding color should serve as initial guidelines regarding the choices offered to the child, but we believe that the child, not the adult, should ultimately make that decision. Information is for both children and adults. But adults should also *listen* to children, not only to children's answers to our questions, but to the questions the child wants answered.

REFERENCES

Adams, F. M., & Osgood, C. E. (1973). A cross-cultural study of the affective meaning of color. *Journal of Cross-Cultural Psychology, 7,* 135–157.

Bibace, R. (1996). What children want to know about medicine. *Proceedings of the United States Pharmacopeia Committee on Children and Medicine.*

Bibace, R., Dillon, J., & Sagarin, J. (1996, September–October). What children what to know about medicine. *Children and medicines: Information isn't just for grownups.* United States Pharmacopeia Conference, Reston, VA.

Bibace, R., Sagarin, J., & Dyl, J. (1998). The heuristic value of Werner's co-existence concept of development. *Journal of Applied Developmental Psychology, 19,* 153–163.

Birren, F. (1950). *Color psychology and color therapy.* New York: McGraw-Hill.

Dillon, J. J. (1998). *The differential effects of four psychological distancing strategies on children's conceptions of biology and the inside of the body.* Unpublished doctoral dissertation, Clark University, Worcester, MA.

Freud, S. (1966). *Introductory lectures on psychoanalysis.* New York: W. W. Norton.

Kitzinger, J. (1995). Introducing focus groups. *Behavioral Medicine Journal, 311,* 299–302.

Rossi, A. F., Rittenhouse, C. D., & Paradiso, M. A. (1996, August 23). The representation of brightness in primary visual cortex. *Science, 273,* 1104–1107.

Saito, M. (1992). A cross-cultural survey on color preference in Asian countries: Comparisons between Japanese and Koreans with emphasis of preference for white. *Journal of the Color Science Association, 16*(1), 1–10.

Sigel, I. E. (1993). The centrality of a distancing model for the development of representational competence. In R. E. Cocking & K.A. Renninger (Eds.), *The development and meaning of psychological distancing.* Hillsdale, NJ: Lawrence Erlbaum.

Werner, H., & Kaplan, B. (1963). *Symbol formation.* Hillsdale, NJ: Lawrence Erlbaum.

7

EDUCATIONAL RESEARCH TRIADS: ACCOMPLISHMENT WITH EFFICIENCY

Roger Bibace
Clark University and
University of Massachusetts Medical School

Nicholas H. Apostoleris
Clark University

James D. Laird
Clark University

ABSTRACT

A format for the functioning of a research group is presented which is designed to encourage a diversity of types of intellectual relationships among faculty members, graduate students, and undergraduates so as to afford maximum opportunities for each group member to attain personally relevant ends. Special emphasis is placed on how the pursuit of knowledge is furthered through the use of Educational Research Triads since even complex, labor- and energy-intensive projects can be conducted with a minimum of funding and a maximum of student enthusiasm and participation. The workings and structure of a currently active research group are described, and feedback from participating undergraduates, graduate students, and faculty is included.

In most universities, faculty involve undergraduates as well as graduate students in their research. However, these activities are usually casually organized on an ad hoc basis. This chapter describes a more formal structure for these interactions and some of the benefits that accrue from being more explicit and clear.

The first and most obvious difference between our practice at Clark University and the norm at many other institutions is that all graduate students are encouraged to participate in "Educational Research Triads" in which the three corners are faculty, graduate students, and undergraduates. A substantial number of undergraduates are involved in these triads. Research experiences of this sort are not reserved for the star undergraduates or the most energetic graduate students, but rather are a common part of many students' experience. We have found that although only a limited number of undergraduate students have the right combination of interests and talents to go on to Ph.D. programs in psychology, all of our undergraduate participants find involvement in serious research both interesting and valuable.

In what ways can a partnership among faculty, graduate students, and undergraduates be facilitated so that a complex research project is carried out so that all participants benefit maximally? The key feature of the triad is the set of values adopted by the members. First, it is understood that all members of the research team bring to bear various skills, outlooks, and limitations, and the faculty must be attuned to these special strengths in the students and be willing to adapt the implementation of the project where appropriate. Second, there is a recognition of the reality of the "division of labor" in the group. Ideally, the very diversity of the group members leads them to take responsibility for tasks in which they have special interest or skills, or which they find personally useful to research. Collaborative efforts extend to participants as well as to junior researchers (Bibace, 1986).

An emphasis on experiential learning leads to the recognition that all participants (faculty, graduate students, undergraduates, and participants) are involved in a series of teaching–learning interactions. The traditional apprenticeship model acknowledges experiential learning in the researcher's world of action (i.e., the laboratory, clinic, etc.), but there is often an assumption of a one-way, asymmetrical relationship wherein the flow of instruction and knowledge is from teacher to student. In contrast, we find that the student-researchers and especially participants often have perspectives that have eluded the faculty and which add to the relevance and power of the research.

Also, we try to take advantage of the special skills and competencies of even the most junior students. For example, if an undergraduate possesses computer skills or knowledge of foreign languages and cultures, an attempt is made to use these skills to further the overall research project. In particular, the special sensitivities of undergraduates to generational differences in the popular culture (when compared to older graduate students and especially to faculty) are used to heighten the relevance and appropriateness of the research whenever this is applicable.

At a more abstract level, the Educational Research Triad is a distinctive way in which the university/college ideal can be put into action. The objectives of creating knowledge (the university ideal) and transmitting knowledge (the college ideal) can be aided by use of the triad.

Team members from all three components of the triad are afforded unusual benefits from the arrangement. Undergraduates are given access to the inner workings of the research process—they can see firsthand how research questions are formed and how methods for pursuing the questions are developed and implemented. Course credit is given for participation and a significant commitment in terms of hours and energy is assumed. Undergraduates are encouraged to choose both the types of work they wish to pursue and the content areas that they find most interesting. Minimally, undergraduates are required to write a substantial paper based on their research in the group. Most commonly, undergraduates take a part of the project as their own, and develop their own research questions. They analyze data pertinent to their questions, present their findings at meetings, and take initial responsibility for writing that part of the project for publication. Because of the responsibility of group membership, we have found that the prerequisites for undergraduates should include junior status with at least a B average. Further, courses taken should include statistics and preferably a laboratory/research course. These are general requirements, however, and several exceptional non-psychology majors have participated fruitfully in triads.

Typically, graduate students assume greater responsibilities for the formulation and implementation of the research design. The weekly research group meeting also affords the graduate students with a regular opportunity to teach the group the elements of the project in which they are invested. The most distinctive feature of this experience for the graduate students is the explicit focus on developing mentoring and team-building skills of their own. The faculty members meet regularly with graduate students. For the faculty, the pursuit of knowledge is furthered since even complex, labor- and energy-intensive projects can be conducted with a minimum of funding and a maximum of student enthusiasm and participation (Apostoleris & Bibace, 1995).

As one symbol of the relatively egalitarian structure of these triads, different members of the team are encouraged to be the primary presenter of the team's findings in diverse contexts. Many students present at professional meetings. Others present at research conferences designed specifically for undergraduates. Finally, in addition to other opportunities to share their work, we have a forum at Clark University called Academic Spree Day. Although developed by a psychologist, this is a universitywide opportunity for students in all disciplines to present their scholarly and artistic work, in a variety of formats. Academic Spree Day provides a friendly environment, but one in which the standards are high and the questions asked are challenging. Graduate students are similarly encouraged to present at appropriate conferences.

To this point, the form and the goals of the Educational Research Triad have been emphasized, but it should be noted that no formal structure or set of abstract goals can ensure that participants will have a worthwhile experience in the group. The interpersonal environment must also be conducive to the sharing of ideas without undue inhibition. The students, both graduate and undergraduate, must feel comfortable that their ideas are truly valued and valuable, and that the making of "mistakes" is understood as the byproduct of effort rather than as evidence of deficiency. A spirit of enthusiasm among the group participants is desired for all concerned. Enthusiasm for the project can help make the many necessary tedious jobs less onerous and can even help soften the blow of disappointing evaluations of papers or, heaven forbid, null results.

A major benefit of this arrangement is that the "work gets out." What is perhaps even more exciting, however, is encouraging and witnessing the process by which some members of the group take on the group's goals as their own, thereby moving a good distance down the path toward choosing psychology as a life pursuit. The Educational Research Triad, therefore, can be seen as having the potential for providing benefits at four levels of analysis: at the level of the individual, the research group, the educational institution, and the field itself.

REFERENCES

Apostoleris, N. H., & Bibace, R. (1995, April). *Educational research triads: Structuring opportunities for the sharing of skills and the pursuit of both group and individual interests.* Paper presented at the 9th Annual Conference on the Teaching of Undergraduate Psychology.

Bibace, R. (1986, May). *The educational research triangle: An alternative to traditional research fellowships.* Paper presented to the Society of Teachers in Family Medicine, Boston, MA.

8

A CYCLE OF ACTIVITIES THAT APPROXIMATES A PARTNERSHIP IDEAL BETWEEN RESEARCHER AND RESEARCH PARTICIPANT

Roger Bibace
Clark University and
University of Massachusetts Medical School

Robert F. Leeman
Brandeis University

ABSTRACT

In keeping with the primary assumption of differentiation between self and other, research according to a partnership perspective is guided by the attitude that the research participant has a unique and important contribution to make to a study. This contribution goes beyond the predetermined expectations of the researcher, because the researcher attempts to understand where the research participant "is coming from" through a cycle of seven steps. These steps are meant to act as a guideline to research from a partnership perspective. It is expected that this cycle would have to be modified from study to study.

The aim in a partnership is to determine what the other person thinks and feels, or what s/he has done or would do. In sharpest contrast, the traditional approach is guided by an attitude of "Do you know what I know?" In common parlance, the aim in a partnership is for the researcher to be able to understand "where the other person is coming from." It is the other person, not a "subject" or even "research participant," that the researcher strives to understand. Optimally, every aspect of the interaction between researcher and research participant should be open to the research participant's choices. The research participant should be able to exercise such choices *before* s/he is asked to answer any questions prepared by the researcher.

While an ideal interaction between researcher and research participant is not always possible, due to some of the limitations discussed in Chapter 21, the implementation of steps such as the ones to be discussed here facilitates an approximation of the "ideal." A partnership in the domain of research is characterized by reciprocity and complementarity between researcher and participant. The principle aim of a partnership approach to research is to move toward symmetry regarding an opportunity for both partners to ask questions, to have one's own questions answered, and to provide feedback to one's partner.

In order for this aim to come about in practice, it is necessary for both partners to appreciate the value of differentiation between the researcher and the research participant, or vice-versa. The researcher and the research participant have divergent and valuable contributions to make to the research project. The researcher presumably has considerable general knowledge of both the topic of the research as well as the process of psychological research. The participant's knowledge of his/her own life, personal experiences, and associations *complement* the researcher's factual knowledge of that domain. While the researcher may have a strong grasp of the research topic in general, the researcher is not an expert on the attitudes and beliefs of *this individual* participant, or on where this person is coming from with respect to his/her responses to questions about the domain being studied.

This partnership approach is discussed and contrasted with traditional, asymmetrical interactions between researcher and research participant. In addition to such attitudinal prerequisites, a set of seven, sequential activities are provided in order to assist researchers in moving toward a partnership approach.

The partnership approach to research is presented in the context of two main types of research project. These alternatives vary with respect to the sequence of steps involved in initiating the study. The first type of study involves topics related to everyday, experiential worlds of research participants. Typically, verbal methods are favored in these types of studies. One such study to be discussed later involves the distinction between living and nonliving objects. While this distinction can be complicated, children are faced with it every day in one form or another. In the second type of study, a researcher seeks to address conceptual distinctions that are important to a researcher, but may not be readily recognizable to others. One example would be the Müller-Lyer illusion in which two lines are presented that are actually of equal length, but appear to be different (see Matlin & Foley, 1992, for a discussion of this illusion).

TRADITIONAL, ASYMMETRICAL APPROACHES TO RESEARCH

In contrast to the reciprocal partner relationship, traditional researcher/research participant dyads are asymmetrical. Researchers in these interactions begin with a previously determined list of questions, which they pose to the participant. The participant answers the questions, with the researcher then evaluating the responses. Therefore, input of the participant is limited to specific questions put forth by the researcher. *After* the interaction is completed, the researcher may ask the participant for his/her thoughts and opinions on the process. However, in all likelihood, the researcher will not have the opportunity to fully appreciate where this research participant is coming from because the parameters of relevance for this study have been firmly set, whether or not s/he realizes it.

This traditional approach to research constrains both parties. It limits the participant because s/he has not been given the opportunity to voice what s/he considers relevant to the domain being studied. Or more specifically, the participant is not encouraged to ask his/her own questions related to the topic at hand. Both of these features are related to a research participant's ability to take an active role in research. In addition, the benefit to the research participant in the traditional research interaction is limited to whatever incentive is offered by the researcher (e.g., course requirement, additional credit, money, a lottery drawing). While such benefits are fine, the traditional interaction severely limits the research participant's chances at benefiting from learning through the comparisons that occur in bilateral questions, answers, and feedback between partners.

The researcher is limited in that s/he only learns the answers to the specific questions asked. The participant is less likely to offer additional, personally relevant information that does not directly pertain to the questions posed by the "expert." It is natural for participants to seek social approval from the researcher. Therefore, many participants purposefully avoid giving responses that could be construed as "weird." Hence, it is possible that a researcher may conduct an interview with a participant that fails to address that which is most pertinent and most relevant to the participant with regard to the topic being studied.

A PARTNERSHIP APPROACH TO RESEARCH

The impersonal counterparts related to beginnings in research are epistemologically known as "levels of organization." Levels of organization are the distinctions or levels introduced by different theorists or disciplines to demarcate one domain from another. The choices made regarding such different levels of organization are determined by the socialization of individuals in different disciplines and to the choices of individuals within a particular discipline. Thus, one's area of focus in research is simultaneously an impersonal *and* a personal issue. The choice is impersonal because the professional groups to which individual researchers belong are typically committed to a particular level of organization.

On the other hand, there are also personal aspects to choices regarding research topics. This is the case because choices of specific topics must still be made within the level of organization favored by the individual's professional group. Further, from study to study, the individual foci selected by the individual researcher will change. For instance, in terms of disciplines, psychology and biology differ in their levels of organization. Within the discipline of psychology, many psychologists study cognition; some psychologists adhere to a developmental orientation, while others prefer a social approach to cognition. Further, within the realm of cognitive psychology, a great deal of variation exists in terms of theoretical frameworks that are studied.

From a partnership approach, a basic assumption is that perennial epistemological/ethical issues constitute a meaningful source of understanding individual differences. Or conversely, all statements of beliefs made by any individual can be "converted upwards" (Burke, 1945) into their epistemological and/or ethical counterpart. From this standpoint, an inability to afford the other the opportunity for "upward conversion" is a failure on the part of the researcher, not the research participant. At times, this shortcoming may be due to the researcher's superficiality. This is particularly the case when the researcher's exclusive aim is the categorization of individual differences. In contrast, a partnership orientation requires an intensive analysis of the person who is the research participant. The aim is to make apparent the kind of variability within individuals that illuminates the possibility for change.

The paradox in this partnership approach to research is that it is only through a detailed analysis and appreciation of this variability *within* a person that we will arrive at generalities that can be validly applied to differences *between* individuals. As Harry Stack Sullivan (1940) stated, "we are all more simply human than otherwise." This idea can be best appreciated through a thorough consideration of variability both within a person and through the study of individual differences. Further, the comparison of "normal" groups with those individuals who are considered to be "deviant" from the norms of society (i.e., psychopathology) has also been illuminating in this respect.

The reason why beginnings are so problematic for a research partnership approach is highlighted by comparisons with a doctor–patient relationship. In the latter, a patient seeks out a doctor and states, at the very beginning of the interaction, their reasons for choosing to see the physician. Of course, the symptoms given by the patient as the reason for the visit may be quite different from the biomedical or psychosocial causes assumed by the doctor. In contrast, the researcher's domain is stated up front as a means of motivating "volunteers." This establishes the expectation that the researcher will initiate questions or experimental procedures.

It is again the sequence of events that is the main issue that differentiates a partnership approach from the traditional, asymmetrical relationship. The problem from a partnership approach is how to disconfirm the volunteer's traditional expectation in order to permit the research participant to ask his/her own questions, which may or may not appear to relate directly to the aims of the researcher. The difficulty throughout is to articulate a partnership approach when the other partner is silent. It should be clear that the following alternatives are merely ways of recognizing the issue, not of solving the so-called problem.

When devising a plan for interview sessions with research participants, deciding on an appropriate way to begin is both important and complicated. A researcher's interview questions establish the parameters of "relevancy" or appropriateness of what is construed as an "acceptable" or "reasonable" participant response. These parameters begin to take shape with the opening question, irrespective of the researcher's intentions. Thus, a set of questions constructs the object of inquiry. The formal, determinative feature of a question has been clearly articulated by Levy (1943):

> An ordinary question intends its answer. It calls for it, requires it. In itself it (i.e., the question) is incomplete and establishes a vector towards completion. Once a proper answer is given, question and answer form a complete closed whole. (p. 61)

In recognition of this problem, a trend has begun in research to start an interview with relatively "open-ended" questions and *then* lead into more specific, structured questions. While this is a useful accommodation, even unstructured questions can influence the way in which the dialog between researcher and research participant takes shape.

The dilemma from a partnership perspective is highlighted from the very beginning of an interaction because it is considered important to try to limit the researcher's own egocentricity. The partnership perspective recognizes the difficulty of this predicament. Indeed, the researcher's own interests, based in part on personal values, have influenced the choice of the research topic in the first place. This is a predicament that can only be limited, not surmounted.

While such selectivity cannot be avoided, an effort must be made to subordinate the researcher's egocentricity in accordance with the primary premise of the partnership model: differentiation between the self and other. Given that no one is a "mind reader," the central concern of the researcher should be to afford the research participant opportunities to express freely and articulate his/her own opinions. Indeed, the expectation of a research participant is that, having volunteered to participate, they are only there to answer the researcher's questions. They do not expect to be asked to generate or attempt answering their own questions.

The researcher either directly or indirectly selects the general area to be studied. No matter how strenuously the researcher attempts to accommodate the research participant, it is the researcher's general domain that is the central focus. The issue is how this general domain is to be studied. The guideline is that researchers should seek to avoid the dismissal of any questions, concerns, answers, or opinions as "irrelevant" or "weird."

It is only during later phases of the research sequence that the possibilities for integration should be addressed. A "negotiated understanding" between partners involves an assumption that both differentiation and integration must be maintained. It is not clear whether coconstructionist nor colearning approaches are conceptually as insistent on the importance of the "formal features" of *both* differentiation and integration. Nor is it apparent whether either of these approaches are as firm in asserting that differentiation must occur *prior* to integration.

A SEVEN-STEP SEQUENCE IN PARTNERSHIP RESEARCH

A partnership approach to research is comprised of a seven-step sequence of reciprocal activities. It is necessary to qualify this presentation by stating that the entirety of this sequence does not apply to all types of psychological research. For instance, work on perception in which a researcher aims to assess participant's visual or aural acuity may require a different framework. However, some components of this sequence may still apply to this type of research, perhaps with some variation in the sequence of activities the researcher relies on in engaging the research participant.

1. The first step involves eliciting the research participant's questions, concerns, etc. with reference to the broad domain, the area of phenomenon that is the researcher's focus. The researcher affords the opportunity to the research participant to give voice to anything and everything related to the specified topic. The research participant's "personal associations" are sought, irrespective of their relevance or veracity, as perceived by the researcher.
2. The researcher compliments the research participant on his/her questions (e.g., their range, their degree of specificity). During this second phase, the researcher asks the research participant to answer his/her own questions. Of course, these responses may not be clear and the participant may have doubt as to the quality of his/her answers. But it is important to assess where the research participant is "coming from" in terms of the ideas and feelings s/he deems relevant. Consequently, both the research participant's questions *and* answers are considered relevant.
3. It is only in the third phase of a partnership sequence that the researcher asks his/her own questions of the research participant. This activity should be prefaced by an impersonal comment such as the following: "Well, psycholo-

gists who have studied this phenomenon typically ask questions such as the ones I will ask you. Not all psychologists, of course, ask the same questions, but I've picked some common questions asked by psychologists for you to answer." The researcher then records the participant's answers. The statements must be made "impersonal" because a participant is much less likely to directly contradict a statement the researcher claims is his/her own.

4. The researcher now solicits the research participant's opinion regarding these questions. In doing so, the participant engages in a high-level distancing act (Sigel 1979, 1993) by comparing, contrasting, and evaluating his/her own questions asked earlier, with those of the researcher (for further discussion of Sigel's psychological distancing acts, see Chapter 10). The researcher should react empathically to the participant's input whenever possible. One such statement could be the following: "It's interesting that you said that, because psychologists don't usually think of that aspect when they are trying to figure out what applies to this phenomenon."
5. The researcher, still relying on Sigel's psychological distancing activities, now asks the participant to evaluate responses given by other groups of research participants. For example, "You've told me what you think. I wonder if you could let me know what you think about other people's answers to the very same questions." This allows the participant the opportunity to respond idiographically to answers that represent normative, nomothetic parameters of answers to those same questions. The researcher will benefit from the opportunity to further understand the participant as s/he responds to a wide, representative range of answers. In effect, the researcher also engages in a psychological distancing activity by classifying this participant with regard to group differences (e.g., differences between this person's responses and those of the opposite sex, other age groups, and members of other cultures), individual differences (e.g., with respect to responses given by other participants pertaining to variables of interest to the researcher), and intraindividual variabilities (e.g., comparing these responses with answers given earlier by the same participant).
6. At another time, focus groups of research participants are conducted so as to give the researcher feedback on the questions raised by either the researcher or each of the participants individually. The group would be instructed to consider how they would go about understanding the phenomenon in question. An important aspect of the focus group is that children and adults can question and contradict one another more easily in this format than in a one-on-one interaction with a researcher.
7. Parallel to the focus groups conducted with the research participants, the researcher provides a group of peers with the entire set of data (collected in steps one through six). This allows the group to provide the researcher with feedback on interpretations and also on what should be included or excluded in the next study.

THE ANIMATE/INANIMATE STUDY EXAMPLE

These seven steps make up one sequence of activities, which approximates a partnership ideal in research for some studies. However, in other studies, it will not be possible to include all of these steps in this particular sequence. A study that requires a different sequence is used as an example to illustrate the fact that this sequence of activities acts as a flexible guideline, rather than a rigid order to be implemented in the same way in all studies. The authors have proposed a study aimed at better understanding the nature of children's concepts of the distinction between animate and inanimate objects.

The claim is that a partnership approach to research requires the partner to generate his/her own questions, as the point of departure. It is relatively easy to meet this goal while researching certain topics, but other studies present definite barriers, due to the limitations of the experiential world of everyday activities of a given research partner. A topic such as "medicine" presents relatively few barriers to implementing a partnership approach. Most children and adults have some experiential knowledge of medicine, either directly or through people they know.

In contrast, it is difficult to ask individuals to generate abstract questions, to propose distinctions that are not aspects of their everyday life. Further problems are likely to arise when a research topic involves contrasting counterintuitive distinctions relied on by scientists. For instance, Wiser (1995) has conducted research on people's understanding of the conceptual differences between heat and temperature. However, even some Ph.D.s and M.D.s are unable to grasp this distinction.

Depending on the developmental status of the child, the animate/inanimate distinction suffers from the same kind of constraint. Scientists and mature adults assume that there is a basic distinction between people, animals, and plants on the one hand and objects such as books, tables, and pens, which are not alive, on the other hand. However, it would be a mistake to assume that this relationship is always a given. Children are not born with the knowledge of what is alive and not alive. Some children, for instance, treat animals as things. Accordingly, they may play in a rough way with their pets without fully understanding the cruelty of such behavior.

It is therefore unreasonable to expect that a child who believes clouds and bicycles are alive will be able to generate distinctions between animate and inanimate objects. A child such as this does not possess the cognitive maturity to spontaneously reason in this way. One approach, detailed in Chapter 3, relies on Sigel's Psychological Distancing Acts (1979, 1993). It has been empirically demonstrated that children are able to appreciate the concrete distinctions made by other children, which are analogous to the abstract distinctions relied on by adults.

In turn, one needs to accommodate the sequence of research activities for such a study. For example, one could begin with step five in the sequence in which participants are given concrete responses provided by peers to similar questions. These concrete responses should again be comprehensive within the entire range of responses that are available to the researcher and ordered developmentally. For the animate/inanimate distinction, the study conducted by Laurendeau and Pinard (1962), with a sample of 500 children, provides useful normative data for this purpose. In this case, the children's answers cover the animate/inanimate distinction with a number of different types of objects. Such comparisons and evaluations help enable children to generate their own questions with respect to the abstract animate/inanimate distinction.

As another step, in a focus group the children would have the opportunity to compare and contrast their own questions and reactions to the exemplar normative responses generated by their peers. Such comparisons should facilitate the dialogicality that is necessary to bring about a negotiated understanding.

A final activity for such a focus group could be to ask children to become scientific partners. Children can be asked to offer suggestions to the researcher regarding the questions to be presented to participants in another research cycle on the same topic.

THE PARTNERSHIP APPROACH AS APPLIED TO STUDIES OF PERCEPTION

The partnership approach to research has only been applied to verbal interactions between researcher and research participant. The question is whether this partnership approach can be extended to traditional experimental analyses of perception. For instance, how might one conduct a study on a developmental analysis of perceptual illusions from a partnership perspective? The following notes are speculative because no actual empirical studies have been carried out. The aim is to explore how the sequence of steps in a cycle of activities might be relied on to contrast the traditional approach, compared with a partnership approach to a developmental analysis of visual illusions.

A traditional experimental approach is based on the basic assumption that legitimizes the questions generated through a researcher's "Do you know what I know?" orientation. Evaluative standards such as "How mature do you have to be before you know what I know?" are used in conjunction with this orientation. From this traditional perspective, the research participant's behaviors are assessed within the scope of the researcher's standards for assessing answers.

In contrast, the basic question involved in a partnership approach is "What do you know?" The research participant is asked to generate the questions that s/he thinks are important, relative to the topic at hand, and is then invited to consider ways to answer or resolve these questions. From this perspective, one needs to determine just what questions the research participant considers relevant. It is thus desirable to determine where the other person is coming from. The discrepancies between the researcher and the research participant's "worlds" are themselves assumed to be rich sources of ideas to be explored.

For our hypothetical study on visual perception, let us return to the Müller-Lyer illusion (Figure 8.1) as an example (Matlin & Foley, 1992). A partnership approach might begin by having the child *experience* what adults have come to know as an "illusion." A participant would first be asked which line is longer and which is shorter. After giving a response that corroborates the illusion, the child would be told that some people say that the two lines are "really" the same, even though they "look" different and that A–B looks smaller than B–C . The type of doubt that is brought on by this type of experience acts "as a spur to inquiry," in the spirit of partnerships (Williams, 1998, p. 123). Such a situation provides the child with an opportunity to experience and resolve an inconsistency and an incongruity, given that some children say one thing and others say another.

At this juncture in the sequence, some children successfully resolve the inconsistency by measuring the lines and discovering that they are indeed equal. However, others may adhere to the wrong solution. If this is the case, the researcher might say something like: "Well let me show you why some kids say that A = B." The researcher could then demonstrate by measuring the two lines. Then, the researcher could follow up by asking the child what they think about what these "other kids" say and how they might have come to figure out the correct solution.

Even after arriving at the correct response, children will still note that line A *looked* longer than line B, even though it turned out that both were equal. At this point, the issue to be explored becomes really interesting. It is interesting because the child has had a chance to appreciate the difference between what psychologists refer to as "perception" and "conceptual knowledge." The child as "scientific partner" is now given various explanations of what they have experienced. The diversity of explanations to which they have been exposed is not based on empirical norms of children's concepts of illusions, with respect to developmental differences in ontogenetic development. Rather, the differences the child as "scientific partner" is asked to evaluate are the "scientific explanations" advanced by different frameworks in theoretical psychology. The researcher should note a child's initial preferences among the psychological explanations followed by the child's understanding of the various explanations grounded in diverse theoretical frameworks in psychology.

The researcher's task here is to articulate and demonstrate concrete examples that are *analogous* to the abstract explanations preferred by psychologists who espouse these theoretical frameworks. This is not an easy task since many theories select

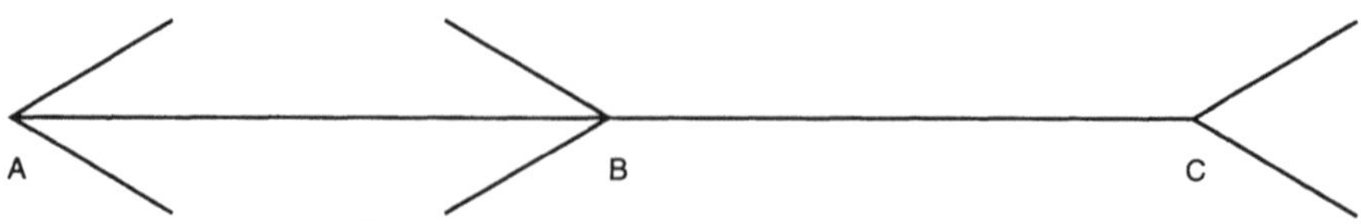

FIGURE 8.1. The Müller-Lyer Illusion

certain phenomena that favor their own explanatory frameworks. Again, the "generalized other" would be involved, but one should avoid invoking the opinions of authority figures, such as: "psychologists say. . . ." Rather, the child should be told that "some people say 'x,' while others say 'y.'"

The child as "scientific partner" could then be engaged in how they would go about figuring out which explanations were better than others (alluding to how the illusion had "looked" one way, but turned out to be different). In this way, the child is asked how to address the issue of individual differences, in terms of this study, or to other phenomena in everyday life. Lastly, the child is asked whether they recognize the issue of variability or of intraindividual differences, both in themselves and in others.

Intraindividual differences, just like other psychological issues, should be translated into the child's world of everyday experiences. For instance, even if a child prefers one candy bar above all others, s/he will not select this candy bar *every* time s/he has the opportunity. The child will no doubt want to have some degree of variety. This type of example could be used in order to demonstrate to a child "how the very same person makes different choices or behaves differently."

From this standpoint, the research partner is given an opportunity to offer questions, suggestions, and evaluations about a general problem in psychology and the particular assumptions of the researcher conducting the study. Hopefully, learning will be facilitated for *both* parties involved in the interaction, through this cycle of activities between researcher and research partner.

CONCLUSION

Of course, the animate/inanimate distinction and the Müller-Lyer illusion are just two examples of domains in which *both* research participants and researchers can benefit from high-level psychological distancing activities. Researchers will have the opportunity to gather useful idiographic "data," related to both individual and intraindividual differences. But ideally, both parties benefit from the dialogicality required for more symmetrical questions, answers, and feedback between researcher and research participant.

However, these benefits can only come about when the value of differentiation is respected. The researcher must view the research participant not merely as someone who will help to verify or refute a hypothesis. Rather, participants must be treated as individuals with their own past history and experiences, who are capable of making a valuable and unique contribution to the research process. Accordingly, the attitudes, opinions, and outlooks of all parties involved in research must be respected at all times.

REFERENCES

Burke, K. (1945). *A grammar of motives.* New York: Prentice-Hall.

Laurendeau, M., & Pinard, A. (1962). *Causal thinking in the child: A genetic and experimental approach.* New York: International Universities Press.

Levy, E. (1943). Some aspects of the schizophrenic formal disturbance of thought. *Psychiatry (Journal of the Biology and Pathology of Interpersonal Relations), 6,* 55–70.

Matlin, M. W., & Foley, H. J. (1992). *Sensation and perception,* (3rd ed.). Boston: Allyn and Bacon.

Sigel, I. E. (1979). On becoming a thinker: A psycho-educational model. *Educational Psychologist, 14,* 70–78.

Sigel, I. E. (1993). The centrality of a distancing model for the development of representational competence. In R. R. Cocking & E. Renninger, (Eds.), *The development and meaning of psychological distance,* (pp. 141–158). Hillsdale, NJ: Lawrence Erlbaum.

Sullivan, H. S. (1940). *Conceptions of modern psychiatry.* Washington, DC: William Alanson White Psychiatric Foundation.

Williams, M. (1998). Doubt. In E. Craig (Ed.). *Routledge encyclopedia of philosophy* (Vol. 3) (pp. 122–124). London: Routledge.

Wiser, M. (1995). Use of history of science to understand and remedy students' misconceptions about heat and temperature. In D. N. Perkins, & J. L. Schwartz (Eds.), *Software goes to school: Teaching for understanding with new technologies,* (pp. 23–38). New York: Oxford University Press.

part II

The Partnership Approach in Educational Settings

9

CONTRASTING TRANSMISSION AND PARTNERSHIP MODELS OF TEACHING AND LEARNING

Laura Johnson
J. Fitzgerald Elementary School, Waltham, Massachusetts

Barbara Noel Dowds
Regis College and
University of Massachusetts Medical School

Roger Bibace
Clark University and
University of Massachusetts Medical School

James J. Dillon
State University of West Georgia

ABSTRACT

The discipline of education has seen numerous shifts in instructional strategy that reflect educational theory and research as well as cultural values, assumptions, and context. One of the most frequently employed models for education in this culture is the transmission model, in which the teacher imparts knowledge to the children. In contrast, the partnership model, which we are proposing, emphasizes the importance of reciprocity. Both teachers' and students' questions, answers, and evaluations of answers are seen as contributing to optimal teaching and learning. After comparing models for classroom teaching, we make connections between the partnership model and current theory and research in education, specifying and building on existing work which is consonant with the partnership model. We also discuss educational partnerships, including how such partnerships have been articulated in some Massachusetts schools with parents and with the larger community.

TRADITIONAL AND CHILD-CENTERED MODELS OF EDUCATION

The transmission model of educational practice, which continues to be used in many classrooms today, has a long history, dating back at least to John Locke's "tabula rasa" conception of the human mind. It places a greater emphasis on the teacher than on the learner because the teacher supplies knowledge to the child's "blank" mind. Mason (1972) suggested that traditional views of education regarded learning environments as a business relationship in which the teacher (agent) does the right things for the students (clients) in order to achieve a profit (learning). Learning is simply viewed as the interpretation of text and rote memorization of facts (Mason, 1972; Michaels, O'Connor, & Richards, 1994) with the primary role of the teacher being to pass on knowledge to those who lack it (Smith, 1986). Illich (1977) argued that socialization trains us to allow the use of transmission models of teaching. We are socialized to believe that teachers are the experts, and students are novices who are not encouraged to think or to generate questions. Smith (1986) suggested that by focusing on instruction, lecture, and repetition of information, students become dependent learners who must constantly ask educators for guidance when making their next move in the learning process.

This traditional view of education also places great emphasis on issues of classroom control (Smith, 1986). Teachers who subscribe to the traditional model of instruction may find comfort in the rigid, ritualistic nature of their classrooms. These teachers are less likely to be able to institute change into their curriculum and are often the educators who suffer "burn-out" (Smith, 1986). This rigidity also places a barrier between the teacher and students and does not foster the sense of reciprocity for which, we believe, classrooms should strive. The prevalence of transmission models suggests that there is little student engagement in the learning process (Herrenkohl, 1995).

The issue of discourse in a transmission model is extremely important. One typical instructional strategy that is used is the Initiation-Response-Evaluation (IRE) sequence (Mehan, 1979). In the IRE sequence the teacher initiates a question, the student responds, and the teacher evaluates the response. The IRE strategy makes little attempt to build on students' existing knowledge, to contextualize the knowledge, or to elicit further evaluation or questions which may help to solidify the learning that is taking place. Thus, from the perspective of the partnership model, it is desirable to move beyond this traditional discourse pattern to a more "thought-provoking" method of instruction.

Although a child-centered model of education has had more limited application in our culture, it gained some popularity in the 1960s. In the child-centered approach to education "the teacher must take her direction solely from the students" (Herrenkohl, 1995, p. 4). While the partnership model emphasizes the importance of the child, it does not presume that the child and teacher are equally expert. Rather it presumes that the teacher has much to offer to the educational process. Thus, while a partnership teacher follows the students' lead at times, the teacher also provides leadership, direction, and knowledge.

THE PARTNERSHIP MODEL OF EDUCATION

The partnership model ideally requires complementarity or symmetry with respect to who asks the questions, who answers the questions, and who evaluates the answers to questions. That is, both students and the teacher ask, answer, and evaluate. Student-generated questions are viewed as important by everyone in the classroom, and teacher-generated questions are likewise viewed as important. In the partnership classroom, students get answers to their questions as well as answering the teacher's questions in the traditional IRE sequence. Finally, in the partnership model, both students and the teacher evaluate the answers to questions. A dialogue in the classroom is more than one complete sequence of asking a question, answering the question, and evaluating the answer. The partnership model presumes that there is not a monopoly of the traditional teacher-driven IRE sequences in a dialogue. It also presumes that there are not many interruptions in the dialogue by either a teacher or a student. Rather, there is respectful listening and collaboration so that, ideally, a synergy occurs, leading to unanticipated approaches and answers, which in turn lead to further questions and additional collaboration.

The partnership model encourages the teacher to rely on "novel" methods to help generate questions by students, especially if the students in the class have been socialized in the traditional model and are not yet confident that their questions are important and will be respected and taken seriously. For example, the teacher could use "focus groups," composed of students in the classroom, to generate questions. This would be consistent with another premise of the partnership model, which encourages peer group interactions among students rather than relying solely on teacher–student dyadic interactions.

Having both students and teachers ask, answer, and evaluate, and using focus groups to help generate student questions, are all means to an end. In the partnership model the ends are specified in terms of reciprocity and of mutuality (Mesterton-Gibbons & Dugatkin, 1997). For reciprocity, the costs and benefits to teacher and student are clear and direct. For mutuality, the costs and benefits are either impossible to ascertain or their assessment is seen as unnecessary by all participants.

Many students and teachers adhere to a reciprocity value orientation. The costs (calculated in terms of time and effort expended) are expected to correlate with the benefits received (grade obtained, amount learned). In contrast, "byproduct mutualism" implies that the cost/benefit ratio for teacher and student may be impossible to assess or it may be deemed unnecessary to determine (Mesterton-Gibbons & Dugatkin, 1997). A teacher and a student may assume that the benefits are vague and long term. The interactions are justified by appeal to "principle." That is, it is good, challenging, and enriching to be involved in the process of learning, even though the outcome remains ambiguous. Thus students may realize, only years later, how much they benefited from a particular teaching/learning intervention or how important it was to learn a particular content.

There are many possible constraints on the enactment of the partnership model, due to its emphasis on dialogue and mutuality. There may be constraints imposed by the school committee or the superintendent of schools, particularly with respect to the resources available. For example, it is difficult to achieve partnerships with students if a teacher has too many students or too diverse a group of students in the classroom. There may also be constraints because of the amount of material that must be covered or the amount of time the teacher has available for training and preparation. These kinds of constraints minimize the likelihood that partnerships can occur in a classroom and maximize the probability that the teacher will rely on the traditional transmission model of education.

THE PARTNERSHIP MODEL AND CURRENT INSTRUCTIONAL APPROACHES

In an effort to revitalize classrooms, educational theorists and researchers have formulated a variety of methods for instruction, some of which include elements that are consistent with what we have termed the partnership model. For example, Bruner (1971) discussed ways to achieve optimum use of knowledge, considering, for example, how one arranges learning to facilitate the recognition of when one should "go beyond" information and make connections to other areas of knowledge. He also stressed that we must afford students the opportunity to make connections and use new information effectively. He believes that in order to encourage learning and thinking, we must define what approaches are successful in fostering intrinsic motivation. Bruner also highlighted the need to give students practice in the process of problem solving and the need to encourage students to try activities that they did not deem possible.

Rogoff (1995) has argued for a process of "participatory appropriation," which involves an active engagement in the learning process. In participatory appropriation, individuals participate in an activity, change as a result of that participation, and then later respond to a different situation in a new way because of their engagement in the prior activity. Rogoff sees this as a process of "becoming"

(p. 142); that is, involvement in an experience helps people handle novel situations. Therefore, the more experiences we have, the better we will be able to adapt to new ones. The partnership model allows for the student and the teacher to engage in participatory appropriation through exposure to novel situations. The partnership model, with its emphasis on student-generated questions and students' evaluations of answers, explicitly argues for "novelty" introduced by students as well as by teachers.

Mason (1972) emphasized collaboration in the classroom. In order for classrooms to be successful, it is necessary that collaboration and sharing of the learning process occur in teacher–student, student–student, teacher–teacher, and teacher–parent relationships (Bruner, 1971). A collaborative approach requires that the school become committed to producing a community of learners (Kelly, 1972) in which every teacher learns and every learner teaches. A collaboration grants teachers the opportunity to model open-mindedness and fosters an environment in which everyone, regardless of "ability," has the chance to learn (Smith, 1986). The partnership model helps to specify how terms such as "collaboration," "cooperation," and "community of learners" can be enacted. That is, the partnership model encourages students, as well as teachers, to contribute to what is learned and how it is learned. In the partnership model, learning frequently occurs through dialogue, because one of the major assumptions in this model is that no one is a mind reader. Thus, dialogue between self and other (student and teacher, student and student) is necessary in order to articulate what each person "means," to check on one another's assumptions, misconceptions, etc. What ideally will be generalized is "learning how to learn," that is, the dialogical processes (the sequences between self and other) that facilitate learning.

The concept of a community of learners also encourages parents to take an active role in the education of their children and insists that the classroom environment be one of mutual contribution to understanding and respect. The atmosphere is less anxiety ridden, and students can feel empowered by the ability to express their ideas and feelings freely without the fear of intimidation that may occur in more competitive, traditional classrooms. There is a greater emphasis on reciprocity rather than repetition of information in a community of learners.

Within the partnership model, there is a requirement that participants generate questions in order to comprehend fully the ideas, opinions, and egocentricities of all people. This concept of questioning highlights the importance of dialogue and discourse in the classroom. Paulo Freire (1970) in his text, *Pedagogy of the Oppressed*, states that:

> *Dialogue* is thus an existential necessity. And since dialogue is the encounter in which the united *reflection and action* of the dialoguers are addressed to the world which is to be transformed and humanized, this dialogue cannot be reduced to the act of one person's '*depositing*' ideas in another, nor can it become a simple exchange of ideas to be 'consumed' by the discussants. . . . It is an act of creation; it must not serve as a crafty instrument for the domination of one man by another. The domination implicit

> in dialogue is that of the world by the dialoguers; it is conquest of the world for the *liberation* of men. (p.77, emphasis added)

This statement rejects the traditional view of the classroom and is consistent with the partnership model which places great importance on reciprocal dialogue. In the partnership model, the symmetrical sequences of questions, answers, and evaluations by both students and teachers facilitates "act[s] of creation." Novelty in the classroom occurs when any of the participants reach a new and, for that person, previously unimagined understanding, conception, or conclusion. The respect for students that is central to the partnership model is consistent with Freire's emphasis on liberation (we believe, were he writing this passage today, he would be speaking of the "liberation of all"). Freire's emphasis on the personal and the particular as important for universal issues that affect all of humankind is consistent with the partnership model. That is, the particular dialogical sequences of individuals will at times address general issues that concern all of us. Thus these dialogues, these creative acts, have the potential to be of value to all human beings, not just those engaged in a particular dialogue.

O'Connor and Michaels (1993) introduced the concept of "revoicing," a method that allows teachers to coordinate academic tasks and social participation while engaging students in intellectual questioning and dialogue. Group discussion, as an instructional strategy, is emphasized as the teacher engages students in the classroom. In an exchange with a student, the teacher may rephrase the student's contribution to provide a more elaborate or abstract formulation of the student's statement and then ask both the student and others to respond. This revoicing can bring strength to a "weak" voice. It also opens up the discussion to others, promotes understanding, and reduces egocentric perceptions. From the perspective of the partnership model, we would emphasize not only the process of "revoicing," but also the particular individuals involved in the dialogue. Thus when "revoicing" makes a "weak" voice stronger, it is the voice of a specific student with whom, at that moment, the teacher is forming a partnership, by trying to clarify or rephrase the student's verbal contribution.

Michaels (1992) noted that when teachers and researchers speak of dialogue, there is a tendency to focus on isolated aspects of language and academics rather than viewing the dialogue as a whole, and, we would add, the persons engaged in the dialogue. This focus on isolated aspects ignores "complex interrelations between the individual, social and textual [which] creates fundamental obstacles to understanding the development and deployment of oral and written discourse in schools" (p. 305).

There is also a tendency to restrict classroom discourse to topics related to curriculum and school-based norms rather than reflecting on cues from students and allowing the discourse to move freely. From within the partnership model, the teacher is attentive to students' interests and questions and to the larger social context of students' lives (what is happening on TV, in the world of science, in their town or city government) and incorporates elements from all of these domains into the lesson plan. The partnership model emphasizes the importance of dialogue in all social interactions. By modeling the desired discourse behavior in the classroom setting, we prepare students to become intellectually engaged in dialogues, language, and culture throughout their lives. Stressing competencies in classroom discourse is a critical mediator between the broader social context and academic content (Applebee, 1996).

FURTHER IDEAS ABOUT INSTRUCTIONAL APPROACHES

Some may question whether the partnership model actually attempts to facilitate learning of content. Learning is maximized when there is an emphasis on both content and dialogue, that is, on knowledge as both product and process. Conversely, there is less learning with an exclusive or primary focus on either content or process alone. Effective dialogue requires as a base some knowledge that can then be enlarged through processes such as dialogue, experimentation, and reading. Teachers who espouse the partnership assumptions are attentive to both content and process because they realize the two are isomorphic. There can be no content without form, and there is no form without content. Dialogue is about a particular content. While it does take effort to achieve an appropriate (and changing) balance, the ability to emphasize curriculum content while also educating students about the process of learning and fostering an understanding of metacognitive processes is both desirable and possible.

When students are placed in small groups and encouraged to work together to solve a particular problem or answer a specific question, they engage in cooperative learning. This instructional strategy has become popular in many classrooms because, by working collaboratively, students can advance their level of inquiry (Martinello & Cook, 1994). In the cooperative learning group, more emphasis may be placed on the process than the final product, which is similar to Japanese educational models (Lynn, 1988). Japanese educators believe that "the important thing is not so much to produce smart children as to produce good children, responsible children, disciplined children. The entire program aims to teach children to work together and to cooperate in solving problems" (Kristof, 1997, p. 40). Cooperative learning encourages students to learn from each other and strengthens the notion of the community of learners within the classroom. The opportunity to evaluate different points of view on the same problem or concept can lead collaborative groups to richer solutions. Learning how to become a productive partner in a cooperative group often enhances the inquiry toward possible solutions (Martinello & Cook, 1994). As Sigel (1981) argued, we must not only foster knowledge and questioning of our physical world, but we must also strive to teach the importance of interaction with others as a basis for understanding the world around us.

Jerome Bruner (1966) popularized the concept of "discovery learning." Bruner suggested that:

> To instruct someone in [a] discipline is not a matter of getting him to commit results to mind. Rather, it is to teach him to participate in the process that makes possible the establishment of knowledge. We teach a subject not to produce little living libraries on the subject, but rather to get a student to think mathematically for himself, to consider matters as an historian does, to take part in the process of knowledge-getting. Knowing is a process, not a product. (p. 72)

Although the name "discovery learning" seems to be more consistent with realist assumptions than constructivist assumptions, we agree with Bruner's assertion that "knowing is a process, not a product." The model of instruction that Bruner describes, when coupled with the partnership model, exemplifies the ideal that students should be active participants in the learning/knowing process. The teacher should provide students with opportunities to have meaningful learning inquiries. The teacher encourages exploration that allows students to recognize that their learning is useful (Bruner, 1971). Cremin (1957) stated that "learning is an active process in which the effective labor must be performed by the learner" (p. 9). Students need to be allowed the freedom to discover their world and to question what they do not understand.

Clegg Jr. (1987), Gall and Rhody (1987) and Wilen (1987) have discussed the importance of questioning in a classroom. Questions are not only used to discover what people know, but also act as motivators, helping people focus their attention on a particular topic (Gall & Rhody, 1987). "The reward for working one's way through the known is to find a new question on the other side, formulated in a new way" (Bruner, 1971, p. 116). Questions also enable us to understand where students "are coming from." Teachers and learners alike must attempt to elicit questions of a "higher order" from each other. Questions that are considered "higher order" require the use of analysis, problem solving, prediction, and evaluation (Gall & Rhody, 1987). However, in order to teach students how to utilize these forms of questioning and thinking, teachers must model the desired behaviors. By using higher-order questions, we activate awareness of metacognitive processes (Nickerson, Perkins, & Smith, 1985) and encourage the use of thinking skills (e.g., making connections, integrating material) as opposed to the traditional method of memorizing, then reciting information.

Some of the concepts and practices that are part of what we term the partnership model are currently endorsed by educators. The National Education Association (NEA) recently published its resolutions for educators in the United States. The NEA (1997) states that "education is a lifelong process" (section A-2) and stresses the importance of parental involvement as well as community support for education. These principles are consistent with the partnership model.

On a more local scale, we looked at mission statements of some of the schools in the Boston area. The goals for which school systems strive are similar to those that we espouse in the partnership model. For example, the Somerville public schools (1992) envision an environment in which "we will base instruction on the strengths of our students, transcending recall of information and mastery of basic skills, to a full engagement in the critical and creative levels of cognition." The Lexington public schools (1997) recognize that their students and teachers should be encouraged to experiment, take risks, and work toward making the school "a positive place in which to teach and learn." These mission statements also expressed the importance of collaboration. Perhaps one of the most poignant examples is that of the Cambridge public school system (1990) which has designed what it has termed "A Shared Vision." This project was initiated in an effort to decrease drop-out rates and illiteracy and to increase achievement levels. The "shared vision" asserts that the improvement of public schools involves "forging of collaborative relationships between schools and businesses at the local level." By engaging the entire community in the formulation of curriculum and allowing the collaboration of schools and businesses, Cambridge demonstrates its creativity as well as its dedication to its community, its economy, and most importantly, its students and teachers. The Watertown public schools (1994) also acknowledge the importance of community involvement and suggest that "education is a community responsibility and excellence can only be achieved through a partnership between school and community." As these examples demonstrate, the desire to implement educational partnerships is indeed present and the benefits have been recognized.

One contribution the partnership model can make to these mission statements is some specificity regarding ways to achieve their stated goals. That is, the partnership model can help to provide the means to the ends articulated in the mission statements.

BENEFITS OF A PARTNERSHIP CLASSROOM

The benefits of a partnership program are many. Students are taught to use their minds in new and exciting ways. They are also given tools to help them continue in a lifelong quest for knowledge. They learn the skills necessary to achieve their highest levels of thinking and also come to an understanding of how and when to apply these skills (Bruner, 1971). Everyone has a chance to learn according to the partnership guidelines. This is perhaps the most important concept for students to understand because it will help them become more respectful of divergent viewpoints, a skill that is necessary for success in any occupation or endeavor.

The partnership model also allows teachers, students, parents, and school systems to focus on current student concerns. Mason (1972) suggested that the problems that are foremost in the lives of students today are the problems that are often brushed aside and removed from discussion. The partnership model makes students feel comfortable asking questions regarding solutions for their problems and concerns and lets them know that someone is "in their corner." If students do not feel that they can approach their teachers or peers about a particular topic, the problem itself may become an intrusion in their ability to learn. Students who are part of a partnership community know that asking a question is acceptable and, in fact, encouraged.

Teachers also benefit from a partnership-based classroom. They are given the opportunity to foster higher-level thinking and creativity that stems from the interests of their students. By guiding students through this type of discovery learning, the teachers also learn and better themselves and their teaching practices. The ability to collaborate with students is one which teachers should not dismiss as unimportant. Students have knowledge to contribute to a classroom as do teachers. Once we realize what a valuable asset our students are to the classroom, our educational system will become stronger.

By using the partnership approach, teachers are less likely to burn-out because each day may present a new and exciting challenge. The mixture of personalities, ideas, and views of students and teacher is a strength for the class and should be considered one of the more intriguing aspects of teaching. A major role of the teacher is to model behaviors that will help students become lifelong learners and thinkers. By modeling such behavior, teachers are actively engaged in their profession, an important principle of the partnership model. The model also encourages the use of innovative, creative teaching practices. Such practices should mitigate against burn-out.

In contrast, if a teacher is unwilling to accept divergent viewpoints, the teacher, as well as the students, lose. Teachers who cannot learn from their students and are not enthusiastic about their profession are seemingly "useless" (Mason, 1972). The teachers who are most likely to burn-out are those who are rigid in their teaching and inflexible in their classroom methodology. These teachers follow the same curriculum verbatim every year and make little accommodation to the mixture of personalities presented to them with each new class of students.

Schools benefit from the partnership model by witnessing and documenting the academic, social, and personal successes of each student. When they engage their teachers, students, parents, and the larger community, there are many exciting possibilities. Community-based problems can be acknowledged, and collaborative efforts to solve those problems can be developed (cf. Chapter 20). As Freire stated,

> we must never merely discourse on the present situation, must never provide the people with programs which have little or nothing to do with their own preoccupations, doubts, hopes and fears. . . . We must realize that their view of the world, manifested variously in their action, reflects their *situation* in the world. (1970, p. 85)

School systems should encourage the active involvement of teachers, parents, students, and administrators in the curriculum planning process. Parental and student ideas are often forgotten when curriculum plans are formulated; however, their input can be far more valuable than many department chairpersons realize. In fact, one of the NEA resolutions suggests that students should be active participants in the deliberative processes of school boards. Seeing the success of the partnership approach would encourage further partnerships among all members of the community of learners.

ACCOMMODATIONS TO FACILITATE IMPLEMENTATION

In order to achieve a partnership-based classroom, teachers need to make accommodations. There is a necessity to refrain from the rigidity of the traditional transmission models of teaching. To achieve classroom success, there needs to be a commitment from all parties involved to become, as mentioned previously, a community of lifelong learners. "The teacher must be a quickener of that impulse life through which thought can grow, indeed a shaper and molder of impulse into the rationality which comes from a healthy craving for contact with reality" (Murphy, 1961, p. 22). However, success with this type of program does not always evolve easily.

One of the difficulties with the implementation of an educational partnership lies within teacher education. Colleges and universities that train prospective teachers need to model the teaching of thinking. A primary goal of college programs should be facilitating growth and change (Dressel & Marcus, 1982). If educators are to produce teachers who will enter the classroom with a willingness to accept divergent viewpoints and encourage self-directed learning, these behaviors and actions must be modeled in the college classroom as well. Many college students and professors become entrapped in what Illich (1977) refers to as a "disabling illusion" (p. 35). Many students view their professors as the "experts" and see themselves as the "novice." This may intimidate students and inhibit them from posing questions or articulating their thoughts and views. If educators remembered what it felt like to be a student, if they formed partnerships with their students, then students would be freer to ask, answer, and evaluate; freer to question and to articulate their views.

One of the major difficulties with teacher preparation programs lies in the fact that a college classroom is often centered around lectures and a more transmission-based model of teaching. Many students read background information in a textbook, memorize that information, and then prepare to be tested on the same information. Professors are often regarded as the experts who dispense their knowledge of a particular topic to the students. In order for prospective teachers to understand how a classroom partnership truly works, it is necessary to see this method of teaching in action. Therefore, we would suggest that students acquiring a degree in education should be given more opportunities to practice what they have read about and should be evaluated on their ability to perform these tasks. Teaching is not a predictable profession. Hence, students of education need to "learn by doing" (Metzger, 1989). By being given these chances to test the scenarios that they have read about in textbooks, future teachers are able to see what works or does not work in various situations. It is our hope that this hands-on approach would allow new teachers to be more flexible in their teaching instruction strategies and more willing to attempt a new method or approach.

THE IMPORTANCE OF IMPLEMENTATION

Research has shown that 80 percent of classroom time is spent on memorization of facts and only 10 percent is spent on critical thinking (the remaining 10 percent is left to other daily tasks such as lunch) (Render, 1989). The partnership model strives to reverse these two percentages. Teachers need opportunities to implement new ideas and to seek out resources for these new ideas. Educators should also be students themselves both by continuing their own education and by allowing themselves to learn from their students. We do not suggest that there are not teachers who currently espouse this tradition. In fact, we are positive that there are many who do implement these strategies.

When parents send their children to a school that embraces the partnership paradigm, they know that their viewpoint and questions are respected. They have become part of the community of learners and are treated as such. Teachers recognize what valuable assets the parents of their students can be (cf. Chapter 13). By making a constituted effort to include parents in many aspects of the educational process, teachers welcome their suggestions, questions, and especially their talents.

The partnership model needs to be adapted to the developmental stages of the children in the classroom. Teachers must appreciate children's current cognitive strengths and strive to provide a learning environment that facilitates further cognitive development. For example, early childhood teachers should take advantage of preschoolers curiosity by designing a curriculum that fosters the ability to question. At this stage, teachers should model how discourse takes place and engage students in discourse as often as possible. With students in the elementary grades, an integration-based model of curriculum instruction is appropriate. The partnership model, with its emphasis on the importance of students' questions and ideas, fosters intrinsic motivation. Students witness their successes and see their "failures" as areas for improvement. In the secondary grades, teachers are often "experts" in one specific topic. Teachers can model a partnership approach to students by collaborating with one another, creatively integrating aspects of the curriculum.

Many college professors have remarked that students are often unprepared for the higher level of thinking that is expected of college students (Dressel & Marcus, 1982; Nickerson, Perkins, & Smith, 1985). The partnership model, if implemented from the primary grades through college, should give students the intrinsic motivation to strive for personal, academic, social, and professional success at the collegiate level and beyond. However, to reiterate what was previously discussed, college professors need to model the same types of behaviors and attitudes that they require of their students. At the college level, especially in the introductory courses, an emphasis on discourse is often not present. Teachers, regardless of what level they teach, when provided with adequate resources, should be models of higher-level thinking.

The partnership model can apply to many social situations. The ability to question and to communicate our thoughts, ideas, and feelings effectively is of great importance to our success as individuals, communities, and societies. If we can reach people through the educational system, we can produce citizens who value thinking, learning, and understanding. If we cannot learn from others, they cannot learn from us.

Throughout this chapter we have attempted to present the partnership model. The implementation of such an approach is not without its difficulties. However, this approach is the most effective means of fostering thinking and learning for all people, not only students in a classroom. We hope we have presented to you, the reader and lifelong learner, some ideas for where we believe the future of education should be heading. It is our hope that with our suggestions, some educators may implement the partnership model in their own classrooms or some may implement the model in other social interactions where an active partnership would enhance communication and facilitate development.

REFERENCES

Applebee, A. N. (1996). *Curriculum as conversation: Transforming traditions of teaching and learning.* Chicago: University of Chicago Press.

Bruner, J. (1966). *Toward a theory of instruction.* New York: W. W. Norton.

Bruner, J. (1971). *The relevance of education.* New York: W. W. Norton.

Cambridge Public Schools. (1990). *A shared vision* [Brochure]. Cambridge, MA: Author.

Clegg, A. A., Jr. (1987). Why questions? In W. W. Wilen (Ed.), *Questions, questioning techniques and effective teaching* (p. 11–21). Washington, DC: National Education Association.

Cremin, L. A. (Ed.). (1957). *The republic and the school: Horace Mann on the education of free men.* New York: Teachers College Press.

Dressel, P. L., & Marcus, D. (1982). *On teaching and learning in college.* San Francisco: Jossey-Bass.

Freire, P. (1970). *Pedagogy of the oppressed.* New York: Continuum.

Gall, M. D., & Rhody, T. (1987). Review of research on questioning techniques. In W. W. Wilen (Ed.), *Questions, questioning techniques and effective teaching* (pp. 23–43). Washington DC: National Education Association.

Herrenkohl, L. R. (1995). *Enhancing student engagement in the context of school science.* Unpublished doctoral dissertation, Clark University, Worcester, MA.

Illich, I. (1977). Disabling professions. In I. Illich, I. K. Zola, J. McKnight, J. Caplan, & H.Shaiken (Eds.), *Disabling professions* (pp. 11–39). London: Marion Boyars.

Kelly, L. (1972). *From dialogue to discourse.* Glenview, IL: Scott, Foresman.

Kristof, N. D. (1997, August 17). Where children rule. *The New York Times Magazine, 146,* 40–44.

Lexington Public Schools. (1997). *1997–1998 Professional development handbook* [Brochure]. Lexington, MA: Author.

Lynn, R. (1988). *Educational achievement in Japan: Lessons for the west.* Armonk, NY: M. E. Sharp.

Martinello, M. L., & Cook, G. E. (1994). *Interdisciplinary inquiry in teaching and learning.* New York: Macmillan.

Mason, E. (1972). *Collaborative learning.* New York: Agathon Press.

Mehan, H. (1979). *Learning lessons: Social organization in the classroom.* Cambridge, MA: Harvard University Press.

Mesterton-Gibbons, M., & Dugatkin, L. A. (1997). Cooperation and the prisoner's dilemma: Towards testable models of mutualism versus reciprocity. *Animal Behavior, 54,* 551–557.

Metzger, D. J. (1989). Challenge to education: A model for individualizing teacher education courses. In J. A. Braun (Ed.), *Reforming teacher education: issues and new directions* (pp. 321–334). New York: Garland.

Michaels, S. (1992). The dismantling of narrative. In A. McCabe & C. Peterson (Eds.), *New directions in developing narrative structure* (pp. 303–351). Norwood, NJ: Ablex Publishing.

Michaels, S., O'Connor, M. C., & Richards, J. (1993). Literacy as reasoning within multiple discourses: Implications for restructuring learning. In *Restructuring learning: 1990 summer institute papers and recommendations by the Council of Chief State School Officers* (pp. 107–121). Mystic, CT: Council of Chief State School Officers.

Murphy, G. (1961). *Freeing intelligence through teaching: A dialectic of the rational and the personal.* New York: Harper & Row.

National Education Association. (1997). *The 1997–98 resolutions of the National Education Association* [Brochure]. Atlanta, GA: NEA Representative Assembly.

Nickerson, R. S., Perkins, D. N., & Smith, E. E. (1985). *The teaching of thinking.* Hillsdale, NJ: Lawrence Erlbaum.

O'Connor, M. C., & Michaels, S. (1993). Aligning academic task and participation status through revoicing: Analysis of a classroom discourse strategy. *Anthropology and Education Quarterly, 24,* 318–335.

Render, G. F. (1989). Research on humanistic education: Implications for the future. In J. A. Braun (Ed.), *Reforming teacher education: issues and new directions* (pp. 233–251). New York: Garland Publishing.

Rogoff, B. (1995). Observing sociocultural activity on three planes: Participatory appropriation, guided participation, and apprenticeship. In J. V. Wertsch, P. Del Rio, & A. Alvarez (Eds.), *Sociocultural studies of mind* (pp. 139–164). New York: Cambridge University Press.

Sigel, I. E. (1981). Social experience in the development of representational thought: Distancing theory. In I. E. Sigel, D. M. Brodzinsky, & R. M. Golinkoff (Eds.), *New directions in Piagetan theory and practice* (pp. 203–216). Hillsdale, NJ: Lawrence Erlbaum.

Smith F. (1986). *Insult to intelligence: The bureaucratic invasion of our classrooms.* New York: Arbor House.

Somerville Public Schools. (1992). *School system mission statement* [Brochure]. Somerville, MA: Author.

Watertown Public Schools. (1994). *The strategic plan: 1995–2000* [Brochure]. Watertown, MA: Author.

Wilen, W. W. (1987). Improving teachers' questions and questioning: Research informs practice. In W. W. Wilen (Ed.), *Questions, questioning techniques and effective teaching* (pp.173–197). Washington, DC: National Education Association.

10

PSYCHOLOGY AND ETHICS: THE DISTANCING STRATEGY AS ETHICAL COMMITMENT

James J. Dillon
State University of West Georgia

ABSTRACT

This chapter explores the relationship between psychology and ethics. It is argued that a much closer relationship needs to be established between these two disciplines. Historical analysis for this estrangement between psychology and ethics is offered. It is argued that an "ethically inspired" psychology is founded on the notion of respect, care, and the "capacity for otherness." Extant developmental theory is evaluated in the light of parameters sketched out for an ethically inspired psychology. Irving Sigel's "Distancing" model of psychological development is presented as an encouraging movement toward an ethically inspired developmental theory.

In our professional training as psychologists, we explicitly, and more often implicitly, accept certain ethical assumptions about human beings and how to relate with them. These assumptions allow us to function smoothly in our various professional practices. Indeed, without codified theoretical and ethical assumptions, practice would be next to impossible. But very often our drive to collect data, test hypotheses, achieve certain therapeutic outcomes, and teach complex concepts, often takes precedence over *serious reflection* on the ethical implications of extant research programs, therapeutic practices, and pedagogic techniques. As Prilleltensky (1997) has recently argued, many psychologists are aware of the role and importance of ethics in psychology, but psychologists lack clear guidelines to appraise the ethical implications of their work. The pages of this chapter seek to provide a clearing wherein certain ethical questions can be raised, options considered, and conclusions/guidelines suggested. I hope to show that in the context of education, Sigel's (1993) "distancing strategy" is most consistent with the basic ethical assumptions behind the partnership model described throughout this volume.

To avoid confusion, I should, at the outset, define what I mean by the term "ethics." I consider the meaning of the term ethics by distinguishing it from its close relative, *morality*. Though the words "morality" and "ethics" are often used interchangeably, there are important distinctions between them. Each is concerned with questions of the good, with what it means to live a good life, but "morality," as I am using it here, refers to the actual *practical activity* of trying to do the good, living as full and authentic human beings, as when one tries to make a "moral" decision regarding love or work. With morality, we are engaged in the struggle to become ever more fully human. Ethics, on the other hand, involves us in specific sorts of *reflective* questions, as when we say to ourselves, "how *should* I have behaved in that situation?" or "What is the *right thing* to do here?" Following Genovese (1987), ethics can be defined as *the study of morality*, "a reflective investigation into what is the morally proper thing to do" (p. 17). So when we systematically consider questions of morality, right living, good conduct, being good, authentic, fully human, we are engaged in the study of *ethics*.

What do I hope to show with such ethical reflection on the assumptions we hold about human relationships? First and foremost, I hope to show that beneath our concrete psychological practice in educational settings lie a number of abstract, theoretical, and ethical assumptions that we may not fully want to endorse. These assumptions rest on completely asymmetrical power relationships and misguided conceptions of human nature. So, broadly speaking, I attempt to argue that psychology generally, and developmental psychology in particular, has become unnecessarily *estranged from ethics* and that a closer alliance between ethics and psychology would highly benefit and improve both disciplines. Specifically, what I hope to do is articulate what an ethically inspired psychology might look like, and then to suggest promising trends in educational theory and practice that are consistent with our partnership model. Let us begin with psychology's estrangement from ethics and then turn to the promising trends in educational theory and practice.

To claim that psychology has become "estranged" from ethics is to say that psychology really does not spend that much time thinking about the good, about what it means to live a full life, to engage in an authentic relationship, to be truly human, and so on. It is to say that for the most part, psychology has attempted, perhaps for quite noble reasons, to bracket questions of the good, the just, the right, and to focus on other types of phenomena. These other phenomena may be valuable in their own right, but the time has come when this bracketing has ceased to be generative and may actually be *occluding* phenomena of great value and significance to human science. I want first to consider some of the reasons why this estrangement has occurred in our discipline in the hope of, if not reconciling psychology with ethics, at least raising the possibility for psychology to entertain certain ethically inspired questions. I sketch out an answer to this question as to how psychology has become so estranged from ethics by exploring what has come to be known as the "Fact/Value" distinction in scientific inquiry.

THE FACT/VALUE DISTINCTION

I begin our discussion of psychology's estrangement from ethics by introducing another term to the discussion, "ontology." Ontology, simply, is concerned with the nature of Being, with the "is." Ethics, as we mentioned, is concerned with systematic reflection on the way things "ought" to be, with just and right action within and between people. It has been noted by many contemporary figures (e.g., Bloom, 1987; Toulmin, 1987) that it is a pervasive facet of the "modern" mind to draw a radical separation between "fact" and "value," between "is" and "ought," or between ontology and ethics. Questions of fact become those to be dealt with by the natural sciences, and as such, are regarded as "objective," that is, out there. Questions of value become those to be dealt with largely by the humanities, and as such, are regarded as "subjective," that is, in here.

Probably the strongest statement of this position comes from the British Empiricists, especially Thomas Hobbes (1650/1840). Hobbes held a view of the universe as basically consisting of matter-in-motion. Physics was therefore held by Hobbes to be the queen of the sciences. Applying this dictum to the psychological realm, it followed for Hobbes that all "mental" activities, including questions of ethics and value, must "really" be the motions of matter on the brain. As such, the psychological and ethical realm becomes "subjective" and "epiphenomenal" (Locke's secondary qualities). Ontology, or the study of what is, gradually becomes separated from ethics, the study of what ought to be.

Though many regard this fact/value distinction as a deeply modern invention, following Lavine (1984), one can see precursors well before the modern period. Specifically, in ancient Greece, there were a group of philosophers now referred to as the "Sophists" who traveled to various cities in the 5th century BC. With their worldly travel, the sophists claimed that since "Reason" produces often contradictory claims from philosophers the world over, one must therefore doubt the power of Reason to lead to truth. On this score, the famous philosopher Protagoras claimed that since there are so many different versions of reality, that reality must be whatever we claim for it, an ancient form of subjective/cultural relativism (Guthrie, 1975).

As Lavine (1984) points out, the Sophists' relativistic claims were in direct conflict with those of Socrates and Plato, who defended Reason's power to discern truth and claimed that Reason can provide a true picture of knowledge *and* objective ethical principles, each of which was seen to be inherent in the structure of the universe. Thus, for Socrates and Plato, the standard of good human living can be found by Reason *in reality itself.* That is, for many of the early Greeks, ontology and ethics were the same thing. As Weinreb (1987) writes, "Reduced to barest, generally agreed essentials, the philosophy of Plato affirms that there is a divinely ordered reality, which is the ultimate good and determinative of the good for human beings. Within limits, human reason can ascertain the good and direct itself toward it" (p. 32).

The prickly question as to when in history ontology became separated from ethics should not concern us here. What I hope the reader will note is that despite the relatively recent eclipse by Enlightenment philosophy, there has been a long tradition in our intellectual history of *not* separating the study of reality (scientia) from the study of the principles of the good (ethica). This long tradition of including the study of ethics in the study of reality is usually not denied by adherents to the fact/value distinction, but is often cast by them as a "backward" and "superstitious" period we have happily transcended. In the pages that follow, I invite the reader to consider whether this characterization of early scientific inquiry is entirely justified.

In considering this issue, one may ask the question as to whether such a separation between "facts" and "values," ontology and ethics, comes easily to the human mind. I draw a central postulate from the work of the medieval philosopher Giambattista Vico (1744/1968) who argued that human beings are concerned the world over with a finite number of fundamental questions, let us call them existential questions. The answers that people give and have given to these questions surely vary from culture to culture and from time to time, but the *provocation* to provide an answer to these questions in the first place is seen *not to vary*. What are some of these questions?

From Vico's (1744/1968) work, we can isolate three such questions. The first I call questions of *origin*. That is, human beings the world over are deeply concerned with questions as to where we come from. Stories are a central means of answering such questions. As Jung (1933) has pointed out, all cultures have creation myths. These diverse myths can be understood as attempts to answer these gnawing existential questions of origin that plague us all.

The second type of question involves human *destiny*. That is, human beings the world over are deeply concerned with questions as to where we are going, to where their lives are leading.

The third type of question involves the aforementioned domain of *ethics*. That is, human beings the world over are deeply concerned with questions as to how they are to get on with one another, with what are "appropriate," "just," "right," "natural" ways to treat one another. Cultures the world over will surely provide different answers to these questions; for example, behavior toward children in one culture is seen to be "just," "natural," and in another culture is seen as "unjust," "unnatural." The central point for our present discussion is that human beings are compelled to ask and answer these questions in the first place. My guiding postulate is thus formulated as follows: It is a central human aspiration to be, in Tillich's (1957) terms, "ultimately concerned." That is, it is a central aspect of being human to try and fit one's life and one's acts into the context of a cosmic and metaphysical narrative of depth, power, and value. Specifically, it is a fundamental human concern to ask ethical questions about life and to see one's own life and acts as being cosmically just, good, right. That is, human beings are at root ethical creatures. From this perspective, separating ethics from inquiry into the nature of human beings is quite an artificial act indeed. In fact, as Chapter 21 notes, the drive toward ethical behavior may just be encoded in our genes.

Assuming the validity of this postulate, the question then becomes, why have the social sciences become so estranged from the ethical disciplines in the first place? Browning (1987) has argued that this separation has occurred in psychology for two major reasons: one is historical, the other is clinical. Let us first turn to the historical factor. A simple survey of any textbook on the history and systems of psychology will show that many influential figures in our field's past, for example, E.B. Tichner, and J.B. Watson, argued strongly and persuasively for the elimination of "intangibles" and "unobservables" like emotion, thought, values, and so forth, from psychological inquiry. Further, many early psychologists, Watson (1913) in particular, argued that psychology is "a purely objective experimental branch of natural science," whose, "theoretical goal is the prediction and control of human behavior" (p.158). This definition of psychology made its way into my undergraduate introductory textbook, most textbooks I have subsequently considered using as a professor for Psychology 101, and it has probably made its way into many of the readers' lives as well. With this definition, take especial note that Watson's goal for psychology is explicitly *anti*-ethical. It can be noted that many attempts have been made, for example, Skinner's *Walden Two* (1976), to put this scientific information to ethical uses, but there is an explicit rejection of the notion of considering ethical questions *in the methodology of psychology* itself. In the act of conducting psychological research, Watson is not concerned with achieving mental health, cultivating satisfying relationships, educating children, the betterment of humanity, and so on. In fact, he views these concerns as *impediments* to the exalted goal of prediction and control. Watson's goal for psychology, in a matter of a few decades in the late 19th and early 20th centuries, quickly becomes "objectivity," "ethical neutrality," and the concern for the tangible. For many, this goal was seen as a valuable corrective to the superstition and prejudice that held sway in the days when ethical and scientific disciplines were more closely allied.

I said that the second reason for psychology's estrangement from ethics is clinical. That is, psychology becomes separated from the normative disciplines of theology, philosophy, and ethics out of a deep and laudable fear of *moralism*. As Browning (1987) points out, with Freud's concept of the harsh and morally punitive superego as being the actual *source* of neurosis and suffering, many psychologists took it as their goal to remove any and all of the moral demands that suffering individuals placed upon themselves. For many psychologists, morality and ethical restraint become equated with *pathogenesis*. The very *last* thing a psychologist would therefore want to do would be to inject ethical concerns into a particular clinical intervention or investigation. For the psychologist, this would be seen as only making matters worse.

The question I raise here is whether the avoidance of ethical questions is the *only* way to avoid the possibility of superstition and moralism that the combination of ethics and psychology presents? I suggest that one can be a tolerant, nonmoralistic, *scientific,* and *ethically guided psychologist.* In trying to persuade you why the extreme stance of ethical neutrality is unnecessary, I want to conjure for the reader what an ethically inspired psychology might look like. I do this by first returning to many of the aforementioned insights from the ancient Greeks and medieval philosophers before turning my attention to certain hopeful exemplars from modern educational and developmental theory.

TOWARD AN ETHICALLY INSPIRED PSYCHOLOGY

As mentioned above, what follows is a vision that I conjure for the reader. As such, it is therefore not intended to convince the reader with its logical and argumentative force, but to appeal to a sense that the reader might have that all is not well with psychology and on that basis, evoke a shared vision. In painting this picture of an ethically inspired psychology, I return for a moment to a few of the insights from the ancient Greeks that we discussed earlier. First, against the rampant relativism of our present epoch, an ethically inspired psychology would hold, with Plato, Socrates, and others, that we inhabit a *normatively ordered universe*, not a universe of blind and random matter-in-motion. Second, against the epistemological skepticism of our present epoch, an ethically inspired psychology would hold that properly instructed human Reason can, within certain limits, ascertain this normative order and direct itself toward it. The question then becomes, where is Reason to look? It is to this third question, with the help of Thomas Aquinas, that we turn now.

Aquinas followed the ancient Greeks in his assumption that human beings inhabited a normatively ordered universe and that it was within Reason's power to ascertain the nature of that order. Aquinas goes much further than this and provides us with some direction as to where to look for this order. In the *Summa Theologica* (1268/1981), Aquinas identifies three types of order in the universe: eternal law, natural law, and human law. *Eternal law*, for Aquinas, is the cosmic, universal order inherent in all things. Special problems arise for Aquinas in considering the eternal law's relationship to the human being. This problem specifically involves human freedom. As Weinreb (1987) points out, "Since human beings are subject to . . . [the] eternal law, there is no need for them to be governed by any other law [in this sense, they are 'instinctive' like animals]. On the other hand, since human beings are free and direct themselves according to their own reason and will, unlike other creatures, they are not subject to direction by nature" (pp. 56–57). Therefore, for Aquinas, human beings are subject to the eternal law in a special way, specifically, following St. Paul, the eternal law is seen to be "written on the human heart" and can be known by human Reason when we are sufficiently present to ourselves. Aquinas calls this law written on the heart the "*natural law*" and notes that unlike animals, human beings are impelled to obey the natural law, but have the capacity to direct their conduct either in accordance with it or not. Weinreb (1987) notes:

> Natural law, then, is the link between eternal law in the mind of God and the moral law for human beings, between nature (providence) and reason. It is a reflection of human nature, the natural human inclinations toward appropriate human ends. Thus far, it is known to all and unchangeable. (p. 59)

Third, *human law* is the codified law of particular groups living in particular times. In the context of natural and eternal law, a human law can be either "just" or "unjust."

Aquinas helps in our search for the normative order with his claim that the natural law is "written" in our innermost being and presents itself to Reason. And what does natural law present Reason with? At the most general of levels, the natural law, for Aquinas, inclines us to *love*, to do what is good and avoid what is evil. In addition, Aquinas notes, the natural law teaches us that we may never do evil so that good may result from it; one must always do the good. Natural law inclines us to abide by the Golden Rule, to live in such a way that, "Whatever you wish that others would do to you, do so to them." Finally, the natural law demands *respect* for one's neighbor and his or her conscience. The particulars and various interpretations of natural law should not concern us here. What we should note in this context are four things:

1. the idea of interiority; that is, the notion not only that a normative order exists, but that this order is "written across the human heart,"
2. this order can be known with the power of the human mind,
3. the normative order impels us to *love* others, and
4. the normative order impels us to *respect* others.

We've explored the scope and implications of the first two propositions, and so we turn now to the last two.

We say that the normative order impels us to love others. In order to avoid confusion with such a loaded term, I should, at the outset, define what I mean by the term "love." I follow Milton Meyeroff's definition from his excellent work *On Caring* (1971). Here he states that to love another person is to act in such a way as to help him or her to *grow*. He writes:

> To help another person grow is at least to help him to care for something or someone apart from himself, and it involves encouraging and assisting him to find and create areas of his own in which he is able to care. . . . I grow by becoming more self-determining, by choosing my own values and ideals grounded in my own experience, instead of either simply conforming to the prevailing values or compul-

> sively rejecting them. I am better able to make my own decisions and more willing to be responsible for them, and I can discipline and limit myself in order to seek out and achieve what is important to me. (p. 13)

So to love another, to care for another, which, following Aquinas is quite "natural" for human beings to do, one helps the other to become the person that he or she is. In love, one facilitates the process of growth. As such, in loving the other, I do not attempt to make the other become what *I* want or need him or her to be. I make no attempt to change the other, to make him or her other than what s/he is. Therefore, intimately connected with this idea of love is the idea of *respect.* When I respect something, I allow it to be what it is and make no attempt to change it. The normative order impels us to develop what I call a "capacity for otherness," that is, the ability to see another, one's child, one's lover, one's neighbor (one's student, client, participant), as a separate and distinct person and not part of a larger narcissistic agenda. As an example of such an agenda, Alice Miller (1981) has persuasively demonstrated, in her clinical work, the consequences of a parent's incapacity for otherness. That is, the parent, Miller says, often *uses* the infant or the child to satisfy his or her own unmet needs, resolve ongoing conflicts, achieve unactualized aspirations. The result of this process is that the child will wall off a huge portion of him or herself for the sake of making the parent happy. As an adult, this individual may have an immense amount of difficulty accessing this repressed portion of the self and will therefore experience "symptoms" of loss, such as depression, mourning, loss of affect, and so forth.

Indeed, in our work as therapists, teachers, researchers, friends, neighbors, parents, and lovers, we do all sorts of things to make the others we deal with understandable and digestible to us. But it is an open question whether we ever *really* know or are open to the other. In this context, I cite the familiar frustrated cries of our students, clients, children, friends, and lovers in our interactions with them: "You're not hearing me!" "You don't understand me!" Who can forget one's own sense of rage as an adolescent at not being seen for who we were? I argue that the more capable we are to experience otherness, the more we can be said to be *respecting* the other, allowing the other to be what s/he is rather than twisting him or her into the analytic categories, images, ideals, wants, and desires that *we* have. Meyeroff writes:

> The union with the other in caring differs . . . from that found in a parasitic relation. Instead of trying to dominate and possess the other, I want it to grow in its own right, or, as we sometimes say, 'to be itself,' and I feel the other's growth as bound up with my own sense of well-being. The worth I experience in the other is something over and above any value it may have for me because of its ability to satisfy my own needs. . . . In caring I experience the other as having potentialities and the need to grow. . . . In helping the other grow I do not impose my own direction; rather, I allow the direction of the other's growth to guide what I do, to help determine how I am to respond and what is relevant to such response. (pp. 8-9)

In sum, to behave ethically toward another is to love and respect him or her as I have outlined it. This, I believe is the ethical foundation for the partnership model. In the remainder of the chapter I turn our attention to certain strands of educational and developmental theory that hold the brightest promise as far as fulfilling these requirements for an ethically inspired psychology.

PROMISING TRENDS IN EDUCATION AND DEVELOPMENTAL PSYCHOLOGY

From the perspective of an ethically inspired psychology, the philosophy of education that comes closest to meeting the aforementioned specifications is one that, in a sense, returns to the classical Socratic model. With this model, education is seen as "educare," or a process of "leading out" rather than "putting in." That is, to educate someone from the standpoint of the Socratic model is, in my terms, to love and respect him or her, to lead his or her nascent capacities into actuality. John Dewey's (1916, 1938; Dewey & Dewey, 1915) many inspiring works on education are excellent modern examples of this philosophy of education. With this understanding of education as a "leading out," as helping the other to grow, in his or her own way, education and *development* thus stand in a very close relationship. If we translated some of our "ethical" terms into "psychological" ones, we might substitute the terms "love and respect" with "educate." We might substitute "growth" with "development."

Crain (1985) outlines two traditions in psychology that nicely illustrate the contrast between an ethically inspired developmental psychology and other approaches. Crain notes that it is quite a common cultural assumption to make that children's development is "in our hands," that children become what *we* make them. Here, as with Marx (1859/1977), Skinner (1972), and others, the child is seen as a "product" of his or her social "environment." Crain refers to this tradition in psychology as "Environmentalism." But there is, he notes, another tradition in psychology. These theorists are often called "developmentalists," and they "are less impressed by our efforts to teach or otherwise influence children. Instead, they are more interested in how children grow and learn on their own" (p. xiii). These theorists believe that "children may have an inner need to seek out certain kinds of experiences and activities at certain times in life" (p. xiv).

John Locke is cited as having begun the environmentalist tradition in psychology, with intellectual heirs such as Pavlov, Watson, Skinner, and so on. Jean-Jacques Rousseau is cited as having begun the developmentalist tradition with intellectual heirs such as Gessell, Montessori, Werner, and Piaget. Briefly, Locke (1965), a 17th century British philosopher, offered the idea that human beings cannot be said to be "innately" good or bad, cannot be said to be "innately" anything. Instead, Locke maintained that the infant's mind is a "tabula rasa" or a "blank slate" upon which life's experiences will impress their form. The 18th-century French philosopher

Jean-Jacques Rousseau (1762/1993), on the other hand, disagreed with Locke and argued that children are not blank slates, but have their own characteristic ways of being. "This is," Crain (1985) writes, "according to Nature's design. Nature is like a hidden tutor who prompts the child to develop different capacities at different stages of growth" (p. 9). Foreshadowing Miller (1981), Maslow (1970), and others, Rousseau argues that the civilized adult is entirely too dependent on other people's validation. "They have forgotten how to see with their own eyes and to think with their own minds; they only see and think what society expects them to" (Crain, 1985, p. 7). Rousseau suggests that instead of rushing in and teaching children the "correct" ways of thinking, parents and teachers should allow them to perfect their *own* capacities and to develop their *own* ways as nature intends.

Rousseau's developmentalism is consistent with the first principle for an ethically inspired psychology, namely, the notion not only that a normative order exists (nature), but that this order expresses itself in the inner recesses of the human being. Indeed, from an ethical perspective, the environmentalistic framework is extremely problematic in that it views the child as nothing more than raw material, "wet clay" to be shaped and molded in any way that the adults in the group see fit. No *respect* is given to the *child's* unique capacities, talents, interests. Development is essentially cast as the process of socialization. For Rousseau, development involves facilitating the process of growth *inherent to the child.* The question I explore for the remainder of this chapter is just how this process of facilitation is to proceed. As I mentioned above, Rousseau's ideas had immense influence on many figures in developmental psychology, including Gessell, Montessori, Werner, and Piaget. I turn now to two of these figures, Werner and Piaget, to help point us in the direction that an ethically inspired psychology might want to go in answering this question.

To begin, the developmentalists Jean Piaget (1985) and Heinz Werner (1948; Werner & Kaplan, 1963) share Rousseau's assumption that development and socialization are not synonymous, that the child has important contributions to make to his or her own growth. What do these two theories of growth involve? For Piaget, developmental change is not simply a process of "accommodating" to knowledge that is already there (realism), nor is it a matter of imposing preexisting knowledge forms upon unformed experience (idealism). Rather, developmental change is seen to be a process of "construction" involving the coordination of simple and uncoordinated action schemes into ever more complex (developed) structures. A person, for example, may be able to employ his or her innate "walking" scheme and his or her innate "chewing gum" scheme separately without any problem. But when the subject tries to complete the task of walking and chewing gum *at the same time*, s/he falls down. The subject is, as we say, "uncoordinated" with respect to walking and chewing gum. For Piaget, in the service of an adaptive function, or the achievement of a particular goal, in this case walking and chewing gum at the same time, assimilatory action schemes (walking, chewing gum) are modified through the process of mutual *coordination*, and eventually come to "accommodate" a state of affairs to which the subject's initial schemes did not apply.

Piaget describes the frustrating initial state in which one's extant schemes do not apply toward the realization of a given end as "disequilibrium." From this state, the subject makes attempts to reestablish equilibrium, or "equilibrates." As Piaget (1985) writes:

> From the point of view of equilibration, it is obvious that one of the sources of progress in the development of knowledge must be sought in disequilibria as such. Disequilibria alone force the subject to go beyond his current state and strike out in new directions. (p. 10)

While it is true that *all* cognitively frustrating or confusing situations, what he calls "perturbations," do not necessarily lead to developmental progress, Piaget notes that there are *certain* perturbations that, as he writes, "give rise to developments that surpass what has previously existed and go on to specific reequilibrations" (p. 10). It follows from this that an individual who, as a result of an action or exercise, is in a state of disequilibrium, may act to modify (coordinate) his or her extant schemes in an effort to establish greater equilibrium. Thus, in certain situations, the individual goes *beyond* what s/he knew before, his/her mental functioning changes, becomes more integrated, develops. The general direction of developmental change for Piaget is from ego, bodily centered, and time-bound modes of cognition in infancy and early childhood to the formal, impersonal, abstract, and timeless modes of cognition in middle childhood and adolescence.

In their characterization of developmental change, Werner & Kaplan (1963) present a similar sequence to Piaget's. Werner & Kaplan employ the notion of "distancing" or "polarization" to characterize developmental change. Development, for Werner & Kaplan, occurs in what they call "symbol-situations." Symbol-situations consist of four basic components: an addressor, an addressee, the object of reference or "referent," and the symbolic "vehicle" employed in referential representation. In the course of development, they note, each of these four components undergoes change. Specifically, there is progressive *distancing* between addressor and referent, between addressor and vehicle, between vehicle and referent, and between addressor and addressee.

Ontogenesis, Werner & Kaplan (1963) note, begins with what they call the "primordial sharing situation." They write,

> the primordial sharing situation may be described as one in which the distancing between the components [of the symbol-situation] has hardly begun to form; it is a pre-symbolic situation in which there is little differentiation in the child's experience between himself, the Other (typically the mother) and the referential object. (p. 42)

Gradually, they continue, a specific kind of relationship emerges, that of "sharing" of experiences, which has its clearest early illustration "in the nonreflexive smile of the infant in response to the mother's smile" (p. 42).

Next, the infant comes to share what they call "contemplated objects" with the Other, for example, looking at the same object, event, and so forth. Gradually a higher stage is reached in which the sharing of contemplated objects takes place through *symbols*, particularly through verbal symbols or names. The mark of a symbol, they say, is its representational function; "a symbol represents a referent" (p. 43). The gradual distancing of the four components of the symbol-situation from the initial "primordial" situation enables the child to transcend the immediately given, to extend the universe into the realms of the nonpresent, for example, the conceptual, formal, general, imaginary, hypothetical, and so on.

The characterization of developmental change offered by Piaget and Werner & Kaplan opens up several interesting possibilities for both the educator and the psychological researcher. Specifically, it becomes both theoretically feasible, and perhaps pedagogically imperative, to construct and present tasks and exercises designed to induce *disequilibrium* so as to facilitate, accelerate, and observe the achievement of increased psychological *distance* (development). The psychologist Irving Sigel has developed a research program that draws together the above components of Piaget's and Werner & Kaplan's theories of developmental change. But contrary to Werner & Kaplan (1963), who, he says, see developmental distancing as being *in* the activity of the addressee, Sigel (1993) sees developmental distancing: a) in terms of the cognitive demands placed on the addressee *as a function of* what he calls the "distancing acts" of the addressor, and b) in terms of the mental activities (reequilibrations) set in motion by said distancing acts.

Sigel thus sees developmental change as induced by the repertoire of psychological "distancing activities" employed by those *interacting* with the child, rather than solely in terms of the mental operations *of* the individual child him or herself. Such distancing activities, following Piaget and Werner & Kaplan, are seen to force a degree of cognitive separation from the immediate behavioral environment, from the here and now, from concrete sensori-motor involvement. Distancing activities place cognitive demands on the child to reconstruct events, to employ his/her imagination in dealing with objects, events, and people, to plan and to anticipate future actions, or to attend to the transformation of phenomena from one symbol system to another (Sigel, 1992).

For Sigel, distancing acts lead to what he calls greater "representational competence," because they induce "decentration" which serves to generate differentiation and reorganization of cognitive schemas. As Sigel, Stinson, and Flaugher (1991) note, distancing strategies generate discrepancies between what is *experienced* and what is *expected* by the subject, creating disequilibrium. It is with an eye toward the resolution of this discrepancy that leads the subject to reconsider prior knowledge, reexamine assumptions, try out alternatives, and, in so doing, *restructure* the extant schema. This restructuring process involves *representational thinking* and transforms the subject's initial response.

So for Sigel, developmental change is understood in terms of specific and identifiable gains in "representational competence," and *not* by further acquisition of knowledge/information *or* by the maturation of innate concepts. Within Sigel's paradigm, representational competence is understood as an individual's awareness and understanding that an idea or an object can be represented in various forms and still retain its essential meaning (Sigel, 1970). For example, Sigel (1953, 1970) presented 8- to 11-year-old middle- and low-income children with three-dimensional objects and pictures of those objects. Instructions were given to classify the members of each set any way that the subject wished. Sigel found that there was no significant discrepancy in the way middle-class children grouped either pictures or objects. The low-income children, on the other hand, had no difficulty in grouping the three-dimensional objects, but they *did* have significant difficulty grouping the pictures. Sigel concludes that the low-income children could not understand that a picture is a *representation* of an object, and hence "symbolically" shares its meaning.

Sigel identifies some 40 distancing strategies that are organized into three hierarchical levels defined in terms of the complexity of cognitive demands inherent in the act. *Level 1* distancing strategies make mental demands for associations, visual observations, or routinized information; for example, "What is the name of this . . . ?" or "This is a boat." Minimal demands are placed on the child to separate him/herself from the ongoing present. *Level 2* distancing strategies make demands to classify and/or to relate disparate events; for example, "Classify these objects" or "How are these shapes like these shapes?" Here, cognitive demands force a transcendence of the immediate environment, but visual objects still form the basis for the mental operations to be performed. *Level 3* distancing strategies make demands upon the subject to engage in causal inferences, to predict outcomes, to employ hypothetical reasoning, to transform from one symbolic medium to another; for example, "Can you show me some different ways to illustrate the concept of . . . ?" or "What would happen if . . . ?" Such strategies are designed to place the subject in a position of maximum distance from his/her extant schemes so as to provide the opportunity for reorganization. In fact, general hypothesis guiding the distancing model of psychological development is that the *frequency* of distancing acts that a child experiences will influence the developing level of representational competence, and the *developmental level* of those distancing experiences will account, to a significant degree, for the variation in representational competencies a child will acquire (Sigel, 1993, p. 146).

In the above mentioned example of picture-object confusion, Sigel (1953, 1970) reasons that certain high-level distancing acts employed by parents and teachers serve to facilitate the child's ability to conserve meaning when moving from one symbolic medium to another. In other words, specific interventions can lead to marked improvements in representational competence and the development of psychological distance. From my own research, I had 100 children between 5 and 10 years of age draw the inside of the body on a blank body outline and respond to a 10-item biological knowledge questionnaire. Participants were then randomly assigned to one of five experimental conditions in which they were asked to respond to questions designed to induce developmental change in biological knowledge. These strategies differed in terms of the cognitive demands placed on the participant to answer the question (Sigel, 1993). Specifically, there was a low-level distancing condition, a medium-level distancing condition, a high-level distancing condition, an analogy condition, and a control condition which had equal numbers of items from each of the above mentioned four levels of distancing strategies, but questions pertained to an entirely different domain, household items. Post-tests were administered to assess advances over initial conceptions. High-level distancing strategies and analogies had a significant effect on pre- and post-test scores for 5- to 7-year-olds on drawings and questionnaires, and for 8- to 10-year-olds on drawings. Further, these strategies significantly reduced the discrepancy between scores on initial drawings and questionnaires for 5- to 7-year-olds, indicating improvement in representational competence. Sigel's hypotheses have been confirmed in numerous other studies.

To conclude, I argue that the distancing strategy is an excellent example of a technique that incorporates the above mentioned parameters for an ethically inspired psychology. In Sigel's work, we see the notions of "interiority" reflected in the Rousseau-Dewey developmental tradition, specifically the idea that development is not simply a matter of socialization, but that the child has important contributions to make to his or her own development. At the same time, Sigel integrates important insights from the Lockean tradition with his idea that the environment is the catalyst for development, but *not* its source or cause. Further, we noted that an ethically inspired psychology would involve us in the difficult project of *loving and respecting* others. The distancing strategy, in this sense, does not seek to *impose* change on the child from without, but attempts to *facilitate* the child's growth (love) by providing verbal catalysts that will impel the child to change on his or her own (respect). It is my sincere hope that my vision conjured in this chapter of a more intimate union between psychology and ethics has been persuasive and would lead others to propose additional directions for an ethically inspired psychology.

REFERENCES

Aquinas, T. (1981). *Summa theologica.* Westminster, MD: Christian Classics. (Original work published 1268)

Bloom, A. (1987). *The closing of the American mind*. New York: Simon & Schuster.

Browning, D. (1987). *Religious ethics and pastoral care.* Philadelphia: Fortress Press.

Crain, W. C. (1985). *Theories of development: Concepts and applications.* Englewood Cliffs, NJ: Prentice-Hall.

Dewey, J. (1916). *Democracy and education.* Toronto: Collier-MacMillan.

Dewey, J. (1938). *Experience and education.* New York: Collier Books.

Dewey, J., & Dewey, E. (1915). *Schools of to-morrow.* New York: E. P. Dutton.

Genovese, V. (1987). *In pursuit of love: Catholic morality and human sexuality.* Wilmington, DE: Michael Glazier.

Guthrie, S. (1975). *History of Greek philosophy: Plato the man and his dialogues.* Oxford, England: Clarendon Press.

Hobbes, T. (1840). Human nature. In W. Molesworth (Ed.), *The English works of Thomas Hobbes* (pp. 134–307). London: John Bohn. (Original work published 1650)

Jung, C. G. (1933). *Modern man in search of a soul.* New York: Harcourt Brace Jovanovich.

Lavine, T. Z. (1984). *From Socrates to Sartre: The philosophic quest.* New York: Bantam Books.

Locke, J. (1965). *An essay concerning human understanding* (Vol. 1). In J. W. Yolton, Ed., *Everyman's Library.* London: J. M. Dent & Sons. (Original work published 1690)

Marx, K. (1977). *Capital* (B. Fowles, Trans.). New York: Vintage Books. (Original work published 1859)

Maslow, A. H. (1970). *Motivation and personality.* New York: Harper & Row.

Meyeroff, M. (1971). *On caring.* New York: Harper Perennial.

Miller, A. (1981). *Drama of the gifted child* (R. Ward, Trans.). New York: Basic Books.

Piaget, J. (1985). *The equilibration of cognitive structures: The central problem of intellectual development.* Chicago: University of Chicago Press.

Prilleltensky, I. (1997). Values, assumptions, and practices: Assessing the moral implications of psychological discourse and action. *American Psychologist, 52*(5), 517–535.

Rousseau, J-J. (1993). *Emile* (B. Foxley, Trans.). Rutland, VT: Charles E. Tuttle. (Original work published 1762).

Sigel, I. E. (1953). Developmental trends in the abstraction ability of children. *Child Development, 24*(2), 131–144.

Sigel, I. E. (1970). The distance hypothesis: A causal hypothesis for the acquisition of representational thought. In M.R. Jones (Ed.), *Miami Symposium on the Prediction of Behavior, 1968: Effect of early experience* (pp. 99–118). Coral Gables, FL: University of Miami Press.

Sigel, I. E. (1992). The belief-behavior connection: A resolvable dilemma? In I. E. Sigel, A.V. McGillicuddy-DeLisi, & J. Goodnow (Eds.), *Parental belief systems: The psychological consequences for children* (pp. 433–456). Hillsdale, NJ: Lawrence Erlbaum.

Sigel, I. E. (1993). The centrality of a distancing model for the development of representational competence. In R. Cocking & A. Renninger (Eds.), *The development and meaning of psychological distance.* Hillsdale, N.J.: Lawrence Erlbaum.

Sigel, I. E., Stinson, E., & Flaugher, J. (1991). Socialization of representational competence in the family: The distancing paradigm. In L. Okagaki & R. J. Sternberg (Eds.), *Directors of development: Influences on the development of children's thinking* (pp. 121–144). Hillsdale, N.J.: Lawrence Erlbaum.

Skinner, B. F. (1972). *Beyond freedom and dignity.* New York: Bantam Books-Vintage Books.

Skinner, B. F. (1976). *Walden Two.* New York: Macmillan.

Tillich, P. (1957). *Dynamics of faith.* New York: Harper Torchbooks.

Toulmin, S. (1987). *Cosmopolis: The hidden agenda of modernity.* Chicago: University of Chicago Press.

Vico, G. (1968). *The new science of Giambattista Vico.* (T. G. Bergin & M. H. Fisch, Trans.). Ithaca, NY: Cornell University Press. (Original work published 1744)

Watson, J. B. (1913). Psychology as the behaviorist views it. *Psychological Review, 23,* 158–177.

Weinreb, L. L. (1987). *Natural law and justice.* Cambridge: Harvard University Press.

Werner, H. (1948). *Comparative psychology of mental development.* New York: International Universities Press.

Werner, H., & Kaplan, B. (1963). *Symbol formation.* Hillsdale, NJ: Lawrence Erlbaum.

11

INTERPRETING EVERYDAY BEHAVIOR USING THE LEARNING TO LEARN CYCLE AS A MEANS TO PURSUE INDIVIDUAL INTELLECTUAL ENDS

Roger Bibace
Clark University and
University of Massachusetts Medical School

Nicholas H. Apostoleris
Clark University

Ximena Soto
Clark University

Patricia Quinn
Clark University

ABSTRACT

A strategy for structuring the learning experiences of students in an advanced undergraduate seminar is presented which facilitates the understanding of personally relevant, complex phenomena. In the process of pursuing increased understanding of the topic of interest, students are asked to examine both the universals related to that topic and a particular exemplar of the topic. Students are provided with strategies for interpreting their intellectual and ethical orientations and are asked to critique the Learning to Learn Cycle and evaluate their own progress in understanding their chosen topic. Student evaluations show that, on a Likert scale of 1–5, the mean score of overall favorableness toward the cycle was $M = 4.03$, $SD = 0.73$, $N = 37$.

The Learning to Learn Cycle has been developed over several years at Clark University as a strategy in teaching psychology. The Learning to Learn Cycle is not a learning theory as such, but rather is an approach to the acquisition of personally relevant and enriching knowledge, a strategy for self-actualization through intellectual enrichment. The goal of the approach is to empower the student with the ability to pursue any area of knowledge that the student finds to be of interest.

The Learning to Learn Cycle integrates some formal features of learning, the cycle of activities to be articulated below, with the particular interests of each and every student. Thus the student is asked to examine both the universals of the area and a particular exemplar of the area. The how of learning is generalizable from the suggested cycle of activities. The what of learning, the topic or content, is selected by the student. Thus, the Learning to Learn Cycle deals with both the diversity of individual interests that students bring to a seminar and the expertise of the teacher in helping them to learn about something that they have selected as a focus for the entire semester. In turn, such an approach draws on the student's motivation and signals a different relationship in learner–teacher interactions.

THE DIALECTIC BETWEEN ACTION AND THOUGHT

Many developmentalists (e.g., Piaget, 1967 and Werner, 1948) and some cognitive scientists assume that knowledge develops from action to thought; from reflexivity to reflection. Thus, for Werner and Kaplan (1963), there is a "shift in function" from "objects-of-action" to "objects of contemplation." Or as Lakoff (1987), an experiential realist, argues:

> Thought is embodied, that is, the structures used to put together our conceptual systems grow out of bodily experience and make sense in terms of it; moreover, the core of our conceptual systems is directly grounded in perception, body movement, and experience of a physical and social character. (p. xiv)

For the seminar, the dialectic between thought and action is assured through the following sequences:

I. Beginnings: Selection of the Phenomenon to be Interpreted
II. Articulating the Universals[1] Relevant to the Phenomenon to be Interpreted
III. Description and Interpretation of a Particular Instance of the Phenomenon

IV. Interpreting the Interpreter
V. Endings and New Beginnings for Further Understanding of the Phenomenon to be Interpreted

The nature of these sections will now be explicated, and this is followed by our suggestions for implementing the cycle within contexts of an advanced-level college seminar.

STEPS ALONG THE WAY

Beginnings

Students are admitted to the course only if they can demonstrate to the instructor that they are personally intrigued by a relevant topic. Students' initial interest must be rooted in their everyday world of action; they should have experienced aspects of the topic in their everyday world. For instance, a student who was an avid cyclist chose to study bicycling as an aspect of sport psychology. It is this initial interest in a phenomenon grounded in the world of action that is to be transformed into an "object of contemplation" by reviews of pertinent literatures. This requirement ensures that the interest is not a superficial one.

This beginnings section is comprised of the student's personal account of the reasons for the interest in the topic as well as a statement of the student's current understanding of the topic. The aim is to clarify the student's preliminary understanding of the topic and to begin the process of relating the self to the learning process. An additional benefit is that it provides students with their own baseline upon which to reflect as the learning cycle continues.

Exploring the Universals of the Topic

Whereas in the Beginnings section the student focuses on the self, a dialectic between self and other develops in the second step of the cycle. This second step, the exploration of the Universals, asks the student to review many literatures, including historical, biological, psychological, sociocultural, and anthropological. The objective is not mere breadth, but rather a perspectivism to make the student aware of how (both in terms of subject and method of inquiry) different experts interpret the same phenomenon or topic. Flexibility is suggested here, in that the student's topic may lend itself to a somewhat different set of literatures to be reviewed. The personal experience becomes the object of reflection.

In addition to perspectivism, the review of the literatures serves as an opportunity for the student to engage in dialogue with the "generalized other" (Mead, 1934), namely the writings of experts in the field of choice. Thus it can be seen as a conversation between one's self and the "generalized other," between one's personal concrete experiences and the abstract, conceptual characterizations of the phenomenon by experts from various disciplines. Biologists, psychologists, sociologists, anthropologists, historians, and other experts are, in effect, making claims for the student's attention. These experts are claiming that their theories "show" something about an aspect of the topic. The student is encouraged to make an informed but personal judgment regarding the relative merits and applicability of the competing claims coming from the diverse perspectives and argue for a reasoned, favored synthesis of approaches based on the student's understanding of both self (through, in part, the Interpreting the Interpreter section) and other (through the multiple reviews of the literatures). In this way the many literatures, that is, the many "generalized others," are funneled to one integrated perspective, as articulated by the learner (self).

A relationship between the learner and a concrete, "personalized other" is encouraged by asking each student to choose a partner with whom they will consult throughout the course of the seminar. Students are encouraged to bring their partner to meetings with the teacher or the teaching assistant, use the partner to evaluate their project critically, and collaborate on projects such as role-playing sketches with the partner. Some flexibility is needed in this partnership approach so that students without preexisting relationships with other students in the class are not placed in awkward and disadvantaged situations.

An additional means by which a broadening of perspectives on the topic is achieved is through a conceptual restructuring via the use of Burke's Pentad (Burke, 1962). Through the use of this flexible tool, the topic is viewed not through the lens of reviews of different literatures, but rather by re-framing aspects of the topic in terms of the Act, the Agent, the Scene, the Means, and the Ends.

The rationale for the inclusion of a Burkean analysis is threefold. First, such an analysis emphasizes the *active* role of the student in the restructuring of the reviews of the literature. Second, the Pentad is a useful tool in characterizing the assumptions that underlie the literatures reviewed. Does an author, for instance, exclusively stress the "ends" or purposes of an Agent? Does such an author emphasize the scene or the means that the Agent relies on in attaining the goal? Class exercises focus on discussions aimed at analyzing any interpretation of behavior through the lens of Burke's Pentad. Third, such a restructuring ideally leads to a critical summary that highlights areas emphasized by the author; the critique would suggest potentially different emphases and more advantageous analyses. While the Pentad has been utilized in the Universals section of several very successful student papers, it forms the dominant tool for analysis of the next phase of the cycle, the Description and Interpretation of a Particular Instance of the Phenomenon, referred to as the Particular Section.

Investigating the Particular

Many undergraduates assume that psychology addresses the topics with which the students are most familiar; that the courses they take will help them to interpret and understand their own or other people's experiences. As is widely known, most introductory courses in psychology explicitly reject such assumptions as naïve. Rather, many psychologists attempt to socialize and induct an undergraduate into our discipline by disabusing them of such "expectations." At best, many textbooks illustrate and concretize concepts and ideas through use of an example. In such instances, the path is from the abstract ideas being discussed to the concrete example.

What is lacking, however, is the converse. That is, relating the concrete example and experiences of everyday life to the relevant abstractions (the concepts, theories, and relevant empirical findings). It is this feature, the interpretation of everyday behaviors through the multiple perspectives of theories, concepts, and findings in the human sciences, that is central to the seminar. Other courses cover theories and research on particular topics. Laboratories deal with the interpretation of experimental results. But undergraduate curricula rarely include seminars that begin with personal concrete experiences, review literatures relevant to such experiences, and then require students to analyze a topic systematically by relying on the concepts and findings from the review.

The Particular section, the third step in the dialectic, requires the student to utilize the concepts and empirical findings they have summarized from the literature to interpret a particular instance of the phenomenon they have selected. That is, the dialectic here is between concepts initiated by others (the literatures) and the utilization of the concepts by the student. The requirement that the student interpret a particular example of the phenomenon has several advantages. The student (and teacher) become aware of the "applicability" of some concepts compared to others, of the relevance of various empirical findings to understand a specific instance or case. In common parlance, the student is required to "use psychology" by "interpreting" something that is of interest to the student.

The interpretation of the particular facilitates the student's critique of the experts. Here, after all, is a concrete example of the phenomenon as chosen by the student. Yet none of the theories may address explicitly the specific aspect of the phenomenon of interest to the student. As opposed to the Universals which emphasize interpretations independent of context, the Particular section tends to result in interpretations that are substantially dependent on context. It is, in large measure, this dialogical tension between the Universals and Particulars that is key to the endeavor, and the disequilibrium thus created can be seen as driving the cycle. Conceptually, this assumption is congruent with Piagetian conceptions of how the disequilibrium between Assimilation and Accommodation leads to new Adaptations. The acquisition of knowledge propels the cycle forward, resulting in a form perhaps best understood as spiral in nature (Werner & Kaplan, 1963).

Tools for interpreting the particular

The Particular section looks at an instance of the topic. The instance need not be the most representative example of the topic, but it should in some way be able to serve as a useful exemplar. The instance should be carefully described and then analyzed in light of the Perspectives used in the Universals section, but with a special emphasis on the use of Burke's Pentad, a tool that serves to provide a multidimensional, macroscopic, contextual grounding to the Particular so that it can, in essence, be located within the Universals of the topic. Appropriate use of the Pentad allows for an adequate description of the specific instance. That is, the Particular section should include a description of the Act, the Agent, the Scene, the Means, and the Ends as they pertain to the specific instance of the topic being studied.

Assessment devices based on the McMaster Model of Family Functioning (MMFF) have been found to be of great value in the microanalysis of families and other small, interpersonally connected groups (Epstein, Bishop, & Baldwin, 1982). The MMFF was chosen because it embeds the interpretation of the individual in a social context, while retaining the individual as a crucially important level of analysis. This "contextualist" world view is deemed advantageous by the authors to counteract the tendency in psychology to focus on processes within individuals (e.g., cognitive processes). In contrast, the McMaster model requires the student to consider *how* the same issue or topic may be viewed differently from the diverse perspectives of family members. We also consider the cross-culturally validated psychometric properties of the McMaster model instruments (Epstein, Bishop, & Baldwin, 1982) to be valuable in educating the undergraduates in the selection of *means* to achieve desired interpretive ends.

Interpreting the Interpreter

The dialectic is furthered with the fourth step in the process when students are asked to impersonalize themselves. Typically the students (who are juniors and seniors) have had at minimum a laboratory course, a statistics course, and a course on quantitative and qualitative research methods in psychology. They are thus familiar with the term "bias" and the many sources of bias in designing an experiment or research project. Here, however, they are asked to Interpret the Interpreter. Or more informally, they are asked to consider: "Where are *you* coming from with respect to your interpretations?" The paradoxical approach to the interpreter is, essentially, to consider the person impersonally. That is, to interpret themselves through lenses that focus on epistemic issues in psychology, on persistent value orientations in our society, and on their preferred world hypotheses.

Tools for interpreting the interpreter

The Interpreting the Interpreter section encourages students to understand better their analyses by evaluating what they themselves bring to the process. This is attempted by including general demographic information and a general description of the sociocultural characteristics of the student in the analysis along with the results of three specific measures intended to suggest the student's intellectual orientation. The interpreter's vision, constrained or unconstrained, is evaluated based on Thomas Sowell's *A Conflict of Visions* (Sowell, 1987), the student's epistemic differential is examined through a questionnaire based on the work of Kimble (1984), and the student's world hypotheses are evaluated based on the works of Pepper (1942) and Laird (1976).

Thomas Sowell's *A Conflict of Visions* is used as a required text and forms the basis of one of the self-assessment questionnaires because it encourages the student to grapple with fundamental issues of the nature of humanity and the assumptions that underlie a wide range of interpersonal and political conflicts. In exploring the nature of these perennial conflicts, Sowell states that:

> Behind the episodic eruptions of specific political and social controversies is a pattern of beliefs about the world, about man, and about causation. These implicit assumptions or visions repeatedly divide controversialists at all intellectual levels, on a wide spectrum of issues, and across the boundaries of the law, the economy, the polity, and the society, as well as across international boundaries. Though these controversies often become emotional, the opposing views tend to cluster, not around an emotion, but around the logic of a vision. Each vision tends to generate conclusions which are the logical consequences of its assumptions. That is why there are such repeated conflicts of visions in such a range of otherwise unrelated issues. (Sowell, 1987, p. 224)

By studying the underlying rationales for conflicting visions, the student is encouraged to use this knowledge to understand better the viewpoints of others with different underlying visions.[2]

Gregory Kimble's epistemic differential research provides the basis for the second instrument used by students in the Interpreting the Interpreter section. Kimble (1984) posits and documents the existence of two distinct cultures within psychology: the scientific and the humanistic. These cultures are seen as based on competing, conflicting, and unreconciled value systems with a splintered field of psychology as the result. Six key dimensions that illustrate the conflicting values of scientific and humanistic psychologists are tapped in the Epistemic Differential questionnaire. These dimensions are:

1. scholarly values (scientific versus humanism);
2. lawfulness of behavior (determinism versus indeterminism);
3. sources of knowledge (observation versus intuition);
4. favored setting (laboratory versus field or case study);
5. generality of laws (nomothetic versus idiographic);
6. appropriate levels of analysis (elementism versus holism).

(Kimble, 1984, p. 833)

The rationale for including this questionnaire is clear: the advanced undergraduate is being asked to begin to think about issues that are hotly debated in the field with an eye toward understanding how the interpreter's values along these key dimensions will influence the analysis of the student's chosen topic.

A questionnaire developed by Laird (1976) and based on the work of Pepper (1942) is included. Pepper posited four main world hypotheses that were "relatively adequate" (p. xii). These are Formism, Mechanism, Contextualism, and Organicism. They share the characteristic that "every consideration is relevant to a world hypothesis and no facts lie outside it" (p. 1). The impact of one's world hypothesis is profound and pervasive. Conflicting world hypotheses can lead to feelings of impatience, disrespect, or incomprehension, yet often the nature of one's world hypothesis is obfuscated by the details of this or that issue or argument:

> It is just because world hypotheses are so intimate and pervasive that we do not easily look at them from a distance, so to speak, or as if we saw them in a mirror. . . . World hypotheses are likely to be studied as creeds to be accepted or rejected, or as expressions of highly individual personalities, or as expressions of epochs, or as objects of historical scholarship to be traced to their cultural sources. (p. 2)

The questionnaire provides a clear method for the student to position himself or herself in terms of the world hypotheses, and the student is encouraged to frame interpersonal or theoretical conflicts with the world hypotheses of the protagonists in mind.

These tools are intended to provide an opportunity for the student both to gain insight and to come to know intimately the limitations of such assessment techniques. Students are encouraged to evaluate their "scores" on these measures from the vantage point of a knowledgeable insider who can see in which ways their own complexities and subtleties might not have been adequately captured by the instruments.

The reflectivity of the self-interpretation seeks contrasts between the initial and current accounts of the phenomenon. Microgenetic aspects of Werner's (1957) orthogenetic principle are used to understand better the developmental changes in the interpreter's understanding of the phenomenon, helping to explain differences in the "then" and "now" from the learner's experiential standpoint.

Endings and New Beginnings

The fifth step in the process, Endings and New Beginnings is intended to give the student the opportunity to reflect on his or her initial learning cycle leading to the beginning of a new cycle. The student is also encouraged to articulate his or her own conceptual schema or variation of the Learning to Learn Cycle in contrast to the instructor's choices. Where appropriate, students might be encouraged to begin designing an empirical study to analyze further their chosen phenomenon. In this final phase the cyclic nature of the process is emphasized and explored.

OSCILLATION BETWEEN ACCOMMODATION AND ASSIMILATION FOR LEARNERS AND TEACHERS: THE FUNCTIONING OF THE SEMINAR

In the cycle, the teacher begins by accommodating to the student's interest in a particular topic or phenomenon. Questions about this topic lead to discussions that can stimulate both the teacher and the student—teachers because they may not know much about an activity, students because the teachers' questions further stimulate the curiosity of the student which is assumed to be the driving force of the cycle.

More generally, the student assimilates and accommodates to the Learning to Learn Cycle of activities and the cyclical relationships of these activities to one another. The teacher, by accommodating and assimilating to the student's interests, learns to modify the cycle of activities or to introduce novel activities or options for students. The teacher will surely be stimulated to learn about sociocultural issues. For instance, a Chinese student wrote about family structure in China. Two Japanese students wrote about gender issues in Japan. Similarly, issues that are quite ordinary yet not usually pursued in depth by at least some teachers in psychology can be stimulating for the instructors. Humor, lying, and altruistic/philanthropic behaviors were all topics chosen by students about which the teachers' knowledge was limited to superficial acquaintance.

In our experience, the students appreciate their interests being taken seriously. They appreciate having the teacher follow their experiential leads. The Learning to Learn Cycle is a means to pursue their own interests. The objective is to get students to internalize the Learning to Learn Cycle, to make it their own, so that they can pursue any (or most) topics that interest them in the future.

The diversity of the topics chosen by any group of students in the seminar in a given semester is also evidence of the generalizability of the Learning to Learn Cycle. The seminar during class time devotes time to articulating each student's area of interest from the multiple perspectives mentioned above (historical, biological, psychological, sociocultural, and so on). Much effort is directed toward providing the student with a working knowledge of the tools of analysis that are suggested for use throughout the cycle. The Pentad and the McMaster Model of Family Functioning mentioned above have been shown to be especially worthy of extensive discussion and explication.

We have found in successive semesters that students need structure for interpreting behavior. It is the hope of the authors that the Learning to Learn Cycle will provide this structure to the learner without imposing constraints that can stifle a productive, atypical learning style used by individual students.

STUDENT FEEDBACK

Student evaluations of the Learning to Learn Cycle were taken from three sources. First, a questionnaire was developed that addressed the following: overall favorableness toward the Learning to Learn Cycle, favorableness toward specific aspects of the cycle and course, and mention of specific problem areas. This questionnaire was administered to the most recent group of students ($N = 10$). Second, copies of the "Endings and New Beginnings" sections of all papers written in the prior three years for this seminar were collected, rendered anonymous, and coded by two undergraduates, who had previously taken the seminar. Third, undergraduates who used the Learning to Learn Cycle in creative and productive ways were asked for their critical comments regarding their own experiences using and helping others to use the cycle.

For the coded sections, interrater reliability for the overall favorableness rating was $r = 0.70$. Including all coded sections and questionnaires, overall favorableness toward the Learning to Learn Cycle was $M = 4.03$ (on a Likert 1–5 scale, with 1 = very unfavorable, 3 = neutral, 5 = very favorable), $N = 37$, $SD = 0.73$. Results for the evaluations of specific aspects of the cycle are found in Table 11.1. All of these results are based on a three-point Likert scale with a rating of "3" signifying the most positive response.

In addition to the overall favorableness rating and the ratings of the different aspects of the cycle, three additional statements were included in the questionnaire

TABLE 11.1.
Student Favorableness Ratings

Aspects of the Cycle	M (1-3)	SD	N
Use of Perspectivism	2.87	0.39	31
Universals/Particular Format	2.53	0.61	33
Burkean Pentad	2.66	0.52	27
McMaster Model of Family Functioning	2.60	0.61	24
Sequence of Activities	2.35	0.76	26
Interpreting the Interpreter	2.47	0.82	22
World Hypotheses Questionnaire	2.17	0.86	15
Epistemic Differential Questionnaire	2.29	0.70	14
Sowell's *Conflict of Visions* Questionnaire	2.06	0.70	16
Use of Role Plays	2.80	0.40	15
Means of Evaluation	2.47	0.75	17

and coded from the papers. These assessed whether students disagreed (scored a 1), were neutral (2), or agreed (3) with the following:

1. The student found using the cycle to be personally fulfilling;
2. The student was at first unfavorable toward the cycle and then became more favorable later in the process;
3. The student had insufficient time to pursue the chosen topic adequately.

Ratings indicated that students did tend to find the process personally fulfilling ($M = 2.62$, $SD = 0.56$, $N = 37$) and agreed that they were more favorable toward the cycle as they proceeded in their research ($M = 2.45$, $SD = 0.60$, $N = 37$). Students also tended to agree that there was not enough time to work properly through the cycle in a one-semester seminar ($M = 2.12$, $SD = 0.70$, $N = 37$).

Discussion of the Student Evaluations

In addition to the students' high level of overall favorableness toward using the cycle, several other findings are of interest. The use of multiple perspectives in the investigation was especially favored by the students; it seems as if this is one of the most widely accessible and least confusing aspects of the cycle. Students also strongly endorsed the Universals/Particular dialogical format. For example, one student reported that

> The exercise of interpreting a particular example of the phenomenon allow one to apply what was learned in the literature review to a more specific occasion or situation. An essential feature of the cycle is that following the interpretation of the particular, one may still change and expand upon the Universals section as one's thinking and views about the phenomenon changes.

Burke's Pentad and the McMaster Model of Family Functioning were also highly rated. As one student commented,

> From working with (the Pentad and McMaster Model), I have taught myself the necessary aspects to consider before making an interpretation of a particular behavior. The skills I have acquired have not only served an academic purpose, but have proven helpful in terms of internships as well as everyday life situations. In a sense, I have been able to make sense out of disturbing or chaotic situations which in the past would have appeared insurmountable.

So, for the investigations of the Universals and the Particular, both the task and the tools (the Pentad and the McMaster Model) were viewed favorably by the students.

This is in contrast to the evaluations of the Interpreting the Interpreter section. While the task was rated relatively favorably, the tools used to aid the interpretation were not rated very favorably (World Hypotheses, Sowell's *Conflict of Vision*

(1987), and Epistemic Differential questionnaires). The students seem to like the general idea of the section but the means are problematic. As articulated by one student,

> At times, they indeed seemed too structured. Once you get wrapped up in the whole learning cycle it is hard to remember that these tests only define PARTS of us and these tools are good to a certain extent. There is life outside this that is not taken into consideration. It was hard to remember that we were learning SOMETHING about ourselves, not our whole selves although that little piece that we learn can open many new doors.

That is, the intention to impersonalize the interpreter may preclude him or her from focusing on individual life experiences which may be highly relevant to achieving a holistic understanding of self as interpreter. Issues of professor/student boundaries are of concern here, however, and our approach has been to dissuade students strongly from revealing details of their personal lives or histories.

Some problems were indicated with the sequence of activities in the cycle. Some students prefer to approach the Universals and the Particular simultaneously, while others prefer sequential investigations. This is a matter that may be best left up to the discretion of the learner. The magnitude of the project and the seemingly daunting complexity of the chosen topic may be responsible for the phenomenon of increasing favorableness toward the cycle the further along the student proceeds. Students (and teachers) may view this information as encouragement to work through the early difficulties with the knowledge that others have found such effort worthwhile. Illustrating the value of the effort, one student observed that

> After making multiple revisions of the particular and the universals, the individual must come to a point in which he or she is satisfied with the interpretation and the answers which have come from the work. It is at this established ending point that one realizes the true cyclical nature of learning. One finds that there may indeed be satisfactory explanations for behaviors and answers to questions but new questions are a natural result of the learning process. The final lesson learned is that learning about any behavior has no definite end, there are only ending points that one can set for oneself.

The theme of reflectivity was prominent in several comments: "The option to develop, reinterpret, and change one's views . . . is a vital characteristic of the . . . Cycle."

> Reflecting back to my original thoughts about a particular instance of a behavior after examining the universals and making a revised interpretation has been a means for me to generate new thoughts and questions. Just as one does not stop learning after the cessation of a formal education, one never learns all there is to know about a particular phenomenon. There are always questions to be generated which turn the learning process into an exciting, thought provoking cycle.

In fact, for some students, a one-semester seminar did not provide the necessary time to work adequately with the cycle, and they have taken an internship or a research practicum which allowed for more of a focus on the Particular.

ON SOME OF THE CHALLENGES

While it is intended that students are not only exposed to a variety of sources of information, a broadening experience, but that they also deal critically with the conflicts and contradictions revealed, this often does not occur. Conflicting views are often reported rather than critically analyzed. It could be that a necessary step in the learning process is the acquisition of sufficient breadth of experiences, which then may or may not result in integration. Integration itself will vary in terms of its comprehensiveness.

The task of encouraging the interpreting of the interpreter cuts at the divide between Kimble's (1984) two cultures of psychology. Students are asked to undertake the sometimes uncomfortable task of impersonalizing themselves. This task is designed to give students a better understanding of the relationship between the self and one's views, between the self and the stance one takes toward the world. Understanding the perennially divisive issues between the two cultures of psychology impersonally has helped many students locate themselves personally. That is, they have been able to locate their own personal stance with respect to the seven divisive issues identified by Kimble.

The assigning of grades to the work of students using the cycle is highly problematic. It counteracts all attempts to encourage an intrinsically motivated learning experience (Bruner, 1962; Deci, 1980). Since the student knows that graduate schools will indeed be looking at the letter grade to assess how the student "did" in this seminar, the degree to which the student's ends can be internally rather than externally oriented is limited. Attempts made to combat grade anxiety have included adhering to the distinction between formative and summative evaluations. Formative evaluations are emphasized by the providing of detailed, ungraded comments as each section of the project is completed; only after the "final" version of the project is evaluated is a traditional grade assigned. Nevertheless, the deleterious effects of the assignment of a final grade has yet to be fully overcome. Students have been offered the choice of taking the seminar on a credit or no-credit basis, but not a single student in our competitive educational environment has exercised this option. We are seeking ways in which to deemphasize the negative effects of the grades which seem so difficult to do without.

NOTES

[1] By "Universals" we refer to the theories, concepts, and generalizations that scholars in different disciplines espouse.

[2] There has been a frequent misapplication of Sowell's analysis on the part of students by which the constrained vision is understood as "bad" or "jaded" while the unconstrained vision is seen as the preferred approach.

REFERENCES

Bruner, J. (1962). *On knowing: Essays for the left hand.* Cambridge: Harvard University Press.

Burke, K. (1962). *A grammar of motives and a rhetoric of motives.* Toronto: Nelson, Foster, and Scott.

Deci, E. (1980). *Intrinsic motivation.* New York: Plenum Press.

Epstein, N. B., Bishop, D. S., & Baldwin, L. M. (1982). McMaster Model of Family Functioning: A view of the normal family. In F. Walsh (Ed.), *Normal family processes* (pp. 115–141). New York: Guilford Press.

Kimble, G. A. (1984). Psychology's two cultures. *American Psychologist, 39,* 833–839.

Laird, J. (1976, October). *World hypotheses.* Paper presented at the New England Social Psychological Association annual meeting, Hanover, NH.

Lakoff, G. (1987). *Women, fire, and dangerous things.* Chicago: University of Chicago Press.

Mead, G. H. (1934). *Mind, self & society from the standpoint of a social behaviorist.* Chicago: University of Chicago Press.

Pepper, S. C. (1942). *World hypotheses: A study in evidence.* Berkeley, CA: University of California Press.

Piaget, J. (1967). *The child's conception of the world.* London: Routledge & Kegan Paul.

Sowell, T. (1987). *A conflict of visions: Ideological origins of political struggles.* New York: William Morrow.

Werner, H. (1948). *Comparative psychology of mental development.* New York: International Universities Press.

Werner, H. (1957). The concept of development from a comparative and organismic point of view. In D. B. Harris (Ed.), *The concept of development: An issue in the study of human behavior* (pp. 125–148). Minneapolis: University of Minnesota Press.

Werner, H., & Kaplan, B. (1963). *Symbol formation.* New York: Wiley.

12

STUDENTS AS PARTNERS*

Barbara Noel Dowds
Regis College and
University of Massachusetts Medical School

ABSTRACT

This chapter describes three approaches toward achieving a partnership between undergraduate faculty and students. The first section describes a study that investigated nursing students' philosophical assumptions in the classroom. The second focuses on independent studies as a way to build partnerships. The third describes the use of interdisciplinary work as a means toward achieving more of a partnership between faculty and students.

Traditionally, faculty at many undergraduate institutions are seen as the "experts" who impart their knowledge to students, the "novices." Within this paradigm, teachers proceed from their own philosophical assumptions. There tends to be a unidirectional (teacher to student) rather than a bidirectional flow of information, questions, and evaluations of responses. This approach does not necessarily encourage "active learning." Further, it may decrease intrinsic motivation rather than encourage it. However, as the zeitgeist has begun to change, some faculty and students are pursuing a partnership approach to teaching and learning, which, though not a relationship between equals, explicitly recognizes both that the student is important in the teaching/learning process and that teaching and learning are bidirectional. This approach acknowledges that students' own philosophical as-

*I thank Barbara Marcel for her comments on an earlier draft of this chapter. Portions of this chapter are adapted from Dowds & Marcel, 1998, and Dowds, 1998.

sumptions are important. It has the potential for a bidirectional flow of information, with teachers learning from (and with) students as well as students learning from teachers. It also has the potential to encourage students to be more proactive and more engaged in the process of learning. Further, it may increase students' intrinsic motivation by building on their own interests.

UNDERSTANDING STUDENTS' PHILOSOPHICAL ASSUMPTIONS: A BASIS FOR WORKING TOWARD PARTNERSHIPS

The study (Dowds & Marcel, 1998) of nursing students' philosophical assumptions arose from the experience of teaching undergraduate nursing students. It seemed that many of them found psychology an intriguing but, at least initially, challenging course that called into question their fundamental assumptions. They were puzzled and frustrated by the ambiguity inherent in the multiple, and often conflicting, theoretical models used to describe and explain behavior. As nursing students, they were more used to clear-cut, definitive answers and wanted the same from psychology. Yet psychology can answer relatively few questions in a definitive manner. In fact, there is often disagreement within the discipline about what questions to pose and what research methodologies to use. We reasoned that some of the nursing students' initial frustration was due to a mismatch of implicit philosophies. Most students socialized in western traditions of thought are more familiar and comfortable with a conclusive, linear understanding of events. However, at least some approaches to teaching psychology derive from a more provisional and relational basis for understanding events.

According to the philosopher Stephen Pepper (1942/1970), there are four world hypotheses, or four "relatively adequate" (p. 141) ways of understanding events. Each of these world views has its strengths and weaknesses, and none is seen as more adequate than the others. Yet adherents of a particular world view are most comfortable with that world view's assumptions. One of these world views, "mechanism," involves understanding in terms of cause-and-effect relations. Much of modern health care is based on this approach. For example, if someone has a sore throat, the question is what caused the sore throat. The underlying assumption is that once the cause of the symptom is determined, an appropriate course of treatment can be devised. Thus, in the ideal situation, there is a specific cause for the symptom and a specific treatment, which produces a remission of the symptom by curing the underlying cause. The health care field's success in discovering causes and cures for many illnesses is often consistent with discrete mechanism's search for linear cause-and-effect relations.

The other world hypotheses that Pepper described are "formism," "organicism," and "contextualism." Formism understands events in terms of their similarity to some ideal or objective standard. Thus understanding is derived from categorization. Much of biology typifies this philosophical orientation. For example, the phylogenetic classification of plants and animals is based on comparisons of similarity.

Organicism understands events through the discovery of patterns and relationships. It is less analytical than either formism or mechanism. Instead it uses a synthetic approach, in which an understanding of the parts is dependent on an understanding of the whole. From this world view, for example, a child's cognitive development can only be understood through consideration of the child's entire developmental history.

Contextualism, like organicism, is synthetic, but the relativity of contextualism separates it from the others. From the contextualistic world view, understanding depends on context. But context is relative, open to change, and dependent on the particular perspective used at the moment. Perspectives can change depending on factors such as historical era and geographic location, or depending on more individual factors, such as motivations and goals.

In many ways, contextualism and discrete mechanism are antithetical world views. Within a mechanistic world view, the critical concept is cause and effect, not context. Thus understanding is independent of time and place. For example, the definitive cause for a strep throat is the streptococcus bacteria, in all times and all places. According to the mechanistic world view, understanding is not aided by a relativistic and changing perspective.

The teaching of psychology lends itself toward a contextualistic approach because there are a number of theoretical models that can be used to explain a single phenomenon. For example, a psychodynamic understanding differs from a behaviorist point of view, and each of these differs from a humanistic perspective. Studying these different models, with their differing assumptions, methods, and realities, may be initially puzzling and challenging, particularly in a society such as ours in which the "hard sciences" are held in high regard and knowledge is frequently presented in terms of linear cause-and-effect relations.

Such a conflict in explanatory styles can be explored by examining students' preferred ways of understanding events. It was hypothesized that nursing students would most prefer a mechanist explanation and least prefer a contextualistic explanation.

Forty female nursing students aged 17 to 46 years ($M = 22.60$, $SD = 6.82$) were recruited from psychology classes in a hospital-based nursing program. Each student signed a statement of informed consent. The mean number of years of prior education was 12.30 ($SD = .76$).

The nursing students completed a modified version of the World Hypothesis Scale (WHS) (Harris, Fontana, & Dowds, 1977). The WHS has 12 items, each with four possible explanations of an event. A sample item follows:

Sue is borrowing a lot of money.

____A. There are several ways to look at Sue's borrowing a lot of money. Economically she feels one way about it, and emotionally she feels another way. There is no one way she sees it. (Contextualism)

____B. Sue is a big spender. She is the kind of person who could be expected to buy things before she's saved up for them. (Formism)

____C. Sue is borrowing a lot of money because she wants to buy a new car. Thus there is a specific reason for her borrowing money at this time. (Mechanism)

____D. Sue's borrowing money now is one stage in the development of her dependability. This development has roots in her past and there are stages in the future through which she will pass. (Organicism)

Nursing students were asked to rank the explanations in terms of their preference for understanding the event. Their first choice for each item received a score of four, second choice a score of three, etc. Thus scores could range from a high of 48 to a low of 12 for each scale.

Data were analyzed by paired *t* tests. Mean scores for each orientation were compared with pooled mean scores for all other orientations. Comparisons that tested the hypothesized relations were students' responses to mechanistic explanations versus all other explanations, and students' responses to contextualistic explanations versus all others. Means, standard deviations, *t* values, and significance levels are presented in Table 12.1.

As hypothesized, nursing students rated mechanistic thinking significantly more positively than all other world hypotheses. That is, they endorsed most positively explanations of behavior that invoked linear cause-and-effect relations. Also as hypothesized, they rated contextualistic thinking significantly more negatively than

TABLE 12.1.
Paired t-tests of Nursing Students on the World Hypothesis Scale

Variable	Mean	Standard Deviation	*t*	*p*
Formist	30.35	6.37	.35	ns
Not Formist	29.88	2.12		
Mechanist	33.68	7.33	3.17	<.01
Not Mechanist	28.78	2.44		
Organicist	29.40	6.66	–.57	ns
Not Organist	30.20	2.22		
Contextualist	26.58	7.50	–2.89	<.01
Not Contextualist	31.14	2.50		

ns = not significant

all other orientations. That is, they least preferred explanations for behavior that relied on multiple perspectives, with no one right way of understanding an event. No other comparisons were statistically significant.

While understanding the principles of cause-and-effect relations is critical for nurses, it is also important for them to be able to understand and accept "uncertainty and idiosyncratic human responses" (Wilson-Barnett, 1983) and to embrace a holistic approach to prevention and treatment (Wells-Federman et al., 1995; Witmer & Sweeney, 1992) because nurses must help individual patients and their families in real life contexts, not just treat patients' diseases as if the diseases were isolated in test tubes. In order to help students achieve these ends, it is useful for teachers to appreciate their students' assumptions and to build bridges from these assumptions. That is, striving for more of a partnership relationship with nursing students requires accommodation by faculty as well as by students.

One such accommodation is to begin a course in psychology for nursing students by discussing specific instances of the interaction of psychosocial and biological factors. An intriguing example is the research investigating the effects of environment on brain structure and function. This introduces the course with content and terminology that are familiar, and hence comfortable, to the student, while also helping to establish the course as one in which multiple perspectives and levels of analysis are investigated.

Another important tool in bridging the distance between teacher and student is the extensive use of concrete examples. Examples help to make theoretical, nomothetic material less abstract and illustrate how diverse theoretical perspectives may be applied to the same behavior, with each perspective adding to or changing the understanding of the behavior. As Clarke (1983) has suggested, whenever possible, the examples should relate directly to nursing issues such as patient care and clinical judgment. That is, it is important, in forming a partnership, for the teacher to meet students "where they're at." For traditionally trained psychology teachers, this may require some "extra homework." However, this accommodation of expert to (relative) novice is very much in keeping with the partnership model.

In addition, students can bring to the classroom their experiences with patients in the "hands on," practicum, component of their training. Again, psychology faculty must make some accommodation to students in this process by learning some of the language used by nursing students. That is, from a partnership perspective, it is helpful not only for students to learn some psychology "jargon," but also for psychology teachers to learn some nursing "jargon." Similarly, just as students can be encouraged to read psychological literature, the psychology teacher can read nursing literature and bring material from those sources into classroom discussions. By discussing their own clinical cases and how these illustrate (or fail to illustrate) a variety of psychological principles, students become more active partners in learning.

Teaching strategies such as these have seemed to reduce nursing students' resistance to psychology as a discipline. Moreover, some students have responded very favorably, commenting that they learned more than they had ever expected they would and that the course had changed the way they think.

In teaching psychology to nursing students, not as a set of incontrovertible facts, but as various possible explanations for behavior that invite exploration, discussion, and critical thinking, students (and teacher) engage in "critical reflection" (Ford & Profetto-McGrath, 1994). Both students and teachers learn from such a process. That is, in a partnership relationship not only will the nursing students learn from the psychology teacher but the teacher will also learn from and with the students.

INDEPENDENT STUDIES: EXAMPLES OF PARTNERSHIP POSSIBILITIES BETWEEN TEACHER AND STUDENT

A number of students undertake independent studies in which course credit is given to a student who pursues an area of interest, conducts a research study, and writes a research report. The student may choose an area in which the faculty member has both interest and expertise or may choose an area, if the faculty member is agreeable, in which the faculty member has some interest but relatively little expertise. In either case, because it is an individualized study, student and teacher have the opportunity to work closely together throughout the semester. The following three independent studies illustrate varying degrees of partnership with the student.

An example of partnership in which the faculty member had both some interest and expertise is one in which a student investigated whether an intervention could be designed to reduce elementary school children's gender stereotypes. A senior psychology major had approached me with the goal of doing an independent study as an elective in psychology. Rather than having a specific area that she wanted to pursue, she wanted the experience of an independent study. I knew she was also in the education program and would soon be student teaching for a semester. I suggested that she design an intervention and administer a pre- and post-test to see if the intervention worked; I thought that kind of research process might be one that she could use throughout her career as a teacher. We were still left with the decision of what content area to pursue, but after a little discussion we decided on gender stereotypes in children, an area in which I had some expertise and one in which she wanted to learn more. Thus this independent study is similar to a traditional tutorial in which the student works with the faculty member on an area in which the faculty member has some expertise. After the student reviewed the literature, we decided on an intervention of children's literature that was counter-gender-stereotypic, and chose a measure to assess gender stereotypes in children. She implemented the study in three separate classrooms, then analyzed the data as planned. We discussed the results and possible interpretations. She wrote a final report and presented it at an undergraduate research symposium. With encouragement, she submitted and presented the results at an annual meeting of the New England Psychological

Association. Although she described the independent study as initially "overwhelming," she also found it "a great new challenge," one that she was "so glad . . . [she] chose to do."

Another basis for an independent study is for a student to take a topic that relates to a faculty member's research but investigate it from a perspective that is of interest to the student. This is more in keeping with the partnership model because it builds on the student's interests and areas of expertise. For example, I was involved in a research project whose participants included bilingual Hispanic women who were asked to respond to questionnaires in English. I wondered if they would have responded differently if the questionnaires had been in Spanish. I approached a bilingual psychology major and asked if she would consider doing an independent study related to that possibility. She responded enthusiastically, but, as we continued to meet, she decided she was more interested in whether the age at which one learns a second language was related to the degree of proficiency one maintains in the original language. We designed a study that enabled us to investigate both of our interests, which she conducted. That is, our partnership enabled us to research not only what I, as a faculty member, was interested in, but also what she, as a student, was interested in. Her literature review focused on her area of interest; the design and data collection addressed both of our interests. She analyzed the data to examine her hypothesis and wrote a final report from the perspective of her interests and research hypotheses, which she presented at an undergraduate research symposium. I have the data available to me to test my hypothesis. During our work together, we discussed both of our areas of interest. We learned more from this approach than we would have had we pursued only one of our interests. In addition, we also made use of the opportunity to converse, in the finest sense of the word. We learned a little about each other's cultures and were each personally enriched by our collaboration.

The final example is of a student who approached me wanting to do an independent study on psychoneuroimmunology. Although I had some expertise in research design and the stress-illness literature, the student and I were both novices on immune system functioning, and therefore partners in learning at a very basic level. At several points we were helped by a faculty member in the biology department whose research interests included the immune system. Thus the student saw me learning from another faculty member, just as she was. We both read some of the literature, discussed all the reading she did, which was more extensive than my reading, and puzzled together about how to go from the literature to developing a project that would be feasible at the undergraduate level. Here my prior interest in stress and autonomic nervous system functioning proved useful. We were able to design a project that incorporated ideas from her reading of the psychoneuroimmunology literature within the constraints of an undergraduate research setting by looking at the relationship between students' stress about writing papers and taking exams and their level of autonomic nervous system arousal, because autonomic arousal has been implicated in immune system functioning. Our partnership enabled the student to learn about an area of interest to her that was not available in any course offerings. I was able to learn a little more about the immune system, which has since been helpful to me in designing an interdisciplinary course on women's wellness. We could come full circle if, after the student completes her graduate work, she would be a guest lecturer in that course.

INTERDISCIPLINARITY: A TOOL FOR FORMING PARTNERSHIPS

Just as the study of nursing students was "inspired" by their puzzlement and frustration with the underlying philosophical assumptions of their psychology courses, the use of interdisciplinarity was "inspired" by undergraduate students (Dowds, 1998). In this case the inspiration was some of the students' "I'd rather be elsewhere" looks and my growing realization that some of them could, and were, performing more competently in contexts other than the psychology classroom (e.g., outstanding written work in a student literary publication but not in papers and essays for their psychology course). Therefore, part of my motivation to become more interdisciplinary came from the students' needs, interests, and dissatisfactions, particularly among students who were not psychology majors and who were taking psychology courses to meet distribution or program requirements. That is, some of the students were not only not interested in psychology per se, they viewed their psychology courses as something they had "to get through" in order to do what they wanted. I wanted to be able to engage them so that they would be likely to put forth their best effort and be motivated to learn because of their own interests. I knew that for them to develop an enduring interest in the field, they would need to become intrinsically motivated (Deci & Ryan, 1992). From a partnership perspective, I needed to begin "where they were at."

In experimenting with ways to engage these students, I decided to try to teach psychology in a more interdisciplinary manner. I believed that if I could encourage students to make connections between psychology and what they were "really" interested in, they would become more involved. Consistent with the partnership model, I accommodated to the students' interests, and by doing so I provided students with more ways to connect with me and the course. I also hoped that they would be more creative by making connections between disciplines in novel ways (Sternberg & Lubart, 1991, 1992). To this end, students were encouraged to use not only psychology journals but also journals from their majors. Similarly, they were encouraged to take ideas from psychology and create connections to their majors. Class discussions were expanded beyond psychology. With an explicit focus on interdisciplinarity and the desire to draw upon students' strengths, I acknowledged both my own limitations and their expertise. As partners in learning, they could initiate new directions for class discussions, I could learn from them, and they could learn from each other as well as from me.

For their individual and group projects, students were asked to consider what topics they would find most interesting to pursue, including those that were not traditionally found in psychology. They were also encouraged to consider making use of drama, music, and literature when presenting their ideas or reviews of the psychological research. Students from other disciplines (e.g., art, biology, language, literature, music, and sociology) were encouraged to take topics from those disciplines and integrate them with the psychology we were studying.

A number of students responded with effective interdisciplinary work. In fact, in watching those students respond with competence, enthusiasm, and creativity, I felt lucky and privileged to have expanded to a more interdisciplinary approach.

A psychology major, for example, used a variety of dramatic techniques from her theater course to present material on gender stereotypes. First she described in some detail the *Hopkins* vs. *Price Waterhouse* case, in which a top manager was denied partnership in the firm, not for lack of competence, but for supposed lack of femininity and interpersonal skills (Fiske, 1993). She then had us participate in a "role on the wall." Specifically, we were to write around the outside of a human figure outline, representing Ann Hopkins, descriptions of what we thought were the external pressures Hopkins experienced in deciding whether or not to pursue a court case. Inside the drawing of Hopkins we were to write adjectives that described how we thought she felt as she was making the decision. After that we divided into groups and enacted tableaus, or still images, of key figures in the case. Finally, the student took the "hot seat," pretending to be Ann Hopkins, and answered, based on her reading about the case, questions from the class. Her presentation was excellent, and she responded to the positive feedback from all of us with increased participation in class discussions throughout the remainder of the semester. She had had the opportunity to use her talents in the classroom, to be an expert not only on Ann Hopkins but also on using dramatic techniques in the classroom. When the student experiences a sense of expertise, the possibility of partnership between student and teacher becomes more alive.

An English major/women's studies minor tried to determine if the books chosen for review in *The New York Times* were particularly likely to have been written by white males. More important than the specific project, she came to appreciate, through discussions with me in developing her project, that she could make connections between psychology and literature and that I could learn from her. That is, she realized that the course could enrich her understanding of literature and that my understanding of literature could be enriched by her analyses, which incorporated both literary and psychological perspectives. She compared her poetry before and after the course and concluded that she was able to probe and explore in ways she had not previously done. A recent poem, influenced by the psychology class she had taken, addressed "the psychological struggle of mothering in the face of questions mothers don't always want to answer or can answer." More generally, she commented that:

> To be encouraged to write from my major (English) into psychology offers me many opportunities to integrate subjects. . . . What is most important is that from the freedom you have offered me to write across subjects, I will be able to develop my future writings, particularly and eventually fiction, with psychology in mind.

Freedom to think about ideas important to oneself is an important component of any partnership relationship.

In papers and presentations, particularly in the developmental courses, students have frequently used literature, including excerpts from novels, plays, and short stories that "embody" psychological theory and research. For some students, literature seems to be the best means to make the material "come alive." That is, literature adds "flesh and blood" to the kind of sparse writing characteristic of psychology. When literature is used in dramatic presentations, the effect can be spell-binding. For example, in a child development course one group of students enacted part of a play that involved a bitter argument and physical violence within a family. Another group enacted a scene of racial prejudice in a child's life, showing the adults' judgments and prejudices, and the child's ensuing confusion and dismay.

In a "Psychology of Women" course, students proposed that the final exam incorporate creative elements. Following a class discussion about possible formats, we decided that each student would give a 5- to 10-minute oral presentation that had to include two or more of the major topics we had studied, had to use some form of creative expression, and could incorporate personal responses to the issues and the course. Thus students initiated the notion that a creative element be required in the final and participated in evaluating possible formats for the final. Three of the better finals, based on the criteria for grading, demonstrated depth of understanding of the issues, clarity of presentation, and creativity. One student presented from a brief book she had written, containing prose, poetry, and pictures, which addressed the issues of adoption, motherhood, and careers. Another student used a collage as an introduction to an articulate verbal presentation on the importance of biology as well as psychology in understanding human behavior. A third student wrote a beautiful and powerful poem about topics important to her including depression, AIDS, and women as resources to one another, followed by a thoughtful discussion of each of these issues.

As students became involved in group projects and final presentations that incorporated their own areas of strength, their relationships with me changed. In contrast to assignments in which I simply told them what was expected of them, these interdisciplinary assignments, with their greater freedom to go in different directions, meant that they were more likely to meet with me during office hours to think about their projects. Moreover, when they met with me, they were less likely to view me as the sole expert with all the answers. Rather than being someone who could tell them what information to incorporate in their presentations and papers or where to find the information, I became more of a sounding board. There was a gradual transformation in our meetings. Initially, for most students, there was a tentativeness in their discussions with me. For example, a typical meeting would begin with the student asking, "Would it be all right with you if I looked at . . . ?" For most of the students who spoke with me several times around a particular project, there was a shift from this initial tentativeness to a more self-assured presentation of their goals and the means for achieving them (for example, "Here's how I'd like to present. . . ." or "I'm also going to include . . . Okay?").

One of the outcomes of incorporating interdisciplinarity in the classroom is that many more students have stayed in touch with me after a course ends. A number (both psychology majors and nonmajors) have returned to tell me what they are doing in other classes, relating their experiences in those classes to what we did in psychology. A few have incorporated some of the psychological literature we read into papers written for other disciplines. Thus they had made the concepts and literature theirs to use. And, I think, they view me as a long-term partner, someone who is interested in their work well beyond the confines of our shared classroom time.

CONCLUSIONS

Examining nursing students' philosophical assumptions and making some changes in the course to accommodate these assumptions, working with students on independent studies that incorporate their interests, and using interdisciplinarity in the classroom illustrate various ways faculty can form partnerships with their students. In these examples, there is a bidirectional flow of information. I learned from the experiences nursing students had in their practicum work; I learned from the "real world" knowledge the bilingual student brought to our research project; and I learned from the students who integrated art, literature, sociology, and biology into their psychology classes. There was in all these examples, at its best, a mutual respect and reciprocity between faculty and student, an appreciation of our differing strengths and our differing, but complementary, roles, and a willingness to work together, to engage in dialogue. I respected their interests, and they responded with questions that were important to them. I taught psychological content and process. They used these to serve their own ends (becoming a nurse, a psychologist, a writer, a teacher). I explicitly valued these ends, and they shared with me their evaluations of our work together and how they used their newly acquired experience in psychology. Their evaluations help me to continue to modify my teaching in order to form more effective partnerships with my students.

REFERENCES

Clarke, M. (1983). Critique of 'Psychology and nursing: The case for an empirical approach' by Lesley Wattley and Dave J. Muller. *Journal of Advanced Nursing, 8,* 338–339.

Deci, E. L., & Ryan, R. M. (1992). The initiation and regulation of intrinsically motivated learning and achievement. In A. K. Boggiano & T. S. Pittman (Eds.), *Achievement and motivation: A social-developmental perspective* (pp. 9–36). New York: Cambridge University Press.

Dowds, B. N. (1998). Helping students make connections across the disciplines. *Creativity Research Journal, 11,* 55–60.

Dowds, B. N., & Marcel, B. B. (1998). Students' philosophical assumptions and psychology in the classroom. *Journal of Nursing Education, 37,* 219–221.

Fiske, S. T. (1993). Controlling other people: The impact of power on stereotyping. *American Psychologist, 48,* 1070–1076.

Ford, J. S., & Profetto-McGrath, J. (1994). A model for critical thinking within the context of curriculum as praxis. *Journal of Nursing Education, 33,* 341–344.

Harris, M., Fontana, A. F., & Dowds, B. N. (1977). The world hypothesis scale: Rationale, reliability and validity. *Journal of Personality Assessment, 41,* 537–547.

Pepper, S. C. (1970). *World hypotheses: A study of evidence.* University of California Press, Berkeley CA. (Original work published 1942)

Sternberg, R. J., & Lubart, T. I. (1991). An investment theory of creativity and its development. *Human Development, 34,* 1–31.

Sternberg, R. J., & Lubart, T. I. (1992). Buy low and sell high: An investment approach to creativity. *Psychological Science, 1,* 1–5.

Wells-Federman, C. L., Stuart, E. M., Deckro, J. P., Mandle, C. L., Baim, M., & Medich, C. (1995). The mind-body connection: The psychophysiology of many traditional nursing interventions. *Clinical Nurse Specialist, 9,* 59–66.

Wilson-Barnett, J. (1983). Critique of 'Psychology and nursing: The case for an empirical approach' by Lesley Wattley and Dave J. Muller. *Journal of Advanced Nursing, 8,* 335–336.

Witmer, M. J., & Sweeney, T. J. (1992). A holistic model for wellness and prevention over the life span. *Journal of Counseling and Development, 71,* 140–148.

13

PARTNERSHIPS IN THE ELEMENTARY SCHOOL CLASSROOM

Joseph McInerney
McCarthy-Towne School, Acton, Massachusetts, and Tufts University

ABSTRACT

There are many possibilities for partnerships with students, parents, and the larger community. Such partnerships can encourage students' creativity, engage them in the tools and techniques of a subject, and forge deep relationships within and outside the classroom. This chapter describes partnerships that have successfully united children around the common cause of learning, and it illustrates how partnerships, which are basically about human relationships, enrich all those involved in teaching and learning.

"OVER BY THE RADIATOR"

Late one night early in my teaching career I came across this answer to a question I had posed to my fifth graders. I had given the class an end-of-the-year self-evaluation paper to complete. One of the questions asked the children to state in what area of the class they had done their best work. Looking, of course, for answers such as math, reading, spelling, or science, I had not quite anticipated this response, "over by the radiator." One of my boys found a solution to the travails of learning in a drafty, old, New England classroom. This answer made me laugh for a long time and then reflect on the importance of posing clear questions. A partnership with students assumes that learning is a two-way street. This confusion taught me a valuable lesson.

Another memorable misunderstanding came while teaching about archaeology. I told the class that despite the "Indiana Jones" movies popular at the time, archaeology was an exacting science. Archaeologists had to engage in extended study and research before they ever put a shovel into the ground. The landscape of archaeological interest is vast, and excavation is very expensive. Careful study always precedes actual digging. Luck was seldom a part of archaeology with two notable exceptions. One, I observed, was the accidental discovery of prehistoric cave paintings in Lascaux, France. These were found by two boys at play. The other was the Dead Sea Scrolls. I explained how these documents changed the direction of biblical scholarship and were discovered in large urns by shepherds who happened upon them in a cave. "Rare luck in both examples," I noted. The next day, Elizabeth, one of my bright young students, came to me with a puzzled expression and said, "Mr. McInerney, I understand about the prehistoric cave paintings. That seems very important. But why would archaeologists be interested in a bunch of dead squirrels?" Either Elizabeth misheard or I misspoke. When I relayed this story to her parents, they laughed and said their daughter was famous for jumping to the wrong conclusions. My brother heard this story and claimed that Elizabeth heard correctly and that I had not completely eliminated vestiges of a Pittsburgh upbringing from my speech. The point is that teaching partnerships require strong feedback loops; otherwise we will hear and not listen, dig and not find, look and not see.

Partnerships in education: this is a wonderful topic, but as you can see from these vignettes, it is important to define terms and to be clear about the subject prior to excavation! My perspective is that of a teacher with 29 years of experience. All of my teaching, save for college and graduate school presentations, has been with students from grades four to six; in other words, children between the ages of 9 and 12. Teaching can be isolating, and teaching in an elementary classroom especially so. Since so much of my teaching life is wrapped up in direct interaction with young children, like the fish in the sea unaware of its medium, a little self-examination helped me realize that partnerships were abundant in my teaching life.

To me, educational partnership means working with others toward the common goal of helping children learn. Be they formal and longstanding, or informal and passing, such relationships are essential to the task of a teacher. I see partnerships as necessary, constant, and generative to my teaching. I will focus on specific examples from my teaching in order to give the reader a sample of the range of collaboration that is possible in an educational setting. Some are examples of stepping outside the classroom in order to join with others, or are examples of inviting members of the larger community inside the classroom in order to share special talents or skills. They are not a panacea for a troubled classroom. Focusing on them, therefore, should in no way diminish the primary partnerships in a teacher's life, that is, the relationships with students, parents, administrators, and support staff. These in-school associations are the fabric of everyday life for teachers. If these relationships are sound and sensible, they clear the way for a teacher to explore partnerships outside the classroom; if they are conflicted and confused, it limits what a teacher can do or even consider. For example, the trust of a principal allows a teacher to navigate beyond the classroom. But it also requires of a teacher the caution to act responsibly, to collaborate wisely. Partnerships in education claim this middle ground of trust and responsibility. It is a balanced and dynamic center and not a static point. It is where real value is added to educational programs, where children actually learn.

Teaching requires learning, character, and imagination. It requires trust because that is the foundation upon which the student and teacher partnership rests. This is hard-won ground. It assumes the authority of the teacher. It assumes that the teacher, by virtue of superior knowledge and understanding, has something of value to pass on to others; that s/he is the author of a narrative that frames knowledge and makes sense of experience. Children relate to a narrative sequence; to cause and effect; to the beginning, middle, and end of the great stories of our culture. They instinctively trust teachers who can lead them to knowledge with understanding, dignity, and conviction. If this authority is acquired and gained by the teacher, it will be understood and felt by the student.

Authority then is built on a foundation of mutual trust and respect between teacher and student. It does not imply that a teacher knows everything, but that s/he has traveled a long way down the road toward mastering a subject, and that students cannot help but want to take part in the journey. Earned authority makes a teacher into a leader. Leaders don't mind retracing steps in order to show others a better path amid a labyrinth of confusing alternatives. I tell my students when we start a new subject that I am an expert on "beginner's mistakes" because I have a clear memory of making so many myself. In fact, I find mistakes fascinating; they are windows to the minds of my students and tell me how to be clearer in the future.

I do not believe in the current educational trend that teachers should be guides at the sides of children as they create their own paths through knowledge. The road to understanding important subject matter is a linear path and mastery for students comes through a clear narrative by the teacher. Therefore, the teaching authority of which I write draws its ancient etymology from the word "author." This means that stories and metaphors are a key to my teaching, as well as honesty about the task at hand. I do not feel that learning is easy. To tell children this is dishonest. Algebra is not easy, nor is learning German or organic chemistry. Children know that tackling any body of knowledge or acquiring any valued skill is hard work. They know that mastering subtraction, fingering on a flute, executing a corner kick in soccer, throwing a perfect spiral in football, or doing long division are not easy; learning is labor of the most intensive kind. They also instinctively understand that good teachers make hard work interesting. Good teachers hook students on the challenge of mastering these tasks. Good teachers awaken the curiosity from within their students to do the hard work necessary to conquer confusion and master the skill, be it learning to read or learning to play the piano. Such teaching engages students in the tools and techniques of a subject and whets their imaginations to do more on their own.

This ethos creates a classroom that places the needs of the whole in front of the individual performer. The classroom partnership is a group dynamic. Individual differences are noticed and understood, but the key is creating interesting tasks that unite children around the common cause of learning. A good group project frames knowledge and structures experience. It creates its own language and vocabulary, generates deep relationships, and forces team members to meet their commitments to each other. What follows are examples carefully drawn and excavated from my own teaching experience. In "Historical Visitors," "Time Capsule Exchange," and "Mock Trials," I detail what such a perspective looks like in a fifth-grade classroom. Finally, in "The Calculus of a Partnership" I reflect on partnerships with a slightly wider compass.

HISTORICAL VISITORS

With grace he received the gift. It was a "poverty blanket" to warm his crippled legs. He thanked the girl who presented it to him and continued to wheel forward under a 48-star flag. "Hail to the Chief" filled the room with music as the jaunty-jawed Franklin D. Roosevelt shook hands with all of the students around him. He appreciated the welcoming "set," designed to resemble his Oval Office in Washington. He warmed his hands by the roaring "fireplace" near the old fashioned radio as a winter storm gathered outside. It was time for a chat.

When the excited crowd calmed down a bit, President Roosevelt updated everyone on the conditions at the front in December of 1943, and hinted that he might run again for the presidency for an unprecedented fourth term. Then, with great humor and nostalgia, he recalled his childhood in Hyde Park, New York, recounted his long struggle with polio and his hope for a vaccine in the future, and remembered how one Christmas he gave his famous Scottish terrier its name, Fala. After an hour of discussion and questions, the president enjoyed the reception that was prepared in his honor, reminded everyone to put their brown-out curtains over their windows at night, and left to the applause of all.

This event actually took place in my classroom in Acton, Massachusetts, 47 years after FDR's death. "President Roosevelt," in real life an Acton resident and the father of one of my students, worked with me for several months to ensure that his portrayal would be accurate. It is important to teach history through a clear narrative and text, but also to flesh out the historical context of the past with a dramatic event. Toward this end, I invite two historical heroes to my classroom each year.

These august figures from past eras have included Isaac Newton, Louis Pasteur, Alexander Fleming, Florence Nightingale, Thomas Jefferson, and Benjamin Franklin. Even the Greek goddess Athena, who gifted humans with the power of invention and creativity, has spoken to the mere mortals of "Class M-10." Last May, Leonardo da Vinci traveled all the way from Italy to present his famous *Notebooks*. The calendar read 1515, and we greeted him in period costume so that he would feel right at home. This visit culminated a unit on optics, was coordinated with a biography of Leonardo's life, and placed history in a living context.

These historical visitors are the most intense partnerships I have been involved with as a teacher. The research has to be extensive. The courage required on the part of the presenter must be considerable. It is a lot to ask of someone. However, I have been fortunate to find quite a few parents who are willing to work up a character. Importantly, the visit must dovetail with our curricular work. FDR visited in 1992, 1996, and promises to return in the year 2000 and every quadrennial election year after that. (In future visits, he assures me, he will not have to use theatrical graying streaks in his hair!) Leonardo da Vinci has come twice, but Isaac Newton was able to visit only once; he now lives out of state. Alexander Fleming was carried on a chair into the classroom in honor of his discovery of penicillin; historical research can produce the most interesting details. I am on the lookout for Descartes, Madame Curie, and a couple of Wright Brothers for future years. Thomas Jefferson would love to return, but, like Issac Newton, he now lives across the country, transferred by his company.

As an extension of a study of microscopes, bacteria, and the great microbe hunters, Louis Pasteur has visited my classroom several times. One year our concentration was so intense that I called this parent only by his stage name when we fine-tuned his presentation prior to his arrival. We left the 19th-century context only to discuss 20th-century logistics—automobile parking and the like. His children got used to phone calls directed to Monsieur Pasteur. This helped both of us to set the mood and stay in character.

The key to this unique educational partnership is to match the effort of the parent actor. With the children in period dress keyed to the necessary country and era, an in-classroom theatrical set constructed to welcome the visitor, a food and beverage reception befitting the occasion, and finally, a thoughtfully selected gift to thank the actor, I know that the historical collaborator felt welcomed and appreciated. They want to volunteer again. Historical visitors are an intense, enjoyable, and memorable bit of living history. It is magic in the classroom and leaves a lasting impression in the minds of all involved.

The coordination with the adult is important, but my parallel partnership with the children is equally intense. Every step of the preparation involves student interaction and involvement. The visit by FDR, for example, came just before a presidential election and related to a long study of microbiology. This two-fold connection to history and science gave added depth to the historical visitor experience.

The microscope unit started with a visit to a nearby pond to collect jars of seemingly lifeless pond water. Using a hay infusion technique, the sample water was soon transformed into cultures teeming with protozoa and microbial life. With 100x-power student microscopes, we were able to see the "unseen life" within the jars. In doing so, we looked upon a world that Leeuvenhoek viewed for the first time in the 1670s in Holland. We sketched and drew as he did and built replica microscopes in his style, using tongue depressors and lenses drawn from modern disposable cameras. For all of his observational brilliance, Leeuvenhoek never understood the even smaller life forms, the bacteria that seemed to swirl under his lens. However, two later researchers in the 19th century, Robert Koch and Louis Pasteur, understood the role of bacteria in life and sought ways to control bacteria-borne disease. We studied the lives of these scientists and replicated some of their simpler experiments in class, using petri dishes and an incubator. But what about viruses that remained unseen until the advent of the electron microscope near the middle of this century? Ironically, this microbial form, so small that light transmission microscopes were too crude an instrument for its detection, was actually detected by Edward Jenner in the 18th century. His smallpox vaccine used relatively harmless cowpox matter; Thomas Jefferson was one of his greatest champions. Children love these stories of the famous microbe hunters and enjoy reading their biographies. Pasteur's inspired conquest of the rabies virus was a favorite story since it involved children and a wild dog. We discovered that Pasteur never actually looked upon this microbial killer the way that he did the bacteria that causes anthrax. He conquered rabies by indirection and by brilliant conjecture. My classroom became a laboratory of experimentation and microscopic observation. Every child took pictures through a classroom microscope using a 35mm camera and a cable release. "Freeze please" became a favorite call for all to stop so a student could click a vibration-free microphotograph of a protozoan's cilia or a bee's eye. To view the infinitesimal virus we visited an electron microscope factory as a field trip.

Perhaps the greatest viral threat to children in the 20th century was polio. It bested the greatest researchers until the development of tissue cultures as a medium and the earlier mentioned electron microscope. These advances opened a route to conquest but a fund-raising champion was needed. That person was President Roosevelt, crippled by polio in the late 1920s but who went on to become governor of New York and the only president to date to serve more than two terms. He started the March of Dimes and generated the political willpower to fund the research that eventually led to Salk's polio vaccine in 1953. So, during an election year with this rich science as a context and background, why not invite FDR to visit our classroom?

"How might we welcome him?" I asked. Suggestions flew about, one after another. Soon we organized into research groups and project teams to prepare an Oval Office complete with a 1940s style "fireside" radio, a Great Seal backdrop, old newspapers and *Life* magazines, brownout curtains, and other related touches. The "poverty blanket" was suggested by a student whose grandmother wove it during the Great Depression. One Thursday after school an eager team of students stayed to do extra work on the set. Every child planned a costume of 1940s attire in order to welcome our honored guest. Students, teacher, and guest were partners in every respect and willingly suspended disbelief. In our minds and hearts the calendar was turned back 50 years.

We learn best through action first. If thought is internalized action, then this experience lets children author the conclusion of the story. They are ready with questions and reflections. No prompting is needed. Roosevelt talked of the two-front war, of his life in a wheelchair, and of his certainty that a cure is "just around the corner." We understood his struggles but shared his optimism because we were partners in a great enterprise.

U.S.–JAPAN TIME CAPSULE EXCHANGE

Louis Pasteur said that in learning, "Chance favors the prepared mind." It is hard not to agree, and when I think about partnerships in education, I feel fortunate that chance placed Mr. Michihiro Shiraishi in my path. Mr. Shiraishi was an editor with the *Yomiuri Shimbum*. This Japanese newspaper has a Sunday circulation of over 14 million subscribers, drawing on the enormous population of the Tokyo metropolitan area.

I first met "Shiraishi-san" in Tokyo during the summer of 1983 when I attended a summer fellowship for teachers sponsored by the Kaizi-Koho Center. Editor Shiraishi covered our visit for his newspaper and liked a proposal I had written called "Time Capsule 2000." Since the idea involved students from both sides of the Pacific, he offered to help. With his enthusiastic aid, we were able to create an international partnership that would continue as long as we were both working. He has visited my home and classroom in Acton several times over the years, and my son was his guest while studying Japanese during college. Our formal partnership has merged into a friendship, but it was an idea that brought us together. We both believe in the value of taking a "long view" when working with children within, or across, cultures.

Twenty years from now, fifth graders will look upon the 1990s as a distant if not ancient era. Perhaps those born in the 20th century will be dismissed as "nineteeners." When I told my class that their children will think of Michael Jordan as a basketball "old timer," they were astonished. (But how many adults realize that King Tut of Egypt was as far removed in time from the great age of pyramid building as we are from Charlemagne?—1200 years!) It is natural to condense and telescope the past. This project helped put time in perspective.

It should be noted that the time capsule idea, as well as the other partnerships described here, would work with children in any setting, be they rich or poor, black or white. These ideas cost very little and were successful when I taught three years in inner-city Boston as well as in one of its suburbs. There are no textbooks that need to be adopted in order to implement these ideas, or expensive programs to purchase. The true cost relates to the demands of teaching—energy, patience, imagination, and perseverance—these are a constant in every good classroom. Teaching is one of the most powerful and responsible of human activities. It is comforting to realize, therefore, that the best ideas and the deepest partnerships that touch and motivate children years into their future, are free and infectious.

Burying a time capsule is archaeology in reverse. An archaeologist has to work from a few fragments of the past in order to piece together a view of the whole. Each clue has great significance. Contributors to a time capsule try to select key fragments from the present that they feel will be representative of our time to a future era. In order to link science and social studies activities each year, I have my fifth grade class prepare a time capsule that will be buried and not reopened until the year 2000, 2010, or 2020 for more recent classes. On July 4th at noon on those years, we will meet and unearth our treasure. All children included a letter to themselves that described how they and the world might have changed in the intervening years. Many parents enclosed sealed letters to their children with special messages that would wait a long time to see the light of day.

The capsule idea is not new, but the strategies I use to lead up to it are. I use a model based on NASA's preparation of the Voyager space message which describes our Earth; this probe will eventually leave our solar system and travel into deep space. Like the Voyager, each capsule has pictures, taped sounds, and music that the children felt told the most about our past and present. We, of course, are able to add real objects and special future-predicting letters. Our planning was very systematic and involved checklists carefully structured to stay within the NASA format and the size limits of the capsule. For my students, the decision making and problem solving was considerable. (Carl Sagan described an intense debate at NASA in his book, *Murmurs of Earth* (1978), as they went through this process of selection.) The effort integrates an entire year of math, social studies, and science curricula. There are no real experts on the future. As we try to decide what to include in the limited space of the time capsule, the children realize that their teacher is one of the many people who does not know for sure about the future. However, prediction was fun and instructive, so the children wrote letters to themselves in which they described their current lives, but also tried to predict the future. Some students wrote one or two pages but the average letter was longer because the students were asked to consider the present in ever-enlarging circles, starting with themselves, friends, and family, and then expanding into the school, community, and the larger world of experience. I told them that this letter, as well as the missives from their parents, were the heart of the time capsule and would be what they would most want to return to see. A small sample from a letter written in the early 1990s:

> Dear Emily,
>
> Hi! How are you? You will be reading this on July 4, 2010. Right now your kids may be with you. Did you become a World Cup soccer player? Didn't think so. Your best friend in 5th grade is writing away furiously. Do you remember her? I hope she is there with you too. . . ."

As mentioned, parents are given their own homework to include a letter. All find it a moving experience. Many have told me they realize that what they write to their child will be read by an adult. Some older parents realize that they might not be alive when the capsule is opened. I hear about drafts and revisions and tears as all of them struggle to express what is in their parental souls. And what about the students? No such worries! With rare exceptions, the ideas flow as they describe themselves, their school, and their town. The collection of objects to be included always exceeds the volume of the capsule. This results in a team of "packers" making some hard choices. Perhaps a few magazine covers would be better than whole magazines. Then again, one whole Time magazine tells a lot about our current world, packed as it is with news, sports, and ads. Should Henry be allowed to put in an entire baseball or would a few baseball cards make more sense? "Measure twice, cut once," says the carpenter. That wisdom must guide the packers as they negotiate these decisions. And where will we plant it? Potential construction or landscape changes turn this question into a lesson about budget issues and long-term school planning. Eventually a spot is found, and the shovels and spades come out. The diggers need more muscle than the packers but their task is just as important. On the last day of school, we all gather around for a ceremony as we bury the sealed capsule. Children never forget this moment and look forward to the prospect of reunion like an inheritance that will come to maturity.

Mr. Shiraishi was moved by this concept, and in 1984 we expanded the capsule idea to be an exchange with a fifth-grade class in Hiroshima, Japan. He coordinated the event on his side of the Pacific. We exchanged capsules and will open them in our respective countries on July 4th in the year 2000. He visited my class and recorded the impressions of my students for several articles he wrote for his newspaper in Japan.

This activity is engaging and fun for students. But in an important way, it is also a metaphor for teaching, and the creating of partnerships in general. I wanted this international Time Capsule Exchange to take place in 1984 because that was the title of a bleak futuristic novel written by George Orwell. Although the author deliberately inverted the 1948 publication date to come up with his title, Orwell's classic projected a desolate political landscape for our then distant future. Fortunately the passage of time has proven his forecast wrong. Vigorous democracies still flourish. Civilization still holds forth the promise of a bright future, even for the bitter enemies of World War II. And this future-seeking hope is no more powerful than in children.

The very formation of an educational partnership is an act of optimism. Pessimists need not apply, for at base their perspective is negative. Pessimists are arrogant because they have "seen everything" and are sure that "nothing will work." Optimists, on the other hand, are sure that a partnership will bring new perspectives. The Time Capsule Exchange was designed to plant the tangible seed of hope for the future in the minds of children. It chases away Orwell's demons and looks ahead.

Partnerships prepare the mind for the blessings of chance. A good idea touches both the mind and the heart of editors and teachers, here at home and across the sea.

MOCK TRIALS

"Psst, psst! Sam, the jury is deadlocked 6–6. I don't know what to tell them. What does it mean? Who wins?"

"Oh, my!" Sam sounded surprised. But he thought quickly and responded, "A tie is not sufficient for the plaintiff to win. Unless they change their minds, the verdict goes to the defense."

So informed by the clerk, the foreperson stood to deliver the verdict of the jury a few minutes later. Attorneys replayed opening and closing arguments in their minds and nervously pawed legal briefs. Witnesses remembered retorts that failed them under cross-examination and wished for a second chance. The audience hushed.

Calling for calm after she struck the gavel and closed the case, the judge presided over the end of the trial. When the verdict came, the defense felt relief and the joy of victory. However, the plaintiff team took solace in the fact that it convinced half of the jury. Most astonishing of all, both sides happily shook hands and repaired to a nearby home for a reception. Hardly typical behavior in an age of legal gladiators and courtroom histrionics!

This scene was from the end of a mock trial held by my class about a dozen years ago. It took place one May evening in a real courthouse in historic Concord, Massachusetts, not far from Acton. It was a civil action and the jury consisted of my former students, all sixth graders. Veterans of two trials the year before, they tried their best to reach a verdict but were deadlocked in their deliberations. When the foreman informed the clerk of the problem, she came to me for advice. Despite the fact that I had conducted several mock trials in previous years, I had never encountered this situation before and sought professional advice; hence the dialogue at the opening of this section.

The person I spoke to is a highly respected lawyer with the Board of Bar Overseers, and the father of three children, two of whom I taught. With his help and guidance, as well as that of other parent attorneys through the years, I have established two mock trials each year as part of my curriculum. The depth and quality of the McCarthy-Towne Courthouse experience is due to my collaboration with these legal professionals.

The law is often an arena of dispute between what is technically possible and what is socially desirable. I developed a strategy of using mock trials to explore scientific and technical ideas. What happens when societal restraints confront the technically possible? Teachers must help students to ask, "Should we do this?" as well as "Can we do this?" Scientific truths and legal verdicts are often in conflict. Mock trials are ideal vehicles to help children view technology with a human face.

Background

The mock trials I use are outgrowths of various math and science units. One trial is based on the geometry of angles, another is an extension of a study of micro-life and diseases, and a third evolved from a unit on the eye and study of light. I designed a special mock trial about the storied construction of Boston's John Hancock Building. Exactly why did all those windows fall out? In May 1996, the mock trial was conducted at Concord Court on the "World Airlines" crash at Logan Airport in 1982. Why did the plane go off the runway and into the harbor? Was the landing angle too steep? Was the pilot too far down the "touchdown zone" to land safely? In each case, the children start from a common database and are then ready for an excursion into another realm.

Balance

I introduce the case with a short lesson about the specific issue at hand and present a brief on the "facts" of the case. We brainstorm the pros and cons of each side, keeping in mind the critical difference between facts and opinions. Advice from the attorney collaborator really helps me here.

Preparation

For the first week to ten days, we write and polish briefs. I select one child to be the judge and each team divides itself into witnesses and attorneys. Each team can do extra research and prepare witnesses for "direct examination," but, of course, each can only guess at what the other side will ask on cross examination. During this time, we discuss legal procedures and specific vocabulary. Our local lawyer visits to aid in this preparation.

Props

A classroom can easily be reorganized into a courtroom but a field trip to a real courthouse is best. Better still, a mock trial in the evening allows all parents to attend. Everyone can dress up "in character" from the judge's black robe (a recycled graduation gown!) to a medical witness's white attire.

Format

The actual format I use is a fast-paced version of the real thing. There are opening statements, a presentation of witnesses with direct and cross examination, evidence and demonstration of exhibits, closing arguments and a live jury (former students of mine) that deliberates in a separate room and delivers a verdict. Each child has a significant role to play that emphasizes both spontaneity and preparation.

Response

But what is the range of response amongst the children, the reader might ask. Do I have doubts and second thoughts about the effectiveness of such a method? These are good questions. In teaching, we initiate activities with students but that is only the beginning. A real teaching partnership with students has built-in evaluation and response loops. Many children take to these mock trials as if they were born in the courtroom. They love the give and take of ideas, the back and forth of debate, the drama of putting on a play without knowing how the last act will end. A few become very nervous at the thought of public speaking in front of a large audience (in the early years of doing these trials, a child cried on the stand). These students become special projects and I have learned how to help them long before we go to court.

One technique is to link lawyer/witness pairs with care. A strong public speaker with a weak one often helps. As they prepare and rehearse the direct examination, the weaker partner almost always rises to the level of the stronger student. Also, throughout the entire year, in book conferences and class discussions, from the first month to the last, I stress the value of a clear voice, eye contact, audience scan, and stand-up-straight projection. Finally, I invite to special lunches the four or five children whom I feel will get nervous at the public speaking prospect. I tell them stories of old trials, model friendly and cross-examination techniques about anything from who made the sandwich they are eating to exactly when they went to bed the night before. We role-play being on the stand; I am cross-examined about the exact number of cookies in the classroom jar, my penchant for drinking Poland Spring water, and why I insist on elevating the "c" in my last name. The tone is light and fun but my purpose is to model and to teach. Proper preparation promotes positive performance. Time, care, attention to details, and hand signal cues, are what really help the students. The cost to the teacher is a few lost lunch periods but the return in terms of student self-confidence in the public forum is priceless.

New Beginnings

This year, for the first time, one of these cases was heard on appeal by a "higher" court. The verdict of our lower court, the jury in Concord, was appealed by the losing team and carried to the Acton Supreme Court. This august body was composed of nine justices, all former students and fully robed, on the morning of their graduation from high school, partners in this effort seven years after their active participation as students in my classroom. The procedure followed the Supreme Court of the United States model and was so well received by my students, both young and old, that a new tradition has been born. As one student noted later, "I thought the hardest part was getting up to the stand and starting to talk, but once you knew that they weren't looking at you weird, you felt a lot better about yourself and you could do it."

I have written 12 such cases over the years. Each requires extensive research, interviewing, and construction of props. I use them with my fifth grade, but they are appropriate up to twelfth grade. It is a powerful science integration tool. The time invested is considerable, but the yield is well worth it. Children talk about these cases years later because they are so thoroughly involving. For the mind to comprehend, the heart must first listen. The seemingly endless questions that flow from each class as a result of this activity has generated in me completely changed expectations toward science and teaching, collaboration and learning, children and ideas.

Advice to other teachers: "Psst! Psst! Try it in your classes. It works! All your children will win."

THE CALCULUS OF A PARTNERSHIP

Over 100 years ago, in 1896, a child was born in Shanavogh East in County Clare on the west coast of Ireland. When he turned seven, he was fortunate enough to enter a one-room school that had just been built. The year was 1903. The teacher at the helm, Master Crehan, could teach children to read at one end of the spectrum and instruct in Shakespeare and trigonometry at the other end. The boy was an excellent pupil and, after 10 years of study, graduated to a life of farming, cattle raising, and fishing.

However, the economic life of Ireland was depressed, so in time this young man told Master Crehan that he planned to emigrate to the United States. His teacher cautioned him that no one should go to America without knowing calculus! (This was not the first time or the last that a teacher has used a little creative exaggeration.) Master Crehan offered to tutor his former pupil in calculus, physics, and chemistry for two years in return for occasional help with the younger ones . . . all this to ensure a smooth passage through Ellis Island!

As you might have guessed by now, that young man was my father. He emigrated to America in 1922 and found himself sweeping floors at Westinghouse's East Pittsburgh plant. When my dad's boss realized that he had much more than a basic education, he helped him to enroll at Westinghouse Tech for night school to study mechanical engineering. His grades were straight As. He spent nearly 40 years working on power projects such as the Grand Coulee Dam, the Hoover Dam, and the Niagara Power Project. As you might imagine, my brothers and sister and I heard a lot about Master Crehan as we were growing up.

It is one of the blessings of our nation that this immigrant story is not atypical. With Master Crehan's collaboration, my father was able to reach beyond laboring jobs and provide a good life for my mother and six children. To me, the story is a metaphor for partnerships in general. A real partnership is a two-way street, giving and getting, an equal sharing of goals and efforts. I had occasion to put that philosophy to work a few years ago in a tangible fashion.

I was the Massachusetts winner of the 1992 Presidential Award for Excellence in Science and Mathematics Teaching. Along with teachers from the other states, I received this honor at the White House in April 1993. With this award came a National Science Foundation grant of $7,500. Traditionally, teachers use this windfall for long-sought equipment, graduate work, fellowships, conventions, travel, etc. With three years to decide how to use the grant, I searched for another idea.

My goal was to leverage the grant and extend its reach. Toward that end, I sought a corporate sponsor to match my contribution so as to create a fund for teacher training in math and science for the Acton Public Schools. To ensure a clear commitment on the part of the teachers toward any training they sought, my proposal stipulated that the teacher would contribute 50 percent of the cost of any workshop or course. I did not seek a corporate handout. I wanted a corporate sponsor on one side and an individual teacher's financial commitment on the other, brought together by the catalyst of the NSF grant. At every step of the way, I sought and received the support and assistance of the Acton Public Schools Development Office.

The NYNEX Telephone Pioneers stepped forward to help in a compelling way. They realized that the ground-breaking preparation for careers in mathematics, science, and technology begins in the elementary grades. They also understood that today's classroom teachers cannot teach tomorrow's workers using yesterday's skills. NYNEX felt that my idea showed a reciprocity of interests, a two-way street of giving and receiving, with students as the ultimate beneficiaries. Their matching grant has now grown and the fund has $30,000 in it. With teachers always contributing half, the buying power of this fund is now $60,000 worth of training. The "seed corn" of enlightened public policy helped create an eight-fold multiple. In this way, a little federal educational policy help went a long way. The fund is named the McInerney-MacKenzie Fund to honor my late father, Michael, and Don MacKenzie, Town Moderator of Acton.

My father touched everyone he met with his strength of character, deep faith, and gentle grace. From him I learned that all gifts carry parallel obligations. All professional partnerships strive for constructive gain while meeting sober responsibilities. Partnerships balance life's burdens and share life's benefits. They are, at root, about human relationships.

REFERENCE

Sagan, C. (1978). *Murmurs of Earth: The Voyager interstellar record.* New York: Random House.

14

MOVING CLASSROOMS BEYOND TRANSMISSION MODELS OF TEACHING AND LEARNING: A TEACHER–RESEARCHER COLLABORATIVE MODEL

Leslie Rupert Herrenkohl
University of Washington

Marion Reynolds Guerra
Goddard School of Science and Technology

ABSTRACT

In this chapter we explore one of the factors, namely teacher–researcher collaboration, that we believe makes it possible to successfully coordinate theory and practice in classroom settings. We describe how a teacher and a researcher worked together to construct a learning environment that provided opportunities for student engagement and discussion of ideas in science. First, we provide the context for the collaboration and the very real problems that drove and motivated the collaboration. Second, we describe the design of the study. Third, we briefly highlight some of our findings. Finally, we conclude by addressing our perspective on what helps contribute to successful teacher–researcher partnerships.

The idea that students should be actively engaged in their own learning is not a new one. Historically, psychologists and educators such as Dewey, Piaget, and Vygotsky have all advocated for educational environments that provide ample opportunities for students to be deeply engaged in making sense of our complex world. Contemporary figures such as Gardner (1991), Moll & Greenberg (1990), and Tharp & Gallimore (1988) also advocate the construction of learning environments that provide more opportunities for active participation on the part of the learner. Although these pedagogical philosophies clearly support the notion of student engagement, there have been few attempts to articulate classroom models that would promote and sustain such engagement. Even with all this theoretical interest in what is typically called "constructivism," transmission models of teaching and learning continue to inform much of the pedagogical practice used in schools. One reason that may contribute to this discrepancy between theory and practice is that constructivism, as argued by Airasian and Walsh (1997), "is not an instructional approach; it is a theory about how learners come to know" (pp. 444–445). In other words, suggesting that human beings construct knowledge through engagement with their environment does not tell one how to create an environment in which that kind of active involvement is valued and encouraged.

In this chapter we explore one of the factors, namely teacher–researcher collaboration, that we believe makes it possible to successfully coordinate theory and practice in classroom settings. We describe how a teacher (Marion) and a researcher (Leslie) worked together to construct a learning environment that provided opportunities for student engagement and discussion of ideas in science. First, we provide the context for the collaboration and the very real problems that drove and motivated the collaboration. Second, we describe the design of the study. Third, we briefly highlight some of our findings. Finally, we conclude by addressing our perspective on what helps contribute to successful teacher–researcher partnerships. Throughout, we write with our individual voices as well as our collective one.

CONTEXTUALIZING THE COLLABORATION: LESLIE'S "RESEARCHER" PERSPECTIVE

Marion and I had known one another for years before we actually collaborated to design what became my dissertation project. I was working in Marion's school as an ethnographer whose primary concern was to document the implementation of a model science program. It was my job to observe what happened as second- through fifth-grade teachers began to use this program. It was also my responsibility to make notes of the comments and questions that teachers raised as they attended after-school seminars designed to help them become more familiar with the content areas they would be expected to teach. Throughout my observations of these contexts, and the ethnography completed by fellow researcher Maureen Reddy (1994), I noticed several things. First, the activities that the students completed in small groups were frequently organized around a "big idea" or theme (such as electricity). However, students worked in small groups on different investigations related to this theme, so that five or six small groups of students each focused on a different activity. Although adults were able to see the connections among these different activities, it was not clear to me that the children even understood that these activities were related. How were students supposed to make connections across activities without knowing what to pay attention to as they completed them? This was a driving question for me. A common focus for all children regardless of activities seemed like a possible solution to this dilemma.

In addition to this observation, I also noted that teachers commented on the challenge of organizing reporting sessions that occurred after the completion of these small-group activities. It is common to organize elementary science lessons into three parts: 1) introductory and orienting remarks from the teacher, 2) small-group investigations, and 3) reporting sessions designed to have students report about what they discovered in the small-group activities. Many teachers reported that as the unit progressed, the reporting sessions got shorter and shorter, not more elaborated and complex as we would have expected. Teachers also noted that it was difficult to get students to ask questions of one another during this reporting time. This comment was corroborated by my observations of actual classroom reporting sessions in which conversations during reporting time were almost exclusively between the teacher and the reporter. This worked well to accomplish some things, like giving specific kinds of guidance to individual students, but it frequently meant that the audience went on what Marion came to call "snooze control."

Teachers tried many strategies to get the students involved in asking questions of one another but felt that this was a struggle. It was clear to me that changing students' implicit assumption that it was the teacher's responsibility to ask questions was not going to be straightforward. How could we try to assist teachers to develop approaches to engage students in asking each other questions and discussing their ideas?

These questions surfaced for me as a researcher, and, as I was just at the point of working on my dissertation proposal, they provided an opportunity to put theory into practice. This is when I consulted Marion, who was the science facilitator at the school. She was a perfect person to consult and collaborate with in order to address these questions. She had many years of teaching experience with special education students where she had focused on using science as a vehicle to get them talking about their ideas. Marion's years of teaching experience, combined with my theoretical background, proved to be interesting complements to one another.

MARION'S "PRACTITIONER" PERSPECTIVE

When Leslie approached me to collaborate with her on her dissertation work, I felt that we shared many of the same concerns with respect to the implementation of the science program at my school. There had been many discussions between practitioners and researchers focused on the reporting portion of science. Both of us had witnessed rich conversation happening within the small groups themselves and could attest to students' active participation during this time. We observed students clarifying ideas through dialogue as well as manipulating the materials that were provided. We also had quantitative data to support these observations as it was a requirement that all teachers receive feedback on their teaching within the new program. Ironically, we witnessed these same lively, engaged children sitting passively during reporting, watching the teacher ask questions and clarify ideas throughout the oral reports. The contradictions between the children's behavior in each setting were staggering. It was even more surprising, given that the design of the science program removed the teacher from a traditional transmission role. Why then did students' active participation in one portion of the lesson give way to passive listening in another? Many of our private and public conversations grappled with the dilemma of how to get students involved in asking questions of one another in this portion of the science lesson.

As a practitioner and the science facilitator at the school, the contradictions of the classroom, given the overarching goals of the program, were intellectually and professionally motivating for me. My personal interests in classroom talk and children's construction of scientific knowledge were also emotionally tied to the children and the teachers at the school. I knew that Leslie's question of how to assist teachers to develop approaches to engage students in each other's ideas was of great significance and was ultimately tied to her deep respect for my colleagues and their students.

LESLIE'S INITIAL DESIGN: THEORETICAL BACKGROUND

The design of the intervention was first formulated based on my observations as noted above and on my background in Vygotskian approaches to learning and development. Before describing the actual design, it is necessary to understand the theoretical perspective that I brought with me as I attempted to think seriously about what I observed in the school.

Literature on classroom discourse suggests that there is one common speech pattern that tends to run throughout much of schooling, namely, Initiation-Response-Evaluation (IRE) sequences (Mehan, 1979; Sinclair & Coulthard, 1976). IRE sequences are different from other types of conversational exchanges that occur outside of school because the third turn involves the teacher's evaluation of a student's response. In order to judge a student's reply, it must be assumed that the teacher has asked a question to which s/he already knows the answer. Therefore, the teacher's question functions as a test question, one that examines and assesses a student's knowledge. This kind of question is not intended to help students build on their beginning knowledge, it simply functions to test what they already understand.

An important assumption that seems to guide the IRE or recitation-based interactions in schools involves the notion that cognitive processes take place in the minds of individuals alone. Therefore, it is necessary to probe and examine individuals' understanding of important facts and information. Recently in psychology and education the perspective of Vygotsky (1987) and neo-Vygotskians such as Rogoff (1990) and Wertsch (1991) have emphasized that this model of cognitive functioning is not the only possibility. Instead, an alternative conception involves viewing cognitive functioning as socially shared (Resnick, Levine, & Behrend, 1991) or distributed (Hutchins, 1995). As a result of this shift from individually to socially oriented perspectives, new alternatives for school practices must be considered.

Vygotsky was specifically interested in educational contexts and spent much of his life theorizing about and researching children's learning within this setting. One of Vygotsky's most crucial claims about human mental functioning is that the social plane of mental life is analytically prior to individual competence. This tenet is the cornerstone of his theory and is manifested in many ways throughout his research. He writes, "human learning presupposes a specific social nature and a process by which children grow into the intellectual life of those around them" (Vygotsky, 1978, p. 88).

Perhaps the most useful general formulation of Vygotsky's claim that the social plane of mental life precedes individual competence can be found in his "general genetic law of cultural development":

> Any function in the child's cultural development appears twice, or on two planes. First it appears on the social plane, and then on the psychological plane. First it appears between people as an intermental category, and then within the child as an intramental category. This is equally true with regard to voluntary attention, logical memory, the formation of concepts, and the development of volition. . . . It goes without saying that internalization transforms the process itself and changes its structure and functions. Social relations or relations among people genetically underlie all higher functions and their relationships. (Vygotsky, 1981, p. 163)

Vygotsky's perspective offers a new way of looking at interactions within school contexts. He suggests that children's mental processes are generated from the outside (through social interaction with more capable cultural members) and only later are they taken on and regulated by the children themselves. Therefore, the basis of human thinking resides in social life.

The work of Wertsch (1991) and Wertsch, Tulviste, & Hagstrom (1993) expands on Vygotsky's notion while at the same time providing a historical context from which to view his perspective. In their writings, Wertsch and colleagues argue that the tendency to view thinking and agency more generally as a property of individuals is a function of "unexamined cultural beliefs held by contemporary western psychologists" (Wertsch, Tulviste, & Hagstrom, 1993, p. 2). They propose that instead of viewing mind and agency as a property of individuals alone, it is necessary to reconceptualize this notion by recognizing the ways in which "mind [and agency] extend beyond the skin" (Wertsch, Tulviste, & Hagstrom, 1993, p. 2). In this regard, they propose that it is possible to view "individual" action as inherently social due to the culturally generated "mediational means," such as language or other tools, that are a crucial part of all human action.

Rogoff (1990) offers a perspective similar to that of Wertsch and colleagues. She proposes that using events or activities as units of analysis is more appropriate than isolating components such as the individual and the social world. She notes that, "Human activity involves the roles of both the individual and the social world, inseparably involved in the meaningful and purposeful events of life" (p. 28). She argues that learning and development take place as children participate in the culturally valued activities within their communities. She notes, "I take the perspective that learning is a process of *transformation of participation*, arguing that how people develop is a function of their *transforming roles* and *understanding in the activities* in which they participate" (Rogoff, 1994, p. 209, emphasis added).

DESIGNING AN INTERVENTION TO ENGAGE STUDENTS IN DISCUSSING THEIR IDEAS IN SCIENCE: LESLIE'S INITIAL PLAN

Although I designed the initial plan for the intervention, Marion and I recognized that if we were going to be able to change the implicit models of schooling that seemed to guide student interaction, we were going to have to work together closely to continue to refine and add to the initial structure that I established. This initial design had two parts, which corresponded to my concerns about giving students guidance across small-group activities and trying to find ways to help them become more engaged in asking questions and discussing ideas during reporting. First, I created a set of intellectual roles to help guide students to use important scientific thinking strategies including making predictions and coordinating claims with evidence. These roles were based on a review of the literature focusing on science teaching. Duschl (1990) and Kuhn (1993) argue that coordinating theories with evidence is an important aspect of scientific thinking; therefore three strategies were developed to support such thinking: 1) predicting and theorizing, 2) summarizing results, and 3) relating predictions and theories to results.

Second, these intellectual roles could become "audience roles" that students could assume during reporting. Thus, some students in the audience would be responsible for checking predictions and theories offered by the reporters, others would examine the summary of results, and the remaining audience members would focus on checking that reporters related their predictions, theories, and results. Using this design, the same set of roles would function to connect the small-group activities to one another and provide continuity between the small-group work time and the reporting sessions. They would also give every student the opportunity to take on the roles, first from the standpoint of building an explanation of their own small-group activity, and then in reviewing the explanations offered by other groups. These two different orientations would help support a more metacognitive stance among the students. Students would be asked to think and reflect on their own small-group work as well as that of others in the classroom. These two elements, in addition to a well-researched and developmentally organized curriculum focusing on balance and building, provided the basic building blocks for the intervention.

The study was organized to examine how the roles used in the small groups alone and the roles used in both the small-group and the reporting time together functioned to support student engagement and discussion of ideas in science. Given what we have already discussed, it might appear that we asked an unnecessary question. One would expect that the roles in both settings would support student engagement better than the roles used only during the small-group work time. This is a reasonable conclusion but one that may be a function of our own ability to see and reflect on the results that we actually obtained. At the time we designed the study, a very real question for us was, "Would the roles used in small-group time transfer naturally into the reporting sessions without the need for explicit role taking?" We also wondered if the role taking during the reporting sessions would function to constrain the conversations in such a way that students would not engage in asking deep and meaningful questions. We felt that there was the chance that students would not be more engaged, only more scripted. Thus, we truly sought to understand how these roles would function in both contexts.

In order to examine this question, two classes of 12 students each were assembled so that they did not differ with respect to gender, race, or standardized test scores. The lessons in both classes were organized according to the common format we discussed earlier. Whole-class introductory comments, small-group activities, and whole-class reporting sessions occurred every day. Students worked in groups of four to complete their small-group activities. Two students in each small group functioned as "reporters" while the other two students acted as "scribes." The reporters were responsible for presenting their group's activity orally to the whole class while the scribes were responsible for using large chart paper or other materials to organize relevant information that could be used by the reporters during the reporting session. These procedural roles rotated so that all small-group members had a chance to be a reporter and a scribe.

At the beginning of the intervention students in both classes were introduced to three intellectual roles mentioned above (i.e., predicting and theorizing, summarizing results, relating predictions and theories to results). These roles were used to guide students to produce explanations of scientific phenomena and provided the framework for discussion in both classes throughout all three segments of each lesson.

The one difference in the two classes focused on the assignment of these intellectual roles to audience members during the reporting segment of each lesson. Class 2 students were each assigned an "audience role" that corresponded to one of the intellectual roles used during the small-group work time. In Class 1 no special roles assignments were given to the audience members. These audience roles rotated such that all Class 2 students had multiple opportunities to adopt each of the roles (Herrenkohl & Guerra, 1998).

IMPLEMENTING THE INTERVENTION: MARION'S PERSPECTIVE

The initial intervention design was based on Leslie's background in a Vygotskian approach to learning and development. As a collaborator and partner in the translation of this theory into practice, it was crucial for me to continue to work closely with Leslie during the actual implementation. I knew that the set of intellectual roles was going to require ongoing thought and definition. The students and I, the collective "we," had the task of collaboratively constructing a common discourse that revolved around these new intellectual roles. The daily journal I kept during this period reflects my understanding of our approach at a theoretical and design level, while also revealing my concerns about how it would play out in practice. I struggled to find a way to make the "theoretical voice," "pedagogical voice," and "student voices" come together. What was it going to mean to construct a common discourse in service of a set of intellectual roles? Would it require both talk and text? Whose voice would get recognized in the restructuring of participants in a classroom? Ultimately, these questions surfaced for us all.

The dilemma of sitting in a practitioner's chair is having faith in children's abilities to rise to the challenge, but knowing that this process takes both time and apprenticeship. I was concerned that we were going to try and accomplish this in just 12 days. Therefore, I had to come up with some way for the students to take ownership of these roles in a relatively short period of time. In order to accomplish this I thought it was best to use "their words" in a public format that could serve them throughout the study. This kind of public documentation of student thinking could be displayed every day to help support the student to assume these new intellectual roles.

So, I began to develop a set of documents with the students, things we called "public text." We had three forms of public text that served important functions. The first and second forms functioned in both Class 1 and Class 2. A document was constructed with the students during one of the first sessions and served as a set of operational definitions for the intellectual roles. The students and I recorded information that would guide them to understand what we meant by prediction, theory, and results. This was an important exercise and the public display of this information helped guide the students as they struggled to put these concepts to work for themselves in their small-group activities.

The second form of public text that functioned in both classes was what we called our "theory chart." This chart helped us keep a running record of what the students were thinking over time. During reporting we recorded all new theories on this chart as they were developed and discussed by the groups. This chart allowed the students to see all of the theories that had been developed and draw on this information as they continued to work in their small groups. It also provided an opportunity for students to add onto or abandon theories over time. It both broadened and constrained the learning space. The theory chart was also another way to address Leslie's first concern about giving students guidance about what to focus on across activities.

The third form of public text was used only in Class 2, as it was related to helping students take on the intellectual audience roles during reporting. In some ways, this was my first concern. I was convinced that the students would develop an understanding of the conceptual content (i.e., theories, etc.) but I was less sure of how they would respond to these new roles during reporting time. I wondered how they would formulate questions and what they would focus on. So, I developed a "questions chart" to help acclimate students to the audience roles. We spent time one day generating questions that students could ask if they were taking on the roles. We went through each of the roles separately and recorded all the questions that the students could generate. This chart was then displayed during every reporting session so that students could use it to guide their questioning.

I really wondered if this public document would act as a mediational tool to change students' assumptions about the participant structure of the classroom. The answer to my question came on May 21, 1994. "Where do you find your theory in your results?" asked Tina. Her words did not originate from me as the teacher, but rather from one of her classmates, Olivia. Olivia had offered this question to the class as one that might be helpful to ask when in the role of checking the relationship between predictions, theories and results. The class had discussed and agreed that this question was a tool that could be used and understood by all. As a result, it was added to the questions chart for that intellectual audience role. In the beginning this questions chart proved to be a crucial resource for the students, but as time passed, the students did not always need to refer to the chart and many students began to ask questions that were not included there. Tina's use of Olivia's question signaled for me that this was to be an eventful collaboration between student and student, student and teacher, and teacher and researcher.

FINDINGS

The findings that we report about briefly here have been discussed in depth elsewhere (Herrenkohl & Guerra, 1998; and Herrenkohl & Wertsch, 1999). Analyses of transcribed classroom discussions during the whole-class reporting time revealed obvious differences between Class 1 and Class 2. Students in Class 2 who were instructed in the use of the intellectual roles during both small-group work time and reporting sessions were much more engaged in discussion and in building scientific explanations. Students in this group were more likely to ask questions of other students; to monitor their own comprehension of the ideas presented by others; to share responsibility for negotiating, defining, and distributing the cognitive work among classroom members; to coordinate theories and evidence; and to challenge one another's explanations. The roles did not function to script the discussion during reporting time, they seemed to provide a focus and direction for more extended and spontaneous discussion of ideas that the students were contemplating (see Herrenkohl & Guerra, 1999, for more extensive discussion of the differences between Class 1 and Class 2).

Class 2 provided a setting in which children took over much of the responsibility for asking questions that the teacher carried almost exclusively in Class 1. Students in Class 2 asked 226 questions over the time of the intervention while students in Class 1 asked only 3. The intellectual roles used during small-group work time were not used spontaneously in the reporting sessions by Class 1 students. Students in Class 1 were never instructed not to ask questions, so this difference between the classes is quite striking and in some ways surprising. It would be a mistake to conclude that the level of questioning that we observed in Class 2 emerged easily and immediately at the outset of the study though. Many students needed a good deal of time to become accustomed to taking on the intellectual audience roles (as the description of the questions chart underscores). Various forms of encouragement and support, including the forms of public text discussed earlier, were necessary for the children to go through this transition. These findings also suggest that a set of "default" audience roles resembling Mehan's (1979) transmission model of "teacher initiation-student response-teacher evaluation" existed for students in Class 1. In this model students are responsible for responding to the teacher while the teacher is responsible for questioning and evaluating student knowledge. Without explicit attempts to guide students to take on other roles during this whole-class time, standard expectations for school-based conversation seemed to guide patterns of student participation.

Through examining the difference in student questioning patterns across Class 1 and Class 2, however, it is obvious that children in Class 2 did indeed come to engage in interaction on the basis of a quite different set of roles than those found in Class 1. The large difference between Class 1 and Class 2 does not derive from instances in which individual children were responding to directives by the teacher to ask questions. Instead, it reflects differences in how children more or less spontaneously posed questions. We take this to be evidence that children in Class 2 came to appropriate the intellectual audience roles provided in the setting, while students in Class 1 did not seem to spontaneously carry the intellectual roles that they used in their small-group work time into the reporting sessions. These findings from the study itself can be understood further by combining them with the observations that Marion made after the study was completed.

MARION'S OBSERVATIONS OF THE STUDENTS AFTER THE STUDY WAS COMPLETED

One of the great advantages of being the science facilitator at a school is that you get to see students in many different settings. I was fortunate because I continued to observe and interact with the students. They were in fourth grade when we began our work. I had two more years to follow their progress before they left our school for middle school. I will share some of the anecdotal findings that I witnessed as I watched these students engage in new contexts.

Olivia and Susan

The summer following our project many of the children attended a two-week Summer Institute for local teachers. During this institute, participating teachers taught a practicum lesson and received feedback from a certified provider. The feedback consisted of using a standardized classroom observation instrument and an instrument that I developed. As a feedback provider for the summer institute, I witnessed the spontaneous discussion and use of the intellectual roles by Olivia and Susan. Olivia was a Class 2 student while Susan was a Class 1 student in our study. Both of them clearly explained the roles to their small-group members. Not only did the children talk about the intellectual roles but they then constructed their oral reports in such a way that they included predictions, theories, and results.

Emma

During our study, Emma was one of the students who remained quiet until the 8th day of our 12-day intervention. She was always cooperative and on task but tended to be more quiet and shy than the other students. Several months after our project was completed, during the fall of the following school year, our school was visited by a NASA astronaut who happened to live in our area. His program was presented to an audience consisting of the fourth-, fifth-, and sixth-grade students. Dr. Sacco talked to the students about his experience by using slides and conducted a question-and-answer period following the slide show. Prior to the session, I introduced Dr. Sacco to the children and told him that from my experience there were many children present who asked very good questions of each other during science and would therefore be able to ask questions of Dr. Sacco as well. Emma raised her hand with a huge smile on her face and asked the first question of the day. There were more than 200 students present, so it took courage for Emma to step forward to ask her question.

Christie

One of the most poignant experiences came two years after the initial intervention. I had the opportunity to work with Christie in science as a sixth-grade student. Her story seems to embody the theoretical underpinnings of the intervention.

Over the course of the spring 1996 semester, Christie became quite intent on the idea that once you had a beginning understanding of the subject matter presented, there was a tension between that conceptual understanding and the role of predicting. It appeared that her initial definition of prediction centered around the notion that a prediction was made without any prior subject matter exposure. In short, it was a guess.

Two years later, many mornings during the semester were spent discussing and exploring the parameters of predicting as a process. Was there a developmental sequence of sorts at work over time in each of the science units being presented? Could we challenge our own definitions in search of a collective one? How were we all going to agree about what it meant to predict? The discussions were written down as public text and used by Christie and the rest of the class as a working document. In some cases the morning discussion spilled over into Christie's small groups. I taped and transcribed these conversations and found that she was concerned with the fact that each new activity was tied conceptually to the previous activity which made it impossible for her to use her model of a prediction as a "guess" more than once per unit. Christie engaged other students in this notion over the many weeks and enriched our thinking greatly. As I reflected on the tapes, I began to think that she had taken seriously her role as an intellectual audience member and had generalized it to include all portions of science classroom experiences. She was actively engaged in thinking and asking questions of other group members. It also struck me that Christie's implicit assumption was that it was the responsibility of students as well as teachers to refine thinking as it became necessary.

IMPLICATIONS OF OUR STUDY FOR UNDERSTANDING PARTNERSHIPS AMONG TEACHERS AND RESEARCHERS

One of the most important ingredients in our ability to carry out an interesting and informative study was our effort to work together as a team, with both of us striving to put theory into practice and then making sense out of what we observed. Typically, research is criticized for small sample sizes and the participation of only one teacher, both of which characterized our work. These critiques are certainly warranted, and we do not claim that one would be able to replicate these results with any teacher in any school with any students. However, these criticisms are also what make this research particularly interesting, not for its power to generalize but for its specificity and example of a successful collaborative research effort between a teacher and a researcher. Collaborations such as ours are not common. They are not easy to establish and maintain; therefore, we would like to offer our own analysis regarding what helped to make our collaboration possible. In some ways these suggestions are not substantially different from those that one would follow to develop any successful relationship, but we think that it is first and foremost important to recognize that in addition to doing research and teaching we were also building a relationship. This process takes time and effort, which might explain why there are not more partnerships like ours, but we feel that the effort is well rewarded.

Factors That Promote Successful Teacher–Researcher Collaborations

Many forces work against those of us who wish to bridge different communities in order to inform both theory and practice. Some of the most fundamental stumbling blocks that we encounter are our own language and cultural practices. As noted in the introduction to this volume, one of the most obvious constraints is the expectation that research is carried out on "subjects," not partners. Mary Catherine Bateson, in her book entitled *Composing a Life* (1990), eloquently comments on the challenges that she faced when trying to capture the essence of the relationship that she had with the women she describes in her book.

> When I search for a word for my relationship with the women described in this book, I feel a need for a term that would assert both collegiality and the fact that the process is made possible by our differences. The thesaurus betrays me, denying me a term that affirms both symmetry and complementarity. The gap in the language parallels a gap in the culture. We are rich in words that describe symmetrical relationships, from buddy to rival to colleague. We are also rich in words that describe strongly asymmetrical relationships, many of which imply hierarchy and have curious undertones of exploitation and dominance. (p. 102)

Whenever we read this quote, we think Bateson must have been thinking about teacher–researcher partnerships like ours as well. We attempt to respond to the gaps in our language and culture, to make a place for our truly complementary relationship. Our interest in recognizing and valuing the different contributions both of us make to the other requires us to remember that we do not have to speak in one voice, but that our voices in dialogue provide a more complete picture than we would have had otherwise. These conversations are steeped in the knowledge, experience, and perspectives of both worlds. Realizing that the richness cannot be found exclusively in either world is perhaps the hallmark of a successful collaboration. Knowing in advance that successful collaborations push the limits of contemporary language and culture, and therefore create new challenges at every turn, is also crucial.

In order to truly appreciate the ways in which our separate perspectives illuminate one another, it was important for us to create a space that was "ours" together. We came to our project from different communities, but worked within a shared context with children that we considered to be "our" students. In this way we could begin to understand each other's perspectives in a context that was meaningful and known to both of us. It is in this kind of setting that we believe it is possible to truly begin to value each other's voices and respond to each other's ideas. This context required us to make sense of what we were saw and experienced together. It forced us to step outside of our own areas of expertise and recognize the blind spots in our own thinking. We had to think hard about the limits of our own understanding and we had to be willing to let the other push those limits. Although we can clearly identify the roles of teacher and researcher in our collaboration, we can also identify that special space defined by what happened to us together in our joint quest for meaning and understanding.

There are at least two essential ingredients, from our perspective, that make this kind of shared space a reality. The first is a personal and professional commitment to education that supports all learners. Without this, our project would never have materialized. We both believed that our efforts were and continue to be directed toward making educational environments better for students.

The second important ingredient is trust. Without this, the whole enterprise falls apart. We both needed to know that in addition to wanting the best for our students, we also wanted the best for each other. Thus, all commendations, constructive criticisms, and challenges could come from the perspective of supporting each other to be better thinkers, teachers, and researchers ourselves. Our comments to one another carried a strong note of appreciation for and open mindedness to the way that each collaborator practiced her individual craft, while at the same time being very honest about our own perspectives and ideas.

Finally, we think that an important part of a partnership is that it continues even when the immediate project is completed. We have both taken so much more from this project than we ever anticipated. It is common for each of us to actually feel the presence of the other in the work that we now do separately over 3,000 miles away from one another. For Marion, the use of intellectual roles and the students' construction of knowledge has inspired her to think deeply about critical assessment issues in science. She has continued to use the theoretical underpinnings of our work together to develop assessment tools for teachers as well as students in her school community. The process of the students apprenticing into their intellectual roles in service of theory construction and conceptual understanding compels her to push further what is commonly defined as "worthy of assessment." Instead of focusing on products alone, Marion now has teachers noting important patterns of talk and interaction in small groups that we have found to lead to a deeper understanding of and engagement in the scientific ideas being discussed.

Leslie's work has continued to examine how to create lively intellectual communities of young science learners. She has relied heavily on the findings of our collective work in designing her current program. She has especially focused on Marion's idea of public documentation, especially the theory chart, and has dedicated days in current programs to a "theory chart review" so that students can actively evaluate their developing theories together.

We do not usually thank one another for relationships and commitments in life, we work at them and hope they flourish. Yet, it is difficult not to write in terms of gratitude toward one another. Research partnerships are no less worthy of the commitment, respect, trust, and hard work than our personal relationships. Marion's mother used to tell her that, "in life we must nourish the soul." Collaborations across professional lines nourish our souls as much as our minds. They create opportunities to find out more about ourselves, our partners, and in our case, our students. They are not easy to develop or maintain, but they are deeply rewarding and certainly worth pursuing.

REFERENCES

Airasian, P. W., & Walsh, M. E. (1997, February). Constructivist cautions. *Phi Delta Kappan,* 444–449.

Bateson, M. C. (1989). *Composing a life.* New York: Atlantic Monthly Press.

Duschl, R. A. (1990). *Restructuring science education: The importance of theories and their development.* New York: Teachers College Press.

Gardner, H. (1991). *The unschooled mind: How children think and how schools should teach.* New York: Basic Books.

Herrenkohl, L. R., & Guerra, M. R. (1998). Participant structures, scientific discourse, and student engagement in fourth grade. *Cognition and Instruction, 16,* 433–475.

Herrenkohl, L. R., & Wertsch, J. V. (1999). The use of cultural tools: Mastery and appropriation. In I. Sigel (Ed.), *Theoretical perspectives in the development of representational (symbolic) thought* (pp. 415–435). Hillsdale, NJ: Lawrence Erlbaum.

Hutchins, E. (1995). *Cognition in the wild.* Cambridge, MA: MIT Press.

Kuhn, D. (1993). Science as argument: Implications for teaching and learning scientific thinking. *Science Education, 77,* 319–337.

Mehan, H. (1979). *Learning lessons.* Cambridge, MA: Harvard University Press.

Moll, L. C., & Greenberg, J. B. (1990). Creating zones of possibilities: Combining social contexts for instruction. In L. C. Moll (Ed.), *Vygotsky and education: Instructional implication and applications of sociohistorical psychology* (pp. 319–348). Cambridge, UK: Cambridge University Press.

Reddy, M. (1994). *Becoming second grade scientists: A discourse analysis of science discussions.* Unpublished doctoral dissertation, Harvard University, Cambridge.

Resnick, L. D., Levine, J. M., & Behrend, S. (Eds.). (1991). *Perspectives on socially shared cognition.* Washington, DC: American Psychological Association.

Rogoff, B. (1990). *Apprenticeship in thinking: Cognitive development in social context.* New York: Oxford University Press.

Rogoff, B. (1994). Developing understanding of the idea of communities of learners. *Mind, Culture, and Activity: An International Journal, 1,* 209–229.

Sinclair, J. M., & Coulthard, R. M. (1976). *Toward an analysis of discourse: The English used by teachers and pupils.* London: Oxford University Press.

Tharp, R. G., & Gallimore, R. (1988). *Rousing minds to life: Teaching, learning, and schooling in social context.* Cambridge, MA: Cambridge University Press.

Vygotsky, L. S. (1978). *Mind in society: The development of higher psychological processes.* Cambridge: Harvard University Press.

Vygotsky, L. S. (1981). The genesis of higher mental functions. In J. V. Wertsch (Ed.), *The concept of activity in Soviet psychology.* Armonk, NY: M. E. Sharpe.

Vygotsky, L. S. (1987). *The collected works of L.S. Vygotsky* (N. Minick, Trans.). (Vol. 1). New York: Plenum.

Wertsch, J. V. (1991). *Voices of the mind.* Cambridge, MA: Harvard University Press.

Wertsch, J. V., Tulviste, P., & Hagstrom, F. (1993). A sociocultural approach to agency. In E. Forman, N. Minick, & C. A. Stone (Eds.), *Contexts for learning: Sociocultural dynamics in children's development.* New York: Oxford University Press.

part III
The Partnership Approach in Clinical Settings

15

STRIVING FOR DOCTOR–PATIENT PARTNERSHIPS IN OBSTETRICS AND GYNECOLOGY

Barbara Noel Dowds
Regis College and
University of Massachusetts Medical School

ABSTRACT

This chapter describes a model for doctor–patient partnerships, argues for the usefulness of such partnerships in the specialty of obstetrics-gynecology, and presents one approach to teaching obstetrical-gynecological residents about their interactions with patients. Then doctor–patient relationships are discussed, using examples of interactions that exemplify the partnership model (either through its occurrence or its absence). Particular attention is paid to communication, mutual problem solving, and educating patients in the partnership model.

Some readers might wonder whether a meaningful partnership with physicians that goes beyond lip-service is even a possibility, especially if they have experienced or heard of horrific doctor–patient interactions in which the patient's views, or even selfhood, seem not to matter. A cardiologist, in front of the patient's family, may refer to a patient as "the MI in room 12, who presents an interesting challenge"; an internist may describe a patient who fears leaving home because of her colitis as "hysterical and lazy"; an obstetrician may reassure his patient that she will still be able to wear a bikini because of the care he took in cutting and sewing her abdomen, somehow ignoring the large, raised, red scar from a prior surgery extending to the top of her abdomen. These examples illustrate the "egocentric predicament" in which the professional is constrained by his/her perceptions, cognitions, and habits. They also illustrate the need for physicians to strive toward a partnership with patients in which the perspective and selfhood of each patient is valued and respected (see Chapter 10 for a discussion of the central role of respect in ethically informed interactions).

PARTNERSHIP MODEL

In the partnership model of doctor–patient relationships, as in research and teaching partnerships, the physician's expertise remains a critical and valued component of the relationship. Physician and patient are not "equal"; rather they complement one another. The partnership model presumes that physicians must be highly knowledgeable about and technically proficient in the biomedical and surgical aspects of their specialty. In addition to this expertise, the partnership model emphasizes expertise in communication and interpersonal skills. Besides increasing the likelihood that patients are satisfied with and actively participate in their health care (e.g., Bartlett et al., 1984; DiMatteo, Hays & Prince, 1986; Squier, 1990), these communication and interpersonal skills enhance the physician's ability to form partnerships with patients. Since physicians are not mind readers, they must elicit the patient's questions as well as feedback on the answers they give and the treatments they recommend. This dialogical back and forth is necessary if physicians are to achieve an effective partnership with their patients.

The partnership model, with its emphasis on communication, explicitly recognizes the importance of the patient's contribution to the relationship. For example, patients must be willing to ask their questions, to give voice to their concerns and fears, to answer honestly and completely the doctor's questions, and to provide feedback to their doctor, especially about proposed and ongoing treatment regimens. Patients' interpretations of bodily sensations; their beliefs about health, illness, and treatment; and their psychosocial context are all potentially important to their medical care. Although physicians are "body readers" and have access to information about the patient's body that the patient may well not know, patients have information, not only about their subjective experience of suffering and illness (Cassell, 1991), but also about their life-world (Mishler, 1984). The attitudinal atmosphere of a partnership relationship makes it possible for patients to share this information with their physicians and to work with their physicians in order to achieve treatment plans that are mutually satisfactory and "do-able." For example, a patient may have doubts about the practicality of the treatment plan suggested by the physician, given that patient's particular circumstances. Or a patient may have fears and worries about the illness and its treatment, based either on misconceptions or on "valid" understandings. Either way, from within the framework of the partnership model, patients need to be able to express these concerns to their physicians.

In brief, I suggest a more symmetrical and reciprocal approach to doctor–patient relationships because such a relationship maximizes the active involvement and contributions of both partners. In these relationships, not only are the physician's questions recognized as important, but so are the patient's questions and concerns. Both the physician and the patient should have the opportunity, and be encouraged, to respond with feedback to the other's answers and ideas. This back-and-forth dialogical process is the physician–patient partnership in action. I believe that such a partnership maximizes the possibility of good medical care and that the resultant mutually agreed-upon treatment plans have a higher probability of being carried out than those that are made without the patient's input. However, it must be acknowledged that achieving such a partnership, given the power differential between physician and patient and their traditional roles, is far from easy; in fact, striving for such a partnership is a radical shift from much current practice in medicine.

NEED FOR PARTNERSHIP IN OBSTETRICS AND GYNECOLOGY

Medical school education and residency training primarily focus on biomedical knowledge and technical skills. Typically, little emphasis is given to doctor–patient relationships, except in a few disciplines such as family practice and psychiatry. Yet good doctor–patient relationships are as important for obstetrics-gynecology as for any discipline (cf. Coonar, Dooley, Daniels, & Taylor, 1991), and especially so to the extent that obstetrical-gynecological physicians provide primary care to patients. Many aspects of obstetrical-gynecological care require patients' active involvement, from following the guidelines for regular pap smears and mammograms, to using reliably several of the available methods of birth control, to keeping prenatal appointments and following current medical recommendations for a healthy pregnancy. Moreover, as Squier (1990) has argued, the doctor–patient relationship may be especially important "in the early stages of a life threatening condition" (p. 325), a situation that occurs, for instance, when a gynecologist cares for patients who are found to have ovarian cancer. Finally, in some clinics, obstetrical-gynecological physicians are now classified as primary care providers and thus must attend to the whole person. From my perspective, however, even without this mandate, a woman is a whole person, not just something to be treated from the waist down, (as if "from the waist down" were somehow disembodied from the woman's selfhood). I believe implementation of the partnership model validates the patient's selfhood, enhances doctor–patient relationships, and increases the patient's participation in her own health care.

TEACHING RESIDENTS

Teaching residents about doctor–patient interactions became an explicit component of the obstetrical-gynecological residency program at the University of Massachusetts Medical School when the chair of the department recruited me to work with residents one half-day a week. I have worked in a variety of the residents' clinics, including continuity clinics in which the residents follow their own patients on an ongoing basis, high-risk obstetrical clinics in which patients have complicating conditions such as diabetes mellitus or substance abuse, and pre-operative clinics in which the residents see patients shortly before surgery to take the appropriate history, perform a physical exam, and obtain informed consent. The residents with whom I have worked have been at all levels of training, from first-year interns to fourth-year chiefs. I typically work with one resident each week for six-week intervals. The resident obtains the patient's permission for me to observe. In four years, only a few patients have chosen not to have me in the room.

After observing doctor–patient interactions, I provide feedback to the resident. Residents are also encouraged to present cases they would like to discuss and we occasionally role-play doctor–patient interactions. My relationship to the residents is more similar to a teacher–student relationship than to a doctor–patient relationship. The residents are learning their specialty, obstetrics and gynecology, and I am a faculty member in that department. However, in some respects, my interaction with the residents models a partnership relationship for the doctor that may be useful in his or her interactions with patients. For example, within the constraints of the resident's and the clinic's schedule, I solicit the resident's questions and feedback, a process that is applicable to both teaching and clinical interactions.

Just as the context of patients' lives is an important consideration in the doctor–patient relationship, the context of residents' lives is important in my relationship with them. Residents have demanding schedules and often report feeling pressured and, at times, overwhelmed. In working with them, I try to minimize their sense of being judged. However, this is somewhat of "an uphill battle" because evaluation is such a prevalent concern in our society. A resident is likely to say "Oh, you're here to evaluate me today." Perhaps one patient best captured the preoccupation with ratings, when at the end of the visit, she jokingly asked me, "What grade does she [the resident] get?" The residents are not graded, which removes one barrier to developing a partnership with them (cf. Chapter 11 for a discussion of grades as an impediment to partnerships). The residents are told, quite honestly, that this is an opportunity for them to receive feedback on their interactions with patients, with the feedback being given to them but not to any of their medical faculty. I believe learning, particularly learning communication and interpersonal skills, is more likely to occur in a nonevaluative context than in one in which the resident feels judged and subject to evaluation.

Another important context is the clinic in which the resident is observed. I must be able to work with the resident without slowing down the clinic. Although this requires some creativity, it can be accomplished. In most clinics, I discuss doctor–patient interactions after all the patients have been seen; in one, feedback was provided between patients. This latter approach requires a high degree of succinctness. It has the advantage of immediate feedback and therefore may be a better teaching/learning strategy. However, it has the disadvantage of potentially disrupting the flow of the clinic.

As is true in all partnerships, working with residents requires mutual accommodation. Residents accommodate to being "shadowed" by someone from a different discipline; I accommodate to their differing individual styles and varying levels of exhaustion and receptivity to feedback. Moreover, consistent with the partnership model, where and with whom I work has been influenced by feedback from the residents. For example, I briefly worked in the "night float" clinic, that is, in the morning clinic with the resident who had been in the hospital on call to see patients the night before and who will again be on call for the next three nights. The residents were quick to let me know that this was the worst time to work with them. Currently I work with "first years." One of the "fourth years," with whom I had worked both at the beginning and end of his training, had suggested this because he thought styles of interacting with patients were less ingrained and more flexible earlier in residency training (cf. Byrne & Long, 1976 for data on and a discussion of the inflexibility of most doctor–patient interactions).

DOCTOR–PATIENT RELATIONSHIPS/PARTNERSHIPS

This section begins with three clinical examples, illustrating 1) a doctor–patient partnership in the context of an ongoing relationship, 2) a doctor–patient partnership in a relationship that consists of a single visit, and 3) a doctor–patient interaction that dramatically portrays the antithesis of a partnership ideal. I then address multiple aspects of the doctor–patient relationship from the perspective of the partnership model and conclude with a succinct summary of what a physician can aim for when working in partnership with his/her patients.

One of the residents had an ongoing relationship with a patient who had a long history of abusing multiple illegal drugs. The patient had first started seeing the physician shortly after becoming "clean." The resident, in the course of the patient's medical visits, had learned about her past struggles and how she had been able to implement some positive changes in her life. Over time, they had developed a relationship of mutual respect and caring. The affective tone of their communication was warm and often humorous. The patient was comfortable asking questions about her own health ("Yeah, but how'd I get it?"), and the physician answered them thoroughly, making sure the patient understood her answers and seeing if her answers generated any further questions. In working with this patient, the physician viewed treatment planning as a "we" process ("Let's see what we can come up with"). She tried to ensure that the patient understood why she was recommending a particular approach. She asked for the patient's feedback on treatment recommendations ("What do you think of this idea?"), and, if the patient indicated that she did not think it would be easy to do, they "brainstormed" about other approaches to the problem.

One resident in the preoperative clinic saw a patient who had been referred by another health facility for a tubal ligation. As the physician began to explain the procedure, she picked up on the patient's ambivalence and probed further ("You look like you're not sure about this"). Although the patient's response was somewhat tentative and inarticulate, the physician took the time to pursue the issue. As they engaged in a mutual exchange of questions and answers, it became clear that the patient had major reservations about the permanency of a tubal ligation and that there were other viable options that were appropriate for the patient. Together they concluded, given the patient's life context and goals, that an IUD would be an appropriate method of birth control for the patient. This one visit interaction vividly illustrates the importance of a bidirectional flow of questions and answers. It demonstrates that productive, mutual problem solving can occur, and, indeed, should occur, in consultation clinics as well as continuity clinics, with or without an ongoing relationship, with or without a warm affective relationship, with or without the patient having a "good" vocabulary, a high level of education, or other "desirable" demographic characteristics.

In the final example, a secretary in the clinic contacted one of the residents because a patient, who had recently given birth, was on the phone and quite upset because she had "lost her baby" over the weekend. In the conversation, the physician assumed, based on what the secretary had told her and the patient's distress, that the baby had died. When the physician asked if the baby had been sick, the patient responded that it was "a long story." The patient continued to describe how upset she was and asked the doctor to prescribe an antidepressant. The patient and doctor talked at length. However, it was a confusing conversation, and the clinic staff suggested that the physician follow up by calling the patient's pediatrician. Neither the pediatrician nor the local hospital in the town in which the patient lived knew anything about the death. A call to the police and to a friend of the patient's revealed that the Department of Social Services had taken the baby sometime during the weekend.

In the first two doctor–patient interactions, which exemplify partnerships, the physicians "heard" the patient's questions, understood the patient's life context, and solicited the patients' feedback on treatment options. The patients were willing to ask and answer questions, to "hear" the doctors' responses (and the doctors' own questions), and to engage in a dialogue about proposed treatment possibilities, going back and forth, with both doctor and patient presenting ideas, questioning, and responding until an option that made sense to both was chosen. In the first case, this was accomplished within the context of an ongoing, positive, mutually caring relationship. Its success was based on this, as well as on the quality of their communication. In the second case, the partnership occurred within a doctor–

patient relationship that consisted of a single visit. Its success was based on careful listening by the physician and on a willingness by the patient to try to express her views. In the third example, which was framed by the initial message from a secretary and the ambiguity of language, neither the doctor nor the patient was able to "hear" the other, neither got feedback from the other, or checked to make sure they were "on the same wave length." There was no dialogue, with mutual give and take. Instead there were two soliloquies.

Verbal and Nonverbal Communication in the Doctor–Patient Relationship

Communication is central to the development of a partnership between physician and patient. In a meta-analysis of the literature, Hall, Roter, & Katz (1988) reported that good doctor–patient communication was strongly related to patient satisfaction. Of particular interest here, Bertakis, Roter, & Putman (1991) found that increasing patient satisfaction was associated with decreasing physician dominance during the medical appointment. It may be that by decreasing the power differential between physician and patient, one obstacle to more effective communication and to a more positive relationship is diminished. In parallel, patients' active participation in the visit has been positively related to patient satisfaction (Brody, Miller, Lerman, Smith, & Caputo, 1989).

Patient satisfaction and recall have been found to mediate between quality of physicians' interpersonal skills and patients' adherence (Bartlett et al., 1984). Other predictors of patient adherence include doctors' providing information (Roter, 1989), physicians' clear, informative communications (DiMatteo & DiNicola,1982), and physicians' communications that are patient centered (Steward, 1984). In general, in a number of settings, good doctor–patient communication has been found to be related to better adherence (Hall, Roter, & Katz, 1988; Inui, Yourtree, & Williamson, 1976; Korsch & Negrete, 1972; Roter, 1977; Schulman, 1979).

Good health outcomes have also been found to be positively related to good doctor–patient communication (Bass et al., 1986; Greenfield, Kaplan, & Ware, 1985, 1988; Headache Study Group of the University of Western Ontario, 1986; Heszen-Klemens & Kapinska, 1984; Orth, Stiles, Scherwitz, Hennrikus, & Valbona, 1987). Finally, more knowledgeable, informed patients who actively participate in the medical appointment are more likely to have positive health outcomes (Brody, Miller, Lerman, Smith, & Caputo, 1989; Greenfield, Kaplan, & Ware, 1985; Kaplan, Greenfield, & Ware, 1989; Speedling & Rose, 1985).

Good doctor–patient communication, including active patient participation, is consistent with the dialogical back and forth between doctor and patient which is the process of partnership. Yet spoken words alone do not fully constitute the communication between two people. In addition to words, we communicate nonverbally, with our eyes, our gestures, and our body language, as well as with the tone of our voice and the speed of our utterances. Physicians' nonverbal skills have been found to be related to patient satisfaction (DiMatteo, Hays, & Prince, 1986; DiMatteo, Taranta, & Friedman, 1980) and to effective patient care (Milmoe, Rosenthal, Blane, Chafetz, & Wolf, 1967). In the partnership model, it is important for physicians to attend to how they communicate with a patient, both verbally and nonverbally, and to attend to how the patient communicates with them, both verbally and nonverbally.

As the example of the patient who was referred for a tubal ligation illustrated, attending to the patient's nonverbal communication can give clues to a patient's ambivalence. Patients are also likely to express fear or lack of comprehension nonverbally. When physicians "see" these communications from their patient, they can respond appropriately. For example, one physician, after a pelvic exam, used the word "disease" in describing a bacterial infection. Fortunately for the patient, the physician was attentive to the patient's nonverbal signals and beautifully picked up on the patient's discomfort with the term "disease." After a brief back and forth, the physician realized that while from the medical perspective, "disease" meant "syndrome," from the patient's perspective, "disease" meant "sexually transmitted disease."

That the patient initially had a different understanding of "disease" than the physician illustrates the importance of the physician's own language. Medical terminology can be confusing. Much of it is also likely to be unfamiliar to the patient. And some of it can sound judgmental. For example, "She failed her diet," may be okay in consulting with other health care professionals, but should be avoided in talking with the patient. Other examples that may seem judgmental to the patient include "incompetent cervix," "advanced maternal age," and "failed Glucose Tolerance Test."

A common finding in a pelvic exam, often reported to the patient as an offhand remark, provides the opportunity either for the patient to become confused and worried or to become more knowledgeable about her body. The physician may comment to a patient, "Your uterus is tipped," and say nothing more about this finding. Using a partnership approach, the physician does not stop here, but goes on to explain that this is normal and that many women have a "tipped" uterus. Without this further explanation, patients may hear the doctor's observation as "oh, there's something wrong with me." In general, there is a greater completeness to the information physicians convey when they strive for partnerships with their patients. This gives the patient the opportunity to learn from her physician, and the physician has shown respect for the patient by more fully engaging her in her own care.

Even in everyday vocabulary, the physician's language influences the doctor–patient relationship. If, for example, a doctor tells a patient that taking an antibiotic for 4 days out of 10 is "not bad," that response does not maximize a partnership relationship. From a partnership perspective, it would be better to let the patient know it was good that she filled the prescription, to explore with her why she stopped taking it, to educate her about why it is important for her to finish all of a prescription, and, depending on why she stopped the medication, to suggest other possibilities than discontinuance. Thus, even a situation that might be viewed as "noncompliant" provides an opportunity for a back-and-forth dialogue between physician and patient, for the development of a partnership between physician and patient.

Although it is good to empathize with patients, it is probably not helpful for the physician to be unnecessarily negative about exams and procedures. For example, describing the cold gel used in a pelvic exam as "torture" is likely to heighten the patient's anxiety without giving her any useful information. From a partnership perspective, the physician is encouraged to reframe such communications in a more positive, yet accurate and informative direction, e.g., "This will feel cold, but it will enable me to. . . ." If the patient has never had a pelvic exam before, the physician might say "Some people feel pressure, some find it uncomfortable, some don't feel any discomfort. Please let me know how you feel. The gel I use is cold, but exam enables me to. . . ." Such an approach provides the patient with accurate expectations, encourages the patient to provide feedback to her physician, and gives the physician an opportunity to teach the patient about her body (by explaining the purpose of the exam). At the end of the exam, the physician can ask the patient if she has any questions about the exam. The pelvic exam thus affords the physician an excellent opportunity to implement the partnership model, by soliciting the patient's questions and feedback and by providing her with information about her body and her medical care. Further, from a developmental perspective, such an approach to the pelvic exam maintains the differentiation of self and other (Werner, 1948; Werner & Kaplan, 1963). That is, although the resident herself may have experienced cold gel as "torture" when she has had pelvic exams, she is not, in the rephrased communication, presuming that her patient will experience it the same way. Rather than an over-identification with the patient, which can be seen as a violation of self/other differentiation, her empathy for the patient's experience now respects the patient's own experience of the exam.

One simple way to enhance communication and facilitate the development of a partnership is to use the patient's words. This lets her know that she has been "heard." For example, if a patient says, "I got this pain an' it's real uncomfortable," the doctor can respond by asking the patient to "describe the 'uncomfortable pain.' What's it like?" Or if a patient says she's "worried sick" about going for a referral, the physician can say, "I'm sorry you're 'worried sick' about going, but it will really help us understand what's happening." If needed, the physician can further pursue the patient's concerns or describe other patients' positive experiences with this kind of referral.

The physician's nonverbal communication is also important. If a patient has, for example, achieved good control of her blood sugars, the physician should ideally make eye contact with the patient, not the chart, when letting her know she did a good job. Moreover, this example presents the physician with an excellent opportunity to develop further a partnership with the patient, by asking the patient how she was able to achieve such good control. When the patient answers this question, she is able to hear herself being "the expert" about controlling blood sugars. The doctor can let the patient know that "Many patients have difficulty achieving such good control. I'll remember to tell them the approach you used. It might help them too." Here the patient is the teacher, the doctor is the learner, and what the doctor learns may indeed be helpful in working with other patients who are struggling to achieve good control of their blood sugars. This exchange illustrates both reciprocal altruism, with its "give and take" between physician and patient and by-product mutualism (Mesterton-Gibbons & Dugatkin, 1997), with the doctor's concern for many patients, not just this patient.

To illustrate further the applicability of the partnership model to doctor–patient interactions, I present several typical interchanges between physician and patient. Then I describe how these typical communications can be changed to increase the information exchanged between patient and physician to facilitate the development of a partnership between them.

A patient is talking about something important to her such as a miscarriage at six months. The doctor, for whatever reasons (time constraints, nonverbal signals from the patient), believes it is important to move on with the office visit. One typical approach is just to begin an exam or procedure. However, from within a partnership framework, it would be better to acknowledge verbally the difficulty of the patient's situation and then provide a transition to what will happen next. For example, the physician might say,

> You have just let me know something that is very important, the miscarriage you had the last time you were pregnant. This is something you and I need to talk about, to make the time to talk about your thoughts and feelings, especially since you've also indicated you want to try again. Do you agree? Unfortunately, my schedule today doesn't give me an opportunity to do this today. Can we schedule another appointment?

This approach acknowledges the patient as a person with important concerns and explicitly recognizes that she and the doctor have further work to do on this issue.

A physician is trying to learn more about a patient's chief complaint. In one approach the physician asks, "You didn't feel any sharp pain, did you?" This question is one which is driven by a disease protocol. That is, the physician has lists of symptoms that match particular problems and, by asking such questions, is trying to "rule out" a specific syndrome. In the partnership approach, the physician's questions, at least initially, are more "patient driven." Thus the physician asks a more open-ended question, such as, "What was the pain like?" This approach invites the patient to describe her experience and conveys the physician's respect for the information she provides. In addition, this second version of the question avoids "leading" the patient in a particular direction and instead increases the likelihood that the information will be her description of her pain rather than her attempts to give the information she thinks the doctor wants because of the form of the doctor's question.

A patient asks her physician about the advisability of exercising while pregnant. Typically a physician might respond, "It's OK to exercise in moderation." Yet if the physician is attentive to his/her language, s/he will realize that is a very general answer which may mean very different things to the physician and to the patient. Instead the physician might ask what the patient has been doing for exercise and what the patient would like to do. This will enable the physician to answer the patient's question both within the context of the patient's life-world and with more precise medical guidance.

A physician, giving a patient instructions to follow before coming into the hospital, says "Nothing to eat after midnight." However, utilizing the partnership model, the physician does not presume the patient knows what s/he knows, and so provides more complete instructions: "I want you to have nothing to eat or drink after midnight. Not even a morning cup of coffee. But you can have a sip of water to swallow your morning medication. Not eating or drinking will make the anesthesia you take tomorrow safer." In the first set of instructions, the physician knows "Nothing to eat" means no solids or liquids. However, the patient is not likely to know this, and may well end up having the surgery canceled when the anesthesiologist learns she has had a couple cups of coffee and an instant breakfast drink before coming into the hospital. In the second version of the instructions, the physician has differentiated her/himself, as someone with good medical knowledge, from the patient who is typically lacking in such background information. The physician, in talking with the patient, is clear and complete about the instructions and their rationale.

Mutual Problem Solving: Taking Into Account the Patient's Questions, Beliefs, and Feedback

Patients may hesitate to ask questions because they do not want to seem "stupid" or "silly" to the doctor. Doctors may find it easy to ignore any tentative questions (and even easier to ignore implicit questions) because there is so much to attend to in such a short amount of time. Yet soliciting and answering a patient's questions are important components of a doctor–patient partnership. Patients need to know that their questions are important. They need to be encouraged to ask them, and complemented, rather than scorned, when they do. One approach that can be successful in eliciting questions is when the physician asks, "What questions do you have about this?" This gives the message that questions are expected. Sometimes "Do you have any questions?" especially if it is asked within an ongoing relationship in which the patient is used to asking questions, is sufficient to elicit the patient's questions. However, it is less likely to work without such a context or when the physician is shuffling papers or heading toward the door.

The antithesis of a partnership response is when the doctor ignores questions. For example, questions such as "Why do I have pain?" or "Is something the matter?" tend to occur when the physician is in the midst of obtaining a history of the presenting complaint or is in the midst of an exam. Unfortunately, it is not uncommon for physicians to ignore such questions. Working within the partnership model suggests a different response; for example, the physician might answer with "Let's come back to that after I get a complete history of the problem" or a "I don't know yet, but after the exam I hope to have a better idea." Responding to patients' questions, even without a definitive answer, and complementing patients for "speaking up" helps to build a partnership relationship. Thus, ideally, a physician might respond, "That's an important question. I'm glad you asked it. After I finish the exam and look at a slide under the microscope, I think I'll have an answer for you." From this kind of response, the patient learns the physician takes her concerns seriously. Then, after the exam is finished and the doctor has looked at the slide, the physician can answer the patient's question (as best as is possible, given the history and physical evidence) and see if the patient has any more questions, including questions about the physician's answer to the original question.

It is important to listen carefully to patients' questions and to answer them at the level of the inquiry. Often patients' concerns and questions are concrete and specific. Thus, for example, besides needing to know the possible side effects of Depo-Provera (a hormonal form of birth control administered every three months by means of injection), patients may want to know the "small details," such as where it will be given and whether it will hurt. After attending to the patient's question at the level of inquiry, the physician can provide additional or more complex information. Thus the physician might say,

> The nurse will give you the Depo shot either in your arm or your buttock. It may hurt a little. The birth control protection will last three months so it is very important to come in for your next shot when you get a reminder postcard. If you have any questions or concerns at that time, or before, please call to make an appointment with me.

It is also important to remember that when a patient is highly anxious, her level of understanding may temporarily decrease. In this case, physicians must temporarily readjust their communication patterns and the level of information they are trying to convey if they want their patient to be able "hear" them. That is, physicians should speak with patients at a level of medical complexity that is within the patient's grasp at that particular moment, striving over time to increase the patient's level of understanding.

Another important component is eliciting the patient's beliefs about her health. That is, in order for physicians to form partnerships with their patients, they must first understand "where the patient is coming from." Understanding the patient's conceptions of her illness (Bibace & Walsh, 1980) is an important step in building the foundation for any treatment plan that requires the patient's cooperation. I encourage residents to elicit and respond to patients' concerns and beliefs about their health early in the interaction, for two reasons. First, if a patient feels "heard," she is more likely to develop a partnership with the physician and to return to that physician for further care. Second, it is more likely that the patient will be able to listen to and hear the physician's perspective after her own concerns have been addressed. That is, once her issues are addressed, she will be less anxious and less distracted by her own concerns and thus more able to "hear" what her physician says.

Frequently physicians simply tell patients what they are to do, without checking to see if the patient understands. That is, they tend to assume that because they have told the patient something, the patient has heard and understood it. This pattern of communication is consistent with a "container" metaphor of the mind. That is, physicians often presume that the patient's mind is an empty container, a blank slate, ready to receive whatever doctors say. In practicing medicine this presumption frequently underlies a physician's exasperated response, "But I told her . . ." to a lack of follow-through on the patient's part. However, because patients' minds are not empty containers, they integrate what the physician says with what they already know. That is, the patient's preexisting schemas, understandings, and beliefs help to shape what the physician says into what the patient hears. Further, both because patients typically lack an understanding of biology and medicine and because they are often anxious about their situation, they are particularly likely to have difficulty assimilating new information. Since communication involves such complexity, at a minimum, the physician would be wise, after explaining something to a patient, to ask for her understanding of what the illness is, what the instructions are, and whether the patient thinks she can implement the treatment plan.

Other times the patient may understand what she is being asked to do, but, because she does not know the rationale, she is not very likely to follow through. This is especially likely if her life-context presents any obstacles to the treatment plan or if she has an alternative understanding (or misunderstanding, from the physician's perspective) of her medical condition, which mitigates against the necessity of following through.

In order to help the patient and address any misconceptions she may have, the physician must first know the patient's definition of the illness, her understanding of what causes her medical condition, and her beliefs about what cures that medical condition. For example, a woman with gestational diabetes may think she does not "really" need to check her blood sugars. Her reasoning is that she would feel badly if her sugars were high and since she feels well, there's no need to check. Once this misconception is articulated, the physician can explain to the patient that her blood sugars can indeed be high even if she does not "feel badly," and further, that if they are elevated, irrespective of how she feels, there is a risk to the baby. With this corrected understanding of her condition and its implications, the patient should be more likely to check her blood sugars. Thus, ideally, after the exam, the physician explains the findings, gauges the patient's understanding (and any misunderstandings), explains the treatment options and their rationale, and negotiates a treatment plan.

It can also be extremely useful to ask the patient if she anticipates any difficulty in implementing the recommendations. That is, consistent with the partnership model, the physician elicits the patient's feedback on the proposed treatment plan. For example, if the physician wants the patient to fill a prescription for an expensive medicine and the patient has no insurance, the patient may take the prescription but have no intention of filling it. Yet if the patient and physician have more of a partnership in which the physician checks with the patient for her feedback or a partnership in which the patient feels free to raise the constraints she faces, the two of them can address the problems and devise an alternative approach. In this example alternative approaches might include a prescription for a less expensive medication or some medication samples if the treatment regimen is brief. Similarly, if the patient must eat on a frequent basis but does not think her employer will be happy about this, perhaps the physician could offer to write a letter to the employer on the patient's behalf.

This kind of mutual problem solving almost always requires an attitude of partnership. On the physician's part this can be demonstrated by an appreciation of the patient's life-world and a willingness to ask if there will be difficulties implementing the recommendations. That is, the physician must be willing to have the treatment recommendation evaluated by the patient, to take into account the patient's feedback. The physician might even role-play various scenarios ("what if . . .") with the patient and help the patient address any anticipated difficulties. On the patient's part, a partnership attitude is demonstrated by a patient's having enough of a sense of trust to volunteer or acknowledge that there are difficulties with the proposed solution. Such an attitude is facilitated by a doctor who welcomes a patient's questions and attempts to make sure his or her answers make sense to the patient.

Educating the Patient in a Partnership Model

In working with the residents, I try to encourage them to help their patients become active partners in, rather than passive recipients of, health care. This is especially critical for female patients, and particularly for females of low socioeconomic status, because in at least some segments of our society, women, especially poor women, are in a relatively powerless and subordinate position and may adapt to this position with submissiveness and passivity (Miller, 1976). Thus, learning to be an active, collaborative partner in one's own health care, for many women means unlearning both the traditional role of patient (who simply does as she is told) and the traditional role of female (who defers to authority figures). Some of the residents, especially the female residents who are typically far from passive, find this a helpful reminder.

In any patient appointment, there are multiple opportunities for educating patients. Physicians can explain the purpose of exams and procedures to patients as they conduct them. For example, when physicians measure their obstetrical patients at each visit, they can explain to the patients why they are measuring their bellies and what they expect to see. If physicians need to elicit pain during an exam, they can explain to the patient how it will help them know what is wrong. If they ask a patient whether she douches, they can also point out the contraindications to this practice. Instructions for breast self-examinations can specify when and how do them, what is normal to feel, what to look for, and when to call.

Physicians, because they are so knowledgeable about health and illness, may tend to overestimate what patients know about their bodies, their health, and their medical care. From my observations, some patients do not differentiate between a pelvic exam and a pap smear, and many do not know why a pap smear is done. Informal surveys with college women showed that more than 50 percent did not know why physicians take pap smears. Perhaps it is no wonder that many women do not appreciate the importance of regular paps. In explaining the purpose, physicians can emphasize that they are looking for precancerous changes. That is, the physician can educate the patient that the goal of the pap smear is to detect changes early and then intervene to prevent cancer because, with regular pap smears, it is more probable to find precancerous changes than cancer. This should help patients appreciate the importance of annual pap smears without generating great anxiety.

In general, as physicians explain exams and procedures at a level commensurate with "where the patient's at," they facilitate the development of a partnership. In this partnership, the patient, over time, becomes more knowledgeable about and more involved in her health care.

The Patient's Larger Social Context

The patient's larger social system is an area that can have a substantial impact on the doctor–patient relationship. In working with residents, I highlight instances in which this seems to be the case. For example, sometimes the patient's family situation may be a factor in the patient's willingness or ability to follow through on treatment recommendations. Or the patient's economic situation may make it difficult for her to enact healthy lifestyle changes. Although most physicians do not have time, as medicine is currently structured in our society, to address these issues in their patients' lives, in a partnership relationship the physician can at least acknowledge a patient's larger social context. I try to encourage residents to develop an empathetic understanding of their patient's life context, so that even if they cannot "cure" that context, they can at least respond empathetically to the patient and encourage her to make use of other resources, for example, by making referrals to appropriate agencies. The physician's interest in the patient's life and willingness to make a referral may facilitate the patient's willingness to address these issues with other caregivers.

There are also times when the physician can be encouraged to have the nurse follow up on psychosocial issues, especially those that immediately impact patient care. For example, one patient was being scheduled for a D & C and planned to take a taxi back to an empty apartment. Although the physician did not have time to problem-solve this scheduling dilemma, she did ask the nurse to sit down with the patient to find a time to schedule the procedure (late on a Friday afternoon) so that the patient would be able to have someone meet her.

Working With Patients When It May Seem Difficult to Strive Toward a Partnership

Residents have presented interactions with patients that did not meet their expectations for good doctor–patient communication. For example, one reported that a patient had insisted that she had had multiple pregnancies after her tubal ligation, yet none were documented in the chart. The physician said the ensuing interaction felt more like an argument ("You couldn't have been pregnant that many times." "Oh yes I was!") than an exchange between physician and patient, much less a partnership. We discussed several alternate approaches, much like a physician might present several treatment options. The physician liked the idea of responding more in terms of the information available ("I can only go by what is in the chart; it says that the pregnancy test last month was negative, as was the one eight months ago"), rather than in terms of whether she thought the patient was being honest or not. Alternatively, the physician may have tried to elicit the basis for the patient's belief, to inquire of the patient what she would like to happen, to pursue with curiosity and empathy the apparent contradiction between what doctors believe (driven primarily from a biomedical perspective) and what the patient believed (driven primarily from a psychosocial perspective).

Another example that sometimes "raises eyebrows" among the residents is the "noncompliant" pregnant patient. This can be a difficult situation because, in addition to being attentive to the patient's perspective, the physician must also be attentive to and care for the fetus. Here, the resident can look for and build on existing strengths of the patient. Though they may not be readily apparent, all of us have some strengths. For instance, if the patient is keeping her weekly appointments, she can be commended for that. If she smiles when she talks about the baby's kicking, she is expressing an interest in the baby's wellbeing. These strengths can be used to build an alliance in which physician and patient share the goal (even if they have not yet managed to find agreed-upon means) to protect the baby's health as well as the patient's.

What to Aim for In Partnership With Patients

The bridge between the biomedical domain of the physician and the patient's subjective construction of reality was succinctly summarized by a faculty member who tells her patients, "I want you to be happy with me, but I also want you to be safe." That is, she wants a treatment plan that works comfortably for the patient, optimizes their doctor–patient relationship, and maximizes the patient's health outcome. Thus the partnership model does not imply giving the patient carte blanche to do as she pleases, ignoring the physician's expertise to the detriment of her health. Nor is it consistent with the traditional approach of the authoritarian doctor "coming down from the mountain with 'doctor's orders,'" which the patient, once out of the doctor's office, is not necessarily likely to follow. To achieve the goals of "safe" and "happy," the patient and physician must engage in dialogue. The physician's questions must be answered, but the patient's questions also must be addressed. The physician must provide feedback to the patient about her health and medical care, and the patient also must provide feedback to the physician on these issues. Even then, hearing each other's perspectives and accepting difference is not an adequate outcome. What is needed is an integration of both the doctor's and the patient's perspectives in order to maximize the probability of a healthy outcome and a positive working relationship between patient and doctor. Working in a relationship characterized by an attitude of partnership and engaging in the process of partnership, a back-and-forth dialogue, physician and patient are more likely to achieve such a goal.

REFERENCES

Bartlett, E. E., Grayson, M., Barker, R., Levine, D. M., Golden, A., & Libber, S. (1984). The effects of physician communications skills on patient satisfaction, recall, and adherence. *Journal of Chronic Disease, 37,* 755–764.

Bass, M. J., Buck, C., Turner, L., Dickie, G., Pratt, G., & Robinson, H. C. (1986). The physician's actions and the outcome of illness in family practice. *Journal of Family Practice, 23,* 43–47.

Bertakis, K. D., Roter, D., & Putman, S. M. (1991). The relationship of physician medical interview style to patient satisfaction. *The Journal of Family Practice, 32,* 175–181.

Bibace, R., & Walsh, M. E. (1980). The development of children's conceptions of illness. *Pediatrics, 66,* 912–917.

Brody, D. S., Miller, S. M., Lerman, C. E., Smith, D. G., & Caputo, G. C. (1989). Patient perception of involvement with medical care: Relationship to illness attitudes and outcomes. *Journal of General Internal Medicine, 4,* 506–511.

Byrne, P. S., & Long, B. E. L. (1976). *Doctors talking to patients.* London: Her Majesty's Stationery Office.

Cassell, E. J. (1991). *The nature of suffering and the goals of medicine.* New York: Oxford University Press.

Coonar, A. S., Dooley, M., Daniels, M., & Taylor, R. W. (1991). The use of role-play in teaching medical students obstetrics and gynaecology. *Medical Teacher, 13,* 49–53.

DiMatteo, M. R., & DiNicola, D. D. (1982). *Achieving patient compliance.* New York: Pergamon Press.

DiMatteo, M. R., Hays, R. D., & Prince, L. M. (1986). Relationship of physicians' nonverbal communication skill to patient satisfaction, appointment noncompliance, and physician workload. *Health Psychology, 5,* 581–594.

DiMatteo, M. R., Taranta, A., & Friedman, S. (1980). Predicting patient satisfaction from physicians' nonverbal communication skills. *Medical Care, 18,* 376–387.

Greenfield, S., Kaplan, S., & Ware, J. E. (1985). Expanding patient involvement in care: Effects on patient outcome. *Annals of Internal Medicine, 102,* 520–528.

Greenfield, S., Kaplan, S. H., Ware, J. E., Yano, E. M., & Frank, H. J. L. (1988). Patients' participation in medical care: Effects on blood sugar control. *Journal of General Internal Medicine, 3,* 448–457.

Hall, J. A., Roter, D. L., & Katz, N. R. (1988.) Meta-analysis of correlates of provider behavior in medical encounters. *Medical Care, 26,* 657–675.

Headache Study Group of the University of Western Ontario (1986). Predictors of outcome in headache patients presenting to family physicians—a one year prospective study. *Headache, 26,* 285–294.

Heszen-Klemens, I., & Kapinska, E. (1984). Doctor–patient interaction, patients' health behavior and effects of treatment. *Social Science and Medicine, 19,* 9–18.

Inui, T. S., Yourtree, E. L., & Williamson, J. W. (1976). Improved outcomes in hypertension after physician tutorials: A controlled trial. *Annals of Internal Medicine, 84,* 646–651.

Kaplan, S. H., Greenfield, S., & Ware, J. E. (1989). Assessing the effects of physician–patient interactions on the outcomes of chronic disease. *Medical Care, 27S,* 110–127.

Korsch, B. M., & Negrete, V. F. (1972). Doctor–patient communication. *Scientific American, 227,* 66–74.

Mesterton-Gibbons, M., & Dugatkin, L. A. (1997). Cooperation and the prisoner's dilemma: Towards testable models of mutualism versus reciprocity. *Animal Behavior, 54,* 551–557.

Miller, J. B. (1976). *Toward a new psychology of women.* Boston: Beacon Press.

Milmoe, S., Rosenthal, R., Blane, H. T., Chafetz, M. E., & Wolf, I. (1967). The doctor's voice: Predictors of successful referral of alcoholic patients. *Journal of Abnormal Psychology, 72,* 78–84.

Mishler, E. G. (1984). *The discourse of medicine: Dialetics of medical interviews.* Norwood, NJ: Ablex.

Orth, J. E., Stiles, W. B., Scherwitz, L., Hennrikus, D., & Valbona, C. (1987). Patient exposition and provider explanation in routine interviews and hypertensive patients' blood pressure control. *Health Psychology, 6,* 29–42.

Roter, D. L. (1977). Patient participation in patient-provider interaction: The effects of patient question asking on the quality of interaction, satisfaction, and compliance. *Health Education Monographs, 5,* 281–315.

Roter, D. L. (1989). Which facets of communication have strong effects on outcome—A meta-analysis. In M. Stewart & D. Roter (Eds.). *Communicating with medical patients.* Newbury Park, CA: Sage.

Schulman, B. A. (1979). Active patient orientation and outcomes in hypertensive treatment. *Medical Care, 17,* 267–280.

Speedling, E. J., & Rose, D. N. (1985). Building an effective doctor–patient relationship: From patient satisfaction to patient participation. *Social Science and Medicine, 21,* 115–120.

Squier, R. W. (1990). A model of empathetic understanding and adherence to treatment regimens in practitioner-patient relationships. *Social Science and Medicine, 30,* 325–339.

Steward, M. A. (1984). Effective physician–patient communication and health outcomes: A review. *Canadian Medical Association Journal, 152,* 1423–1433.

Werner, H. (1948). *Comparative psychology of mental development.* New York: International Universities Press.

Werner, H., & Kaplan, B. (1963). *Symbol Formation.* New York: Wiley.

16

PEDIATRIC ASTHMA: ASSESSING AND CHANGING BEHAVIOR*

Roger Bibace
Clark University and
University of Massachusetts Medical School

ABSTRACT

The health care professional's expertise with respect to the biomedical aspects of pediatric asthma should be complemented by the patient's understanding of his/her own prior experiences and personal associations. Partnerships provide a framework to bring about a greater degree of complementarity and reciprocity among health professionals, parents, and child asthmatics. Specifically, five practical, "take-home" messages are delineated, that can assist professionals in better understanding where their patients are coming from and how best to communicate with them. Given the particular importance of self-management in asthma care, it is essential for all parties involved to work together if optimal treatment is to take place.

Several groups have emphasized the importance of educating patients for self-management of asthma. Of course, this is not always an easy task. As one

* Portions of this chapter were adapted from a talk given at a meeting sponsored jointly by the American Academy of Allergy, Asthma, and Immunology and the National Heart, Lung, and Blood Institute on "Pediatric Asthma: Promoting Best Practice," May 2–3, 1998, Washington, D.C.

I am very grateful to Virginia S. Taggart, and also to Ronald Adler, James J. Dillon, Barbara Noel Dowds, Michael Ennis, and Elizabeth L. McQuaid, for their helpful suggestions.

8-year-old put it, "my mind sometimes helps me—but I don't know how it works!" I have five take-home messages related to implementing this goal of assisting patients in self-management:

1. Health professionals should appreciate that the health beliefs of children and parents may *not* be based on biological or medical concepts of illness generally or of asthma in particular. Instead, children and many adults often rely on *personal* associations based on their past experiences and everyday activities. More mature children and adults are likely to make use of concepts of the body as a container, and rely on *mechanical* causes and effects. These two stages, personal associations and mechanical explanations, precede a biological understanding, according to the developmentally ordered levels of concepts of illness devised by Bibace and Walsh (1980).
2. One needs to assess the individual child and the parent because *chronological age* is not equivalent to the *developmental status* of a child or an adult's understanding of illness. Immature beliefs coexist with mature beliefs even in "normal" adults. Indeed, not only immature beliefs but irrational behaviors occur where least expected—for example, some surgeons in the operating room do not consistently observe universal precautions.

   Both of these points underline the need for clinicians to ASK, DON'T ASSUME. One must *ask* for the child and the parent's *own* beliefs about the definition, the cause, and the treatments for illness or asthma. Again, this is important because the beliefs of patients and parents may differ widely from those of health care professionals.
3. There are at least three different channels or modes to communicate and represent ideas to children and parents: through words, through pictures, and through the body. Understanding is *minimized* when child or parent merely repeats what has been said to them, using the same mode. Most commonly, health care professionals and patients rely solely on the mode of words in their interactions.
4. The possibility of active learning is maximized when health care professionals employ one mode (e.g. words, pictures, or body) to explain, and then ask the child to *represent* the idea in a different mode. If for some reason the use of multiple modes is not possible, patients may be asked to put the explanation into their own words. This step not only facilitates understanding, but it also allows doctors and nurses to verify whether what the patient *heard* corresponds to what the health professional *said.*

   In the examining room with a resident and patient I have, many times, asked the patient toward the end of the visit, "Your doctor covered many points and I'm not sure I got all of them. Could we go over those together?" inviting the patient to explain what s/he heard. Residents are often surprised with the discrepancies between what was said and what the patient heard.

TABLE 16.1.
Bibace and Walsh Developmental Levels of Conception of Illness*

Magical Level—Explanations Bases on Association	
Phenomenism	The child describes the illness in terms of any phenomenon s/he experiences as associated with the illness, without clear differentiation of cause and effect. "A cold is from . . . it's when your nose runs."
Contagion	The child describes the illness in terms of body experiences or symptoms. S/he associates a specific external cause with the illness, but cannot explain how the cause leads to the effect. "A cold is a runny nose and it's like from going outside in winter." (How?) "It's from being out in the winter time."
Concrete Level—Explanations Based on Sequence	
Contamination	The child describes illness in terms of experienced symptoms and explains its cause as originating in external acts or situations. The child explains how a sequence of causal events leads to the illness by contacting or involving the body as a whole. "A cold is from when you're swimming in cold water or out in the snow. It stays in your body . . . it goes up into your chest."
Internalization	The child describes the illness and explains how a sequence of mechanical actions leads to changes in specific internal body parts. "A cold is when your nose gets stuffed up and you can't breathe. It's from the germs getting into your nose and lungs and clogging them up so you can't breathe. You sneeze to get the germs out."
Abstract Level—Explanations Based on Interaction	
Physiological	The older child or adult describes an entire internal disease process involving the interaction of multiple cause and effects on multiple body parts. "A cold is a change within the body resulting in symptoms like coughing, sneezing, running nose, headaches, and stuffed-up sinuses. You catch the germs that are all around us. Coughing and running nose are the side effects of the body's fighting them off, it makes mucous to carry away the dead germs."
Psychophysiological	The older child or adult explains how multiple causes and effects interact by describing transformation at the cellular level. "A cold is the collection of symptoms that define the immune system's response to an invading virus. The white blood cells. And this happens when the person is experiencing a lot of stress."

*Adapted from Bibace, Schmidt, and Walsh, 1994.

5. A reliance on partnerships among physicians, children, and parents requires that the child/parent be encouraged to a) ASK the health professional questions and b) give the health professional feedback regarding ANSWERS to these questions. By taking such steps, health professionals facilitate self-management and satisfaction in their relationship with patients.

When entering the world of patients and their parents, which is not steeped in biology, it is necessary to address a major source of confusion: the blurring of the physical and psychological boundaries between oneself and the outside world. In a study conducted by Dillon (1998), this was illustrated when 5- to 10-year-old children were asked to "draw the inside of the body including all the parts" within an outline of the body supplied by the researcher. Some 5-year-olds included objects like a baseball, his/her house, and that most important person—Mom—all inside of the body! Adults make a mistake along the same lines when they fail to make a clear distinction between their own thoughts and feelings versus those that are attributed mistakenly to others. In fact, the process of differentiation is a cardinal dimension of developmental psychology. With increasing maturity, there comes a greater degree of differentiation within the physical body and the psychological self, and also *between* the self and others.

Many children and adults do not believe that a cold occurs as a result of germs or any other biological basis. According to this outlook, a cold is an effect of "touching snow" or going out in the cold with wet hair. In fact, a faculty colleague of mine adamantly rejected germs, bacteria, or viruses as the cause of *his* cold. Rather, his cold was strictly due to the weather in southern Italy!! One must keep in mind that no *biological explanations* are required when *personal associations* are used in order to account for an illness.

A college student who participated in a research study was asked "How do people get sick?" He replied: "I think a lot it's in your mind and I think if you just think, 'I'm not gonna get a cold,' you won't get a cold." Another college student was asked "What causes a heart attack?" to which he responded: "You dream that you see yourself in a casket. . . . I can see how with some people it can happen that way." These examples point to the fact that chronological age and developmental status are not equivalent.

By entering the world of the child, by participating in their everyday world, many medically desirable outcomes may be possible without any knowledge of medicine on the part of the child. A nurse at a local hospital has a four-year-old son who is asthmatic and enjoys fairy tales. This very perceptive mother was able to devise a way for her son to actually enjoy using the peak flow meter. She accomplished this by making its use part of a fairy tale. The story resembled "The Three Little Pigs." When it came time for the wolf to blow the pigs' house down, the mother instead told the story in this way: "I'll huff, and I'll puff, and I'll blow . . . into the peak flow meter!!" This fairy tale has another important benefit in that children usually enjoy repeating their favorite stories and the activities associated with the story. The mother was then able to use this story as a way of monitoring her child's asthma on a regular basis.

The next developmental markers are mechanistic explanations. At this point, a clear differentiation is observable in the person's beliefs between cause and effect. The metaphor of the body as a container is typically relied upon. The person explains how specific causal factors act on the body, through a sequence of mechanical actions, to produce *passive* changes in specific internal body parts or processes:

Interviewer: "What is a cold?"
Child: "When your nose gets stuffed up and you can't breathe. Sometimes you sneeze."

I: "How does someone get a cold?"
C: "From cold air and germs."
I: "How do cold air and germs make someone get a cold?"
C: "The germs get in your nose and lungs and clog them up so you can't breathe."
I: "What makes you sneeze when you have a cold?"
C: "To get germs out."

The child described a sequence inside the body in which the external cause (cold and germs) performs a concrete action (clogs up lungs) which results in an impaired function (you can't breathe). Note that there are *no* biological processes involved in these explanations. This particular child cited only mechanical activities as resulting in a cold. Here is an example given by a college student that relies upon a hydraulic, mechanical metaphor:

Interviewer: How do you get a headache?
College student: The thoughts and everything are just too much and they are crowded in your head. They don't have enough room. They try to push out and need to escape.

The same container metaphor applies to the taking of medicine. In a collaborative study (Bibace et al., 1996; Menacker, Aramburuzabala, Minian, Bush, & Bibace, 1999), one hundred children in kindergarten to sixth grade in Baltimore, New York, and Worcester, Massachusetts, believed (with only one exception) that medicines for adults and for children were intrinsically different. One kindergartner added "If you take medicines and its not for kids, then the kids die." A second grader gave this rationale for the difference: "The body is not big enough to hold a lot of germs in a little body, so you only need a little medicine."

The transformative power of taking something into the body has been a persistent belief in many cultures and in different historical eras. In preparing for battle with another tribe one could transform oneself into a ferocious fighter by swallowing powdered tiger's teeth. Advertisers understand this principle very well (e.g., "eat Wheaties and you too can be an Olympic athlete). In an extension of this psychological principle, some children confused the symptoms of a disease with the medicine taken for that disease. As when children said: "If you take someone else's medicine then you get what they have."

Clearly, "giving" patients information should not lead one to assume that they have understood. Patients may listen intently, but that does not mean they understand. This is the case because the mind also is *not* an empty container into which information can be poured by a health professional. Ordinary people, including children and adults, may be ignorant of biological processes. But one should be aware of Mark Twain's definition of ignorance: "Ignorance is not, NOT KNOWING, it is knowing things that ain't so." Remember how adamant my faculty colleague was about the nonbiological origins of his cold!! What the child or parent can take away from a medical interaction is also based on where they are coming from.

This is especially the case for concepts of the interior of the body. In Dillon's study (1998), in which children aged 5 to 10 were asked to draw the inside of the body including all the parts, there was a wide range in what normal children included. As expected, very few 5-year-olds included lungs, but some 6-, 7-, 8-, and even 9- and 10-year-olds did not include lungs either. One must then question how a child who is not aware of his/her lungs can make sense of a picture of *normal* compared to *asthmatic* bronchial tubes.

Sigel's (1978, 1993) Psychological Distancing Activities (PDA) provide a mechanism to help children and parents progress toward a higher level of maturity, with respect to a given concept. In his study, Dillon made use of innovative and powerful analogies for the purpose of improving the maturity of children's concepts of the body interior. Within a single, 30-minute session, Dillon was able to trigger dramatic changes in the participants' concepts of the body, through the use of analogies.

In order to better explain the workings of the lungs in asthmatic and normal patients, I created the analogy of an open and closed fist. There were two main reasons why I arrived at this particular analogy. First, Sigel's psychological distancing activities have been demonstrated to be empirically effective in producing changes in behavior in parent–child and teacher–student interactions over the last three decades. Second, I wanted, for practical reasons, an analogy that did not require any equipment and that relied on two modes of communication: words and the body as a vehicle to experience the idea of normal versus constricted bronchial tubes. This analogy relies on the use of one part of the body, the fist, to explain how another part of the body, the lung, functions. I believe that the experiential, psychological understanding of how air can flow or be stopped through the open or closed fist may be a useful adjunct that complements and supports the verbal explanations given by health professionals.

The following hypothetical interaction between a clinician, Joe (a child asthmatic), and his mother illustrates the usefulness of the fist analogy in clinical settings:

> Joe, please tighten your fist, like this (demonstrate a clenched fist). Tight, real tight. Okay, that's great. Now try to blow air through here (the middle part of the fist). Can you feel any air coming through? See, it's the same for me. When I blow either in or out with my fist tightly closed . . . nothing, no air comes through, even though I blow or try to suck in air real hard. But what happens when we open our fists? We can feel the air going in or out now, very easily, can't you?! And that's what the medicine does, when you use the inhaler, it opens up the tubes inside your lungs, like we opened up our fists. And so it makes it easy to breathe in and out. Well that's kind of how it works. Does that make any sense to you Joe? How about you Mrs. Smith? Do you have any questions about this example?" (approximately one and a half minutes).

Of course, the analogy can be elaborated on subsequent visits. One can also *contrast* a hard tube like the cover of a pen, which cannot be squeezed, to a muscle which is elastic like a rubber band. Muscles are like rubber bands, in that they can be longer and thinner or bunched up. It is due to the psychological activities involved in comparing, contrasting, and evaluating that meaningful changes in behavior—both cognitive and affective—come about.

On yet another visit, one could check on *how* these ideas had been assimilated, how Joe and his mother had made sense of the analogy for themselves, and make any clinically useful corrections. Then, a clinician might add that when the fist is closed and tight, when it is difficult to breathe easily, that's when one hears some noises when one breathes.

> What do you call these noises, Joe? . . . Well, doctors and nurses call those sounds that people with asthma make wheezing. Further, sometimes when things are quite *tight* here (tapping the chest), and breathing is difficult, a person coughs. And you know, Joe, what many people don't know, the cough sometimes is *not* because you have a cold, the cough *is* the asthma.

This clinician is thus teaching the child and the mother to make this distinction, which is a frequent source of confusion, namely, coughing as a symptom of a cold versus coughing as symptomatic of asthma.

There are a number of practical steps being employed in Worcester that you may want to implement in your own practice. Patients in our clinic are told that there are three activities that will occur every time they come to see their doctor:

1. Activities occurring *before* the exam with the clinician:
   a. Ask your questions of the clinician.
   b. Answer the six questions (see below), that help your clinician know you as a person, and better understand *your* experiences with asthma.
2. The exam with the clinician.
3. Activities occurring *after* the exam, but *before* you leave.
   a. Write down, *in your own words,* what the clinician said to you regarding:
      i. your medical problem.
      ii. what you should do about it.
   b. Supply your opinions and reactions to the visit and list any unanswered questions.
   c. Review any relevant educational materials suggested by the clinician.

I have included six questions, that you will adapt as you see fit, to be answered by children and parents separately if possible, depending upon the child's ability, *before* their visit. These are patient-centered questions.

1. What things do you do to make yourself breathe well?
2. How do you know when your breathing is bad?
3. What things make your breathing more difficult?
4. What do you do when breathing becomes difficult?

5. How well does it work?
6. What can I do, as your doctor, to make things better for you? (To physicians: note use of word "things" not "asthma" because it allows for replies such as: "Tell my mother to stop nagging me," or "Tell mom I can play ball," etc.).

Partnerships benefit both patients and physicians, but they require you to recruit your patients as active partners, who can take responsibility in managing their asthma. Statements such as the following may be helpful in conveying the idea of a partnership:

> You know, Joe, as your doctor, I will tell you what you should do to keep you breathing as well as possible or what you should do when your breathing gets worse. But I need to learn from you, because only *you* know, what is easy or hard for you to do. It isn't always easy for any of us to do all the things we know we should do. I think that goes for most people; I'm sure it's true for me and maybe even for you and your mom.

A statement such as this one is an acknowledgement of the principle that no one is a mind reader. This principle may mitigate the omnipotence and omniscience attributed to doctors by patients because doctors often must do and tell patients things about their bodies that are surprising and anxiety provoking. "So, as your doctor, I need to learn from you, Joe, because only you know what is easy or hard for you to do when you are in school, when you are playing, and so on."

Clinicians also must let patients and their parents know that repeated assessments, made possible through continuity of care, are needed if the child's asthma is to be treated optimally. These repeated assessments can be obtained each and every time before seeing the doctor. It should be helpful to assess what makes breathing *easier*—from both the patient's and his/her parents' perspectives, not just what makes breathing harder. Such repeated assessments should help to establish individual *base rates*. So one might say:

> Joe, we need to know what is going on—what you are doing and where you are when your breathing gets worse (ideally a description of WHERE, WHEN, WHO, HOW, and WHY, leading to the WHAT of difficulty breathing). People usually call their doctors when they are sick. But I also want you and your mom to help us figure out what is going on when your breathing is better or your breathing is quite okay. If we can do that I think it will help *us* to figure out how to help you breathe better more of the time.

Repeated assessments can be summarized and shared with Joe and his mother to demonstrate, through their own *words and observations,* behaviors that facilitate or hinder breathing. Feedback rooted in their own comparisons, their own evaluations, of everyday experiences that facilitate or hinder breathing should be persuasive and constructive. One might say the following to a parent/child dyad:

> You know, Joe, I'd like you and your mom to help us figure out, more specifically, what everyday activities help or hinder your breathing. I'm going to give you copies of what you and your mom wrote down when you've come to the clinic and before you see me. Remember the six questions you always fill out? Well now we have to figure out if there are some things that *usually* make you breathe harder or more easily. Do you think you and your mom could do that for our next visit? And remember, it's quite all right if you and your mom don't agree on some things. We can put our heads together to check it out. So, not to worry!

In other words, this dyad and family are actively engaged in comparing, evaluating, or in other words, problem solving.

Let's summarize: What psychological activities are involved in partnerships?

1. Patients ask questions and express their concerns and beliefs *before* they even see their doctor.
2. This is a time-saving procedure that furthers patient-centered interactions between doctor and patient.
3. Patients let the doctor know what they think and feel about the doctor–patient interaction *after* the visit.
4. Patients let the doctor know what they *heard* the doctor say regarding their diagnosis and treatment.
5. Patients keep track of *what* hinders and facilitates breathing—the six questions answered on each visit.
6. *Tracking* over time clarifies problem solving by patients as well as physicians.

Exemplary child/parent dyads can provide clinicians with information that may be useful for other dyads as to how they should organize their everyday lives to accomplish the optimal management and coordination of what one wants to do, what one knows one should do, and what one *can* do to lead a healthier life. Of course, partnerships do not merely rely on questions, answers, and feedback from all the people involved. The symmetrical, complementary activities of a partnership rely on a dialog among the people involved, based on an attitude of responsive, relational understanding (see Chapter 21). The complete antithesis of this attitude is illustrated by the physician who talks about a patient, not as a person, but as a "53-year-old chronic lunger" or a physician who described her afternoon with patients as "boring; I just saw one URI after the other." One general practitioner, William Carlos Williams (1984), had a fascinating way of entering his patients' world:

> But the actual calling on people, at all times and under all conditions, the coming to grips with intimate conditions of their lives, when they were being born, when they were dying, watching them die, watching them get well when they were ill, has always absorbed me. I lost myself in the very properties of their minds: for the moment at least I actually became them, whoever they should be, so that when I detached myself

> from them at the end of half-hour of intense concentration over some illness which was affecting them, it was as though I were re-awakening from a sleep. For the moment I myself did not exist, nothing of myself affected me. As a consequence I came back to myself, as from any other sleep, rested. (p. 119)

Note the paradox: Williams too is violating the boundary between himself and his patients ("I actually became them."). I think you will agree, however, that this is creative empathy. And I have been fortunate to see the consequences of such empathetic encounters between doctor and child. One 12-year-old, in a different context, put it most beautifully:

> I shook his hand
> How good I felt.
> He said "Hello" softly
> I lost my voice,
> But in my mind I said
> everything

REFERENCES

Bibace, R., Aramburuzabala, P., Bush, P. J., Dillon, J. J., Green, D., McNeil, J., Menacker, F., Minian, N., & Quinn, P. (1996, September–October). What children want to know about medicine (pp. 49–53). *Children and medicines: Information isn't just for grownups.* United States Pharmacopeia Conference, Reston, VA.

Bibace, R., Schmidt, L. R., & Walsh, M. E. (1994). Children's perceptions of illness. In G. N. Penny, P. Bennett, & M. Herbert (Eds.), *Health psychology: A life span perspective* (pp. 13–30). Philadelphia: Harwood Academic.

Bibace, R., & Walsh, M. E. (1980). The development of children's concepts of illness. *Pediatrics, 66,* 912–917.

Dillon, J. J. (1998). *The differential effects of four psychological distancing strategies on children's conceptions of biology and the inside of the body.* Unpublished doctoral dissertation, Clark University, Worcester, MA.

Menacker, F., Aramburuzabala, P., Minian, N., Bush, P. J., & Bibace, R. (1999). Children and medicines: What they want to know and how they want to learn. *Journal of Social and Administrative Pharmacy, 16,* 38–52.

Sigel, I. E. (1978). The development of pictorial comprehension. In B. S. Randhawa & W. E. Coffman (Eds.), *Visual learning, thinking, and communication* (pp. 93–111). New York: Academic Press.

Sigel, I. E. (1993). The centrality of a distancing model for the development of representational competence. In R. R. Cocking & E. Renninger (Eds.), *The development and meaning of psychological distance* (pp. 141–158). Hillsdale, NJ: Lawrence Erlbaum.

Willams, W. C. (1984). *The doctor stories.* New York: New Directions.

17

SOME PSYCHOLOGICAL PROCESSES INVOLVED IN MANAGING PEDIATRIC ASTHMA

Roger Bibace
Clark University and
University of Massachusetts Medical School

Robert F. Leeman
Brandeis University

ABSTRACT

Like the previous chapter entitled "Pediatric Asthma: Assessing and Changing Behavior," this chapter articulates the psychological processes through which pediatric asthma may be managed, in keeping with a partnership perspective. While the preceding chapter addressed physicians and allied health professionals, the current chapter is aimed primarily at social and behavioral scientists.

A number of concepts relevant to a partnership approach for managing pediatric asthma are discussed. These include the primary assumption of differentiation between the self and other (Werner 1948, 1957), developmental approaches to symbol formation (Werner & Kaplan, 1963), and Sigel's Psychological Distancing Activities (1979, 1993), that address changes in both intrapsychic representations and interpersonal processes.

Asthma has been a worldwide problem since the early 1980s, particularly among children. In fact, asthma has become the most common chronic disease among children (Platts-Mills & Carter, 1997), affecting approximately 5 million young people (Cowley & Underwood, 1997). Asthma continues to be associated with increased incidents of morbidity and mortality, according to studies cited by Larsen (1992).

Improved self-maintenance through education has been a solution advocated by several groups, most notably the National Heart, Lung and Blood Institute (National Institutes of Health, 1997). While the majority of experts are in agreement that self-management is the ideal treatment objective for pediatric asthma, scientists and practitioners disagree on the best ways to help patients reach this goal.

For instance, "evidence-based medicine" originates from group findings that, according to the Agency for Health Policy and Research, are *not* uniformly and systematically applied by clinicians with their individual patients. One of the main reasons for this lack of widespread application, according to clinicians, is that these results, derived from groups, are not consistent with their "clinical experience," of treating individual patients. This longstanding debate between group- and individual-based orientations reaches far beyond the realm of psychology and can be generalized to another common disagreement that reaches across domains, between the relative importance of "theory" versus "practice."

The preceding chapter, entitled "Pediatric Asthma: Assessing and Changing Behavior," and this one represent an attempt to bridge this gap between theory and practice, with relation to pediatric asthma. The previous chapter was targeted specifically at health professionals, namely pediatricians, family physicians, pediatric pulmonologists, and allied health professionals. In short, it represents an attempt, on the part of a psychologist, to communicate some basic assumptions regarding partnerships, in a manner that is relevant to the everyday practices of clinicians, and provided five "take-home" messages that clinicians were advised to implement.

While Chapter 16 provided clinicians with suggestions relevant to their concrete, day-to-day experiences, the present chapter addresses psychologists and other professionals in the behavioral and social sciences. This chapter provides an overview of current medical findings related to pediatric asthma. A number of relevant concepts are then articulated, including the primary assumption of differentiation between the self and other (Werner 1948, 1957); developmental approaches to symbol formation (Werner & Kaplan, 1963) and Sigel's Psychological Distancing Activities (1979, 1993), which offer an approach aimed at changing both intrapsychic representations and interpersonal processes.

Even though theoretical information cannot be directly "applied" to work with individuals, it can be used as a normative basis for concrete practices, which can then be implemented in clinical settings. To that end, this chapter provides a theoretical background for each of the five "take-home messages," offered in the preceding chapter, related to the implementation of a partnership model between health professionals and patients.

Several applicable, concrete ideas may be derived through a consideration of a partnership model. One objective of a partnership model in the context of pediatric asthma treatment is to modify the Initiation-Response-Evaluation sequence (IRE) (Cazden, 1988; Mehan, 1979; O'Connor & Michaels, 1993; Sinclair & Coulthard, 1976). In this traditional sequence, physicians or allied health professionals typically initiate questions, patients answer, and the medical experts then evaluate the patients' responses.

The principle of differentiation between the self and the other, which is central to developmental psychology, is the key factor in this movement from traditional, asymmetrical relationships to more symmetrical partnership interactions in pediatric asthma treatment. A clear separation between self and other is essential in order for a partnership model to be implemented successfully. The expert must view the counterpart as an individual, different from him or herself, with personal beliefs and attitudes, who most importantly is capable of making a valuable contribution to the partnership.

In the case of pediatric asthma treatment, further complications exist in that a partnership in this domain involves three or four main participants—the health professional, the patient, and his/her parent(s)—rather than the typical partnership with only two chief parties. Health professionals often address their questions to the parent of the asthmatic child and not to the child. As a result, the patient in such encounters does not occupy the role of an active participant or partner. A partnership model, in contrast, would allow for *both* the child and the parent to initiate his/her own questions, to which the health professional would respond. Mutual participation and the arrival at a negotiated understanding should lead to a greater sense of responsibility on the part of the patient and will, most likely, increase the likelihood of compliance with the appropriate practices recommended by physicians, nurses, or other health care professionals.

MESSAGE 1: BELIEFS OF PATIENTS AND PARENTS MAY BE BASED UPON "PERSONAL ASSOCIATIONS"

Physicians make use of information related to medical and biological norms in deciding on treatment recommendations for patients. For instance, Larsen (1992) reports that guidelines for the pharmacotherapy of asthma are based on both the age of the child and the severity of the disease. Both of these regulating factors involve comparing an individual child's case of asthma with normative data based on groups of asthmatic children of different ages.

Similarly, developmental psychologists consider norms in order to situate a particular child's development in comparison with the typical progression displayed by other children of a similar age group. The vast majority of developmental psychologists are in agreement that the maturation of thought throughout the life span follows an invariant sequence. In other words, a normal child begins using mainly less sophisticated concepts and gradually matures to the point when s/he relies primarily upon more complex, abstract conceptions. While most psychologists agree on the existence of such a sequence, there is a considerable disagreement as to what age children typically begin making these progressions.

Two commonly accepted findings based on numerous studies in developmental psychology, that are of particular relevance to the treatment of pediatric asthma are: 1) the general tendency toward absolutistic thinking, especially in areas that individuals have little knowledge, and 2) the immature conceptions of illness that characterize the thinking of many individuals, both children and parents. A consideration of such facts may help to clarify the reasons why patients and parents often make use of health-related beliefs that are centered around "personal associations," rather than information considered by health professionals to be "factual." Individuals outside of the medical field, particularly children, are not familiar with the ways in which the body functions in general or with the biological basis of asthma.

Many people, especially children, exhibit absolutistic thinking, particularly with regard to causation and sequencing. From early on, children are conditioned to believe that if they do x, the result will be y. "Eat all of your dinner, and then you can have dessert." "Be good and you can stay up a half hour later."

Developmental psychologists have empirically demonstrated the use of absolutistic thinking by children in a number of ways. One example is the classic conservation experiment, formulated by Piaget (1952). In this experiment, two short, wide beakers are presented to a child. These beakers are each filled with water to approximately the same level. The experimenter then pours the water from one of the beakers into a taller, thinner beaker. The child is then asked to determine which beaker has more water.

According to Piaget, children are incapable of determining that the amount of water in the two beakers is the same until they reach the concrete operational stage. At this point children normally gain an understanding that some properties of a substance may remain consistent even if its *appearance* is somehow changed (Cole & Cole, 1993). This lack of understanding on the part of children is an example of absolutistic thinking in that the child conceives of something that is taller as *always* being capable of containing more of a substance than a shorter object. Of course, the use of absolutistic thinking is not limited to children. For example, the prevalence of stereotypes and prejudices are illustrative of absolutistic thinking in adults. In general, appearance and perception should be subordinated to a concept. However, the "immediacy" of perception often leads individuals (both children and adults) to "jump to a conclusion."

Children learn cause-and-effect sequences, implicitly or explicitly, in order to avoid adverse situations. For instance, a child learns not to touch a hot stove. A simplistic conclusion would be that this association involves a straightforward cause-and-effect relationship, namely that *if* the stove is touched, *the effect* will be a burn and pain. However, children touch stoves when they are turned off as well.

In such instances, the association would not confirm the earlier parental dictum, nor the child's previous experience. A child's conclusion, based upon absolutistic thinking, could be that "Mom was wrong" about the stove and that touching it does not actually lead to any adverse effects. What such a child cannot understand at this point in her development is that numerous factors, rather than one single factor, play a part in whether or not the stove is hot. Absolutistic thinking relies on single cause, single effect reasoning.

Notwithstanding such exceptions, these types of rules related to causes and effects often help children to avoid trouble. However, such absolutistic approaches create difficulties in the child's understanding of the ambiguities involved with a chronic, variable illness such as asthma. While pediatric asthma is treatable, symptoms may still manifest, even if the individual has taken appropriate preventative measures such as medicating, exercising, and so on.

The story of Keith Brantley, discussed in *Asthma and Exercise* (Hogshead & Couzens, 1989), offers a good example of this variability. In the spring of 1986, Brantley, a world-class road racer and an asthmatic, was to compete in a major race, taking place in Eugene, Oregon. According to Brantley, "the pollen in Eugene is so bad that some people have to wear surgical masks when they run. You can actually see pollen floating in the air" (Hogshead & Couzens, 1989, p. 53). Normally, the best option for an asthmatic would be to avoid such a situation, but given Brantley's profession, this course of action was simply not an option.

Brantley made certain that he took extra dosages of all of his medications prior to race time. But nonetheless, Brantley faced extreme difficulty in trying to breathe: "I couldn't go another foot and had to drop out of the race. It was just too difficult to breathe" (Hogshead & Couzens, 1989, p. 53). It was certainly not Brantley's *fault* that he could not complete the race. He had made every attempt to comply with preventive measures to control his asthma. Not only did he take his medication beforehand, but furthermore, as a highly successful runner, he was in peak physical condition. But in the end, the environment in which the race occurred acted as a precipitating factor for an asthmatic episode. The point is that though such preventive measures are typically sufficient to control the symptoms of asthma, prevention is not *always* possible.

Adults, including parents of asthmatic children, have a difficult time understanding and accepting this degree of variability. It is even harder for children to make sense of such variability. If asthma is to be treated optimally, preventive efforts are needed. Asthma is a chronic illness, unlike a cold, for instance. When one catches a cold, one may take medicine and would continue to do so until the signs of the illness are gone. In contrast with an episodic illness, the treatment of asthma is more complicated because while the repeated onset of symptoms can usually be minimalized, at this time the disease itself is not considered "curable," according to the majority of medical experts.

Hogshead and Couzens (1989) provide another example that speaks to the tendency to view illnesses as "curable." Bill Koch, an asthmatic who won a silver medal in cross-country skiing, had developed a warm-up regimen that helped a great deal with his breathing. However, Koch admitted that at a certain point, he became overly complacent and overconfident with his warm-up routine. Due in large part to his belief that he had "outgrown" asthma, Koch began to forsake his warm-up regimen. As a result, Koch became ill after competing in a race just prior to the 1984 Winter Olympics. Despite his best efforts from that point forward, Koch was not able to compete successfully at full strength during the Olympics and he did not win any medals.

The preventive medicine required for proper treatment of asthma is not linked to the type of "immediate gratification," to which children and many adults are typically accustomed. Children who regularly use inhalers and avoid allergens may not *immediately* see the positive effects. Furthermore, given the unpredictability of the course of asthma as a disease, the child may still experience occasional symptoms, despite making use of these types of preventive efforts. Both the lack of *immediate, observable effects* and the *variability of results* combine to create *doubt* in the minds of both children and parents regarding the effectiveness of such preventive medications.

To consistently take medicine several times per day, especially when one is not experiencing any symptoms is a daunting task for anyone. It is therefore easy to understand why the immediate benefits of not taking medicine (i.e., eliminating a "hassle" in one's daily routine) could outweigh the long-term goal of preventing the onset of asthma-related symptoms.

In keeping with Piaget's findings regarding the invariant sequence of development, Bibace and Walsh (1980) found that children cannot comprehend the idea of prevention until they reach the stage of internalization, the fourth out of the six developmentally ordered stages of concepts of illness developed by these researchers. This increase in the understanding of prevention is correlated to a greater ability to take personal control in treatment.

It is important for health care professionals to understand that successful prevention requires a mature concept of time. Patients must fully appreciate the importance of not only the immediate present, but the distant future, as well. A number of studies (e.g., Shure & Spivack, 1979) have contrasted impulsivity with consequential thinking. Unlike impulsivity, consequential thinking requires an ability both to anticipate and to imagine future consequences for actions beyond the present—both in terms of time and context.

Another manifestation of absolutistic thinking is the grouping of cause and sequence, by adults as well as children. An experience faced by a professor of logic offers a concrete explanation of the assumption that even mature individuals are prone to spuriously relate cause and sequence. This professor was on his way to deliver a lecture and running late. The situation was made worse when he was not able to start his car. After trying several times without success, he got out of the car, walked over to the hood and in disgust, slammed it with his umbrella. When the professor tried to start the car again, it worked.

His mechanic later explained that the professor had flooded the engine with his multiple attempts at starting it. But the time he spent getting out of the car, lifting the hood, closing it, hitting it with his umbrella, and getting back into the car allowed the engine sufficient time to dry and start again. This professor, like many other people, did not understand how a combustion car engine works. Instead, by calling upon personal associations, rather than factual working knowledge, this professor in effect blurred the distinction between cause and sequence, thus leading him to believe, at least momentarily, that hitting the hood caused the car to start!

Many parents as well as patients make use of magical thinking, which derives primarily from personal associations, rather than factual information related to biology or medicine. Crider (1981) cites Schilder and Wechsler (1935) who discuss the importance children place upon the things (e.g., food) that they have put into their bodies in their conceptions of the body interior. To illustrate this point, Crider provides a picture drawn by a seven-year-old girl of the inside of her body. In this picture, the girl has included, along with organs such as the brain and liver, food items such as cabbage and milk. The girl explained that after it is consumed, food travels "into the stomach, down to the leg, then to the little toe, then it stays in the toe" (p. 50). Clearly then, a child with this type of image of her body interior would not assimilate information in a way that is compatible with the physiology of digestion.

Adults make use of immature conceptions of illness as well. An adult college graduate, who participated in a focus group on asthma conducted by Munro and colleagues (1996), displayed immature thinking with regard to his condition. These misconceptions arose from a historical, familial association.

> I expect to outgrow mine [asthma]. My uncle had it and he outgrew it. They have this saying that if you take a Bible and hammer the nail over your head—once you outgrow that nail your asthma will be gone. My grandmother said once my uncle passed that nail his asthma was gone. . . . my mother never got around to doing that for me [laughter]. I don't think I got too much more growing to do. (p. 318)

Further complications arise given that the variability of the course of asthma over time may facilitate such absolutistic ways of thinking. It is a fact that an individual may experience the effects of asthma as a young person, then go through a period in which few or no symptoms occur. However, at a later point in life, the effects of asthma will often resurface, given that the disease is never completely eliminated.

Previous studies conducted by Bibace & Walsh (1980, 1981) and replicated by Susman, Dorn, and Fletcher (1987) and del Barrio (1988) have demonstrated how very general developmental theories of cognitive development, such as those of Piaget and Werner have been applied to an understanding of children's concepts of illness. In particular, a developmental study of children's concepts of illness is in congruence with Werner (1948), given his insightful question regarding human development: "How does *it* develop?" This question allows for a developmental consideration of any behavior.

Bibace and Walsh (1980) and Bibace, Schmidt, & Walsh (1994) created a series of items aimed at assessing concepts of illness. This protocol now includes questions pertaining to the definition, cause, and cure for six illnesses: general "sickness," the common cold, headache, heart attack, cancer, and AIDS. The responses provided by participants were scored according to the system of levels of conception of illness, developed by the same researchers. This system is comprised of six "developmentally ordered explanations for the definition, cause and treatment of illness" (Bibace, Schmidt, & Walsh, 1994, p. 18). These six levels can be collapsed into three main categories of thinking, in ascending order of cognitive maturity: magical, concrete, and abstract.

MESSAGE 2: CHRONOLOGICAL AGE AND DEVELOPMENTAL STAGE ARE NOT NECESSARILY RELATED

For many stage theories, there is an implication that developmental progressions should occur within delineated time frames. Such theorists have argued that a similar correlation between age and stage exists in Piaget's theory. However, Piaget has consistently argued that stage and age are not necessarily congruent. In a chapter entitled "Development and Learning," Piaget argued that "although the order of succession is constant, the chronological ages of these stages varies a great deal" (1978, p. 230).

As discussed in the previous section, scientific psychologists make use of a number of norms in the assessment of child development. Stage theories, such as Piaget's, have been especially popular. Piaget successfully generalized the sequence, but not the rate of development. Indeed, Piaget's influence on the field of developmental psychology has been profound. According to Flavell (1996) "Piaget's greatest contribution was to found the field of cognitive development as we currently know it" (p. 200). "Almost everything people think about and do in this field has some connection with questions that Piaget raised (Flavell & Markman, 1983, p. viii).

However, in the past several years, stage theories have been challenged on a number of accounts. Some of these criticisms are indeed valid. Siegler (1994) states that a major limitation to many stage-oriented models of cognitive development is the implication that a normal child undergoes a "brief, rather mysterious, transition" (p. 1), after which s/he thinks or acts in a different way for an extended period of time, before arriving at another period of change. In contrast, Siegler argues that children's development occurs in a more continuous way, involving considerably more variability than was previously thought.

Stage theory is also vague as to what happens with previously held, less mature concepts, after one progresses to a more sophisticated developmental stage. A "co-existence concept of development," articulated by Bibace, Sagarin, and Dyl (1998) and Bibace, Dillon, and Sagarin (Chapter 3 in this volume) represents an attempt to account for such limitations in stage theory.

Bibace, Sagarin, and Dyl (1998) argue that a coexistence concept of development accounts for both the "expectable order in normal ontogenesis (life-span development)" (p. 154), that typifies stage theories, such as Piaget's, and "the variability which individuals demonstrate regarding the maturity of the cognitive processes relied upon by the same individual . . . in the same domain" (p. 154). This concept was derived from Werner's notion that "a child of a certain age or an adult, depending on the task or on inner circumstances, may qua normal, perform at genetically different levels" (1957, p. 138).

In a study related to concepts of illness, Bibace, Sagarin, and Dyl (1998) provided empirical evidence for a coexistence concept of development. The sample for this study involved three different age groups: 7- to 9-year-olds, 10- to 12-year-olds, and college students. The researchers found that after considering a range of participant's scores, a great deal of intraindividual variability could be observed. In fact, among the college students (the most cognitively sophisticated group), 80 percent gave a response that could be considered magical, at some point during the interview. These magical responses draw mainly upon personal associations from the individual's own experience, rather than upon biological knowledge.

The results of studies conducted by Siegler and colleagues (e.g., Siegler & Crowley, 1991) provide further empirical evidence for a coexistence concept of development. In these studies, a particular child may make use of both correct as well as incorrect methods for solving the same problem twice, even within the same trial.

As older children and adults grow in cognitive maturity and advance to higher levels of cognition, their previous magical or concrete concepts are not replaced. Rather, these less mature concepts coexist alongside the more mature ideas. This would explain the finding that a normal child will often make use of both advanced as well as previously employed, less mature means in a given domain, within the same session.

A lack of consideration of the idea of coexistence may lead to an erroneous assumption on the part of health professionals that the parent is *always* better equipped than the child to assimilate information regarding treatment. Pantell (1996) cites an interaction he observed during a follow-up visit involving a resident, an eight-year-old female patient, and her father.

Resident to father: "What medicine has she been on?"
Father: "Let's see, I think it's ampicillin."
Girl: "Nope, it's amoxicillin."
Resident to father: "And for how long has she been taking it?"

Father: "Oh, it's about five days."
Girl: "Nope, it's ten days."
Resident to father: "And how much is she taking?" (p. 12)

In this example, the resident continually directs his questions regarding the girl's medicine use toward the father, even though the child consistently gave the more valid responses. In a contrast with this particular example, Pantell explains that a number of the physicians he studied did allow children to give much of their own information. But the preponderance of physicians he observed gave about "four times as much information" (p. 15) regarding treatment to parents, as opposed to children. The assumption that parents are more readily equipped with the ability to assimilate information is problematic not only because of individual differences among adults, but also because the same adult will demonstrate intraindividual ability (Bibace, Sagarin, & Dyl, 1998).

A coexistence concept of development allows for the possibility that a child may have a more cognitively mature conception than his/her parent, on a given topic. Some parents may reject this possibility, due to the position of authority they occupy vis-a-vis the child. In a clinical interview, a child contradicted a statement her mother had made earlier. The child asserted to his therapist that the Callahan Tunnel runs under the Charles River, contrary to what her mother had said previously. The parent objected to the child's statement. She again argued that the Callahan Tunnel does not run under the Charles River. When the therapist pointed out to the mother that the child was correct, the mother argued that "correctness" was irrelevant. A child should never contradict a parent!

The authority of a parent over a child is very important in terms of discipline. However, a degree of empathy is needed as well, not only between parent and child, but also among parent, patient, and health care professional, if optimal care in pediatric asthma is to be achieved. The coexistence concept of development provides a basis for this needed degree of empathy.

Baron (1981) discusses the difficulty many physicians have in empathizing with their patients. He argues that the main reason for this lack of empathy lies in the fact that physicians, once fully socialized into the field of medicine, have a difficult time recalling the ways in which they previously conceived of illness and biology. Yet such memories would allow health professionals to emphasize more readily with their patients. Thus, the emphasis of modern medicine upon objective diagnoses, results in a "separation of the patient from the disease" (p. 7).

To illustrate his point that physicians lose touch with intuitive means of conceiving of illness, Baron (1981) offers a telling example of a doctor informing a young lab technician that her uncle recently died:

> The intern, Dr. Jacobs, assured her that everything possible had been done and that no effort had been spared. Sobbing, the niece asked the intern "But I don't understand! What did he have?"

> Dr. Jacobs began to give a simple-minded explanation of TTP; but noticing the white lab coat of Mr. Lee's niece, Dr. Jabobs stopped and asked "Do you work in the lab here?"
>
> "Yes," replied the niece.
>
> "Oh," said Dr. Jacobs, "then you'll be interested in this. You see he. . . . " (p. 14)

The patient's condition in this story was an extremely rare disease that, according to Baron, Dr. Jacobs is "unlikely to see again in his entire career" (p. 14). Unfortunately, Dr. Jacobs allowed his fascination to outweigh the importance of empathizing with the patient's niece. As a result, Dr. Jacobs addressed the niece as a medical colleague, not as the relative of a person who had just died! An appreciation of a coexistence concept of development could help health professionals to gain a better sense of commonality between themselves and patients.

Roter and Hall (1997) also emphasize the importance of a sense of mutuality between a health care professional and a patient. They state that "mutual participation in medical visits is enhanced when status congruence is greatest . . . congruence is highest when the gap between professional and lay status is narrowed" (p. 67).

Even though a health professional is developmentally far more mature than a child, some experts still occasionally make use of less than mature concepts. To reiterate an example provided in the previous chapter, some surgeons fail to adhere to all of the required universal precautions in the operating room. This behavior is indicative of "noncompliance" by physicians even when such professionals "know" that there are very serious morbidity and mortality risks associated with departures from these precautions.

Professionals sometimes exhibit absolutistic thinking in a number of other contexts. These include the penchant on the part of health care professionals to organize patients into categories of "compliant" and "noncompliant." As a consequence of these overgeneralizations, the multitude of reasons for doing or not doing what health professionals prescribe are overlooked. Such a simplistic approach neglects a major requirement of a partnership approach, which stresses the importance of intraindividual variability, in that both patients and health professionals vary in their "adherence" behaviors.

Many health professionals admit to not doing what they know they should do regarding adherence to prescribed medications. A degree of awareness on the part of health professionals of their own noncompliance, should facilitate empathic understanding of their patients. Such an empathic understanding is a component of successful partnerships between professionals and their patients.

MESSAGE 3: MULTIPLE MODES OF COMMUNICATION EXIST

An understanding of multiple modes of communication can be a valuable tool for health care professionals in their attempt to account for where patients are coming from. Often, the mode of verbal expression is relied on exclusively in medical communication. The use of multiple modes of communication can facilitate explanations of illness and treatment in a manner that each individual patient is able to comprehend.

Given the wide variation in maturity of concepts observable both between and within individuals, one cannot assume that medical information, like any other type of information, will be readily assimilated by patients. This assumption regarding the transfer of information has been referred to as the "conduit metaphor" by Reddy (1979). According to Budwig (1991), "the conduit metaphor follows from an assumption that *language transports ideas* from one person to another. . . . Communication then, is the transmitting of ideas from a sender to a receiver" (p. 314, emphasis added). This notion of information transfer thus "views participants stripped from their vantage points" (p. 313). The individual is stripped from the particular place where he is "coming from"; his history, ethnic background, socioeconomic status, and familial contexts.

Several researchers have conducted empirical studies on the difference between presenting information and promoting understanding. Specific to the domain of asthma treatment, Snadden and Brown (1992) cite studies conducted by Hilton and colleagues (1986) and Jenkins and colleagues (1988), that involved the administration of educational materials to asthma patients. In both studies, patients' grasp of information about asthma improved significantly. However, this increase in knowledge was not found to be correlated with significant improvements in self-management behavior or a decrease in patient morbidity.

Ideally, a health professional should recognize that the patient is *different* in many ways from those groups of individuals who are educated in medicine. These differences cannot be glossed over by simply "telling" a patient what to do. The reactions of some health professionals to so-called noncompliant patients includes expressions of frustration and anger. Indeed, some of these patients are now assigned to yet another category—that of "difficult patients." Such emotional reactions may demonstrate the commitment of the health professional to the "conduit metaphor." Reliance on the "conduit metaphor" violates the assumption of differentiation between the self as health professional and the other as patient. Scientific psychology now recognizes that all individuals are *active interpreters,* not passive recipients of "information."

The fact that all persons actively construct meaning is congruent with the differentiation principle. Contrary to the conduit metaphor, the patient who listens may not truly hear what the health professional said. Hence, from this perspective, the health professional needs to verify, to check on whether or not the patient understands the information as intended by the professional.

According to the principles of informed consent, the clear presentation of medical information to a patient is not only preferred, it is required. In drawing up a set of principles for teaching children about medicine, the United States Pharmacopeia Ad Hoc Panel on Children and Medicines (1998) made a similar mention of variability in understanding between individuals: "Recognizing that children of the same age vary in development, experience, and capabilities, these principles do not specify children's ages." Accordingly, the USP panel also requires that professionals relate the child's understanding to his/her ability to give informed consent: "Children in clinical trials have a right to receive appropriate information to promote their understanding before assent and participation in the trials."

In *Symbol Formation,* Werner and Kaplan (1963) provide a useful framework of the multiple ways in which communication can be formulated by a sender and comprehended by a receiver. According to Werner and Kaplan, there are a number of possible modes that may be used for the purposes of creating a symbol to be communicated. Each of these modes makes use of different means of representation. While qualitative differences exist between these various means, each of them can be used with the same objective: the representation of an idea or concept.

Five possible modes of communication include:

1. representation of ideas through bodily activities, experiences, sensations, internal bodily perceptions, and gestures;
2. representation of concepts through imagination of an activity—the creation of an internal image;
3. pictorial schematic representations rather than literal representations of an idea, that are analogous to abstraction;
4. representations through physiognomic perceptions—fusion of perception, action and image; and
5. representations through expressive language—affect-laden language rather than abstract language.

Examples of the simultaneous use of multiple modes are common in special education. Tactile, kinesthetic and visual perceptions have been employed simultaneously in order to teach children the letters of the alphabet and their corresponding sounds.

Linguistic modes of expression are typically abstract and may be ineffective in promoting understanding. Analogies involving the body and other types of images are often useful in making difficult concepts understandable. Hadamard (1949) quotes the great scientist Albert Einstein, who explained his preference for the use of the body in promoting his own understanding of concepts:

> The words or the language, as they are written or spoken, do not seem to play any role in my mechanism of thought. The psychical entities which seem to serve as elements in thought are certain signs and more or less clear images . . . of visual and some of muscular type. Conventional words or other signs have to be sought for laboriously only in a secondary stage. (pp. 142–143)

In his statement, Einstein spells out his preference for imagery in general ("certain signs and more or less clear images") and specifically, of bodily sensations ("some of muscular type"), as opposed to verbal expression ("the words or the language"). Clearly, Einstein understood that there are multiple modes for creating a symbol, beyond just words.

MESSAGE 4: THE USE OF MULTIPLE MODES OF COMMUNICATION

Ideally, a health care professional presents information initially using one communicative mode and then asks the patient to explain the situation him or herself using another communicative mode. This diversity is useful because it allows the professional to observe the degree to which the patient has assimilated the information provided. The use of the second mode also leads to an avoidance of simple repetition, which confounds understanding with immediate recall.

Clinicians can gain a better assessment of the patient's degree of understanding by:

1. asking the patient to put the medical information provided into her *own words,*
2. allowing the patient to transform the medical information, provided through the verbal mode, into a second mode, such as a pictorial representation, or
3. engaging the individual in a "role play" activity in which she acts out the part of the expert, explaining her medical situation to an imaginary patient.

Given that language is so much easier for the expert to use, it is understandable why they rely on linguistic modes of communication so often. But with the potential benefits of employing other modes of communication in promoting patient comprehension, it is worth the extra effort (e.g., discussing ideas for analogies with colleagues, etc.).

Bibace and Walsh (1982) provide an example of the usefulness of pictorial representations in addition to verbal communication. A 40-year-old male was hospitalized with his second heart attack. Despite the seriousness of his condition, the patient insisted on getting up out of bed in order to go to the bathroom, against the strict advice of medical personnel. These professionals could not understand why they were having such a difficult time getting through to this patient, since they explained his condition to him and were convinced that the patient fully understood his illness.

The psychologist on duty asked the supervising nurse on duty how she could be so sure that the patient comprehended his medical condition. The nurse stated that she was certain "because I asked him to repeat it to me. And he got it!" (p. 391). The consultant recommended that the nurse instruct the patient to draw a picture of his heart, for the purpose of illustrating what she had told him. The patient agreed and drew four ovals. He then explained his condition in the following way: "There are four chambers. I've had two heart attacks. I've got two more to go. After I've had the third attack, I'll listen to you; but not before" (p. 391).

Clearly, this patient did not understand that a heart attack affects the entire organ, rather than just a single chamber. Through the use of verbal explanations and a three-dimensional model of the heart, the nurse was now able to successfully communicate with the patient. After gaining a clearer understanding of how the heart works, the patient complied with the recommendations of the doctors and nurses. Through the drawing activity, the patient was able to externalize his *schema* of how the heart functions, derived from personal associations, rather than biological knowledge. It was *through* this representation that the nurse could specify, concretely, the patient's misconceptions.

This story emphasizes the fact that analogies are extremely useful when explaining complex information to people who are nonexperts in a particular discipline. This is especially true in the medical realm, in which health professionals, who are adept at providing biological explanations, repeatedly face the task of explaining complicated issues to patients who are more likely to rely upon "personal associations," in their thinking, rather than biomedical knowledge.

A nurse affiliated with a local hospital created a fairy tale to help her four-year-old son monitor his condition on a regular basis. The story resembled the "Three Little Pigs," except instead of "huffing and puffing and blowing the house down," the young boy would "huff, and puff, and blow" into his peak flow meter. Here, the bodily activities of blowing and the words of the story are combined to provide the child with an opportunity to act out the part and benefit medically in the process.

This nurse intuitively understood that young children live in a "world of action" (Werner, 1948). Many parents are tempted to explain the benefits of relying on the peak flow meter to gauge airflow into the lungs. But such abstract ideas with future benefits are not an optimal way of communicating with children. Keil (1998) provides another example of a couple, both of whom are academics, who attempted to explain to their two-year-old son precisely how a grasshopper jumps. "He hops because he has muscles inside the legs that contract. Do you know what contract means?" (p. 149). This example illustrates how even highly intelligent adults grossly misjudge a child's abilities. Such poor judgment is common among many adults, including some health professionals.

The fairy tale was a particularly effective analogue because the activity of "blowing the house down" was simultaneously an aspect of the child's world of story telling and assessed his lung capacity at the same time. Further, the nurse wisely selected an everyday activity that children would enjoy repeating. Thus, this mother did not burden herself by having to create a novel activity for the child on a daily basis.

While such analogous activities are extremely valuable, they are often difficult to create. The development of an analogy involves breaking down a complex series of events in a way that is understandable, but not simplistic. Because this is a difficult task, it is valuable to consult with colleagues when attempting to create a relevant analogous activity. Collaborators can provide feedback with respect to the appropriateness, or the fit between the representation of the concept and the concept itself. Such collegiality is yet another aspect of the "give and take" intrinsic to partnerships.

The "fist" activity discussed in the previous chapter came about not only through the efforts of the individual researcher, but also from information and ideas provided by a number of clinicians who regularly treat asthmatic children. The "fist" analogy, as a bodily activity, is an example of a high level Psychological Distancing Act (PDA) (Sigel, 1979, 1993). For a more detailed discussion of PDAs, refer to Chapter 10.

The bodily activity of the clenched versus open fist is analogous to constricted versus unconstricted bronchial tubes. The child is asked to compare and contrast blowing into and inhaling from a closed, versus an open, fist. It is readily apparent to even a young child that inhaling and exhaling is possible when the fist is open and impossible when it is tightly closed. This type of comparison and evaluation is precisely what enhances understanding and perspective because it provides a degree of psychological distance between the individual and the concept in question. Concrete, bodily *representations* of the insides of the body are desirable since neither children nor adults can concretely *see* or manipulate the insides of their bodies. This analogy allows the child or patient to better understand *how* the lung and bronchial tubes function *through* the bodily activities of clenching and unclenching their fist.

It is hoped that patients who are given information in this sort of understandable way will take greater control for themselves in treatment, thus leading to greater compliance with the recommendations of health professionals. However, taking an active role and having open communication with health care professionals are values that are not embraced by all patients. The empowerment of the patient and the parent to ask their own questions and provide feedback to health professionals are viewed as necessary in a partnership model. A negotiated understanding between parties is an important aspect of partnerships to be discussed in the next section.

MESSAGE 5: THE IMPLEMENTATION OF PARTNERSHIPS IN PEDIATRIC ASTHMA TREATMENT

The overarching concept behind the partnership model is the idea of differentiation between self and other. In other words, "no one is a mind reader." Thus, the essence of a partnership model is a shift away from treating the patient as a "case," or as a member of a homogeneous class of "patients with asthma." The objective is a symmetrical relationship in which patients, parents, and health care professionals respect the *individuality* of their partners. A number of psychological activities related to achieving these goals of partnerships can be implemented before, during, and after medical visits. These activities were presented as six "summary points" in the previous chapter. Here, we elaborate on these activities and the manner in which they relate to the partnership model.

The traditional IRE sequence (Cazden, 1988; Mehan, 1979; O'Connor & Michaels, 1993; Sinclair & Coulthard, 1976), as it pertains to the interaction between health care professional and patient, needs to be modified if partnerships are to succeed. In this traditional sequence, it is the medical expert who commonly initiates questions, to which patients respond, with the health care professional then evaluating this response.

As an alternative, children should be encouraged to pose their own questions to health professionals. In turn, it is the responsibility of the medical expert and the parent to respect the outlooks and beliefs of the child, no matter how greatly they may differ from their own conceptions. Making this effort toward breaking the static IRE sequence requires an appreciation of the "ask, don't assume" idea. Physicians and parents must ask and not always assume that they know what is best, because they cannot possibly be aware of everything about a child's condition. For instance, even a parent cannot know for sure what a child does on the playground at school, simply because they are not there and children are often not forthcoming with this information. By acknowledging that treatment cannot be successful without the participation of the child, the health care professional acts in a manner that negates the myths of omnipotence and omniscience that are sometimes either *assumed by* or *attributed to* medical experts in our society.

Another common assumption made by both health professionals and parents is that children's goals in treatment are similar if not identical to theirs. As part of the McMaster Model of Family Functioning, Epstein, Bishop, and Baldwin (1982) delineated seven steps in problem solving, the first of which is "identification of the problem" (p. 120). It seems that many patient–physician interactions occur without a clear recognition of the respective goals of all parties involved. While children certainly want to feel better, they may also favor more immediate goals, such as being able to play with their friends in as normal a way as possible. In such circumstances, the child may engage in activities that run counter to the recommendations of a physician or nurse. While the health professional or parent may consider the child to be either noncompliant or disobedient, these categorizations may mask the true problem.

The second step in the application of the partnership model in the realm of pediatric asthma is a negation of the conduit metaphor (Reddy, 1979). In relation to pediatric asthma treatment and pediatrics in general, explanations and treatment recommendations are often directed solely toward parents, according to the empirical evidence offered by Pantell (1996). For several reasons discussed earlier, it cannot be assumed that parents have the ability to act as "transmission belts" between the health care professionals and children. Information related to asthma and its treatment should instead be directed at both children and parents. This information must be presented with the attitude that verbal language does not constitute an enabling of the counterpart to understand in and of itself, but rather, it serves as a means toward this end. As discussed in an earlier section, the use of multiple modes of communication serves to accentuate the ability of a counterpart to gain a more complete grasp of medical information provided by health care professionals. In all cases though, what is crucial to the promotion of partnerships is an attitude of empathetic consideration of where the individual patient and/or parent is coming from, in relation to the expert.

The psychological activities involved in applying the partnership model to pediatric asthma treatment are summarized by the six points provided at the conclusion of the preceding chapter. These activities may be divided among those occurring before the medical visit, during the visit, and afterward. To reiterate, the six summary points were:

1. the importance of patients asking questions and expressing concerns and beliefs before meeting with a health care professional;
2. time is saved by eliciting these questions beforehand;
3. patients let the health professional know what they think and feel about the interaction *after* the visit;
4. patients let the health care professional know what they *heard* the expert *say* regarding their diagnosis and treatment;
5. patients keep track of what hinders and facilitates breathing; and
6. tracking over time clarifies problem solving on the part of patients, as well as physicians.

The first summary point applies to the activities occurring *before* a child asthmatic's medical visit. The following six questions may serve as examples for children and parents to consider before meeting with a health professional. These questions center around the child's *own experience* of what makes breathing easy or hard. The maintenance activities employed by children and parents are addressed as well. To reiterate, these six questions are:

1. What things do you do to make yourself breathe well?
2. How do you know when your breathing is bad?
3. What things make breathing more difficult?
4. What do you do when breathing becomes more difficult?
5. How well does it work?
6. What can I, your doctor, do to make things better for you?

In the case of a young child, the parent and child will discuss the questions, with the parent writing down the responses. But with an older child, it may be best to have both parent and child write down his/her own responses. That way, the child's ideas as to what makes breathing easy or hard and the ways in which these experiences should be addressed through maintenance can be compared and contrasted with her parent's outlook on the same topics.

One might immediately question how this approach relates to partnerships. If the physician supplies a set of questions to the patient and parent beforehand, how does this suggestion differ from other protocols in which physicians specify the sequence and type of questions to be asked? Certainly, the ideal of more symmetrical sequences in which patients *initiate* their own questions is not met through the use of these questions. The formal organization of structured questions to be considered prior to the doctor–patient interaction is in fact a compromise. However, these questions are patient-centered in nature, rather than physician-centered, in a number of ways. These questions elicit descriptions of events, rather than evaluations. Burke (1945) posits five very general criteria for a comprehensive description, including what, where, when, and how it occurred, and lastly, the reasons why the occurrence came about.

Further, the six questions allow for descriptions of both the patient's positive (i.e., "What things do you do to make yourself breathe well?") and negative experiences (i.e., "What makes breathing more difficult?"). The rationale for these questions is to encourage patients to provide a comprehensive description of their breathing experiences. In a medical context, the tendency with a question such as "How has your breathing been?" is to focus solely on difficulties in breathing. Further, individuals who are socialized into a "no pain, no gain" philosophy concentrate on difficult situations as offering potential for growth. However, in asthma treatment, it is equally important for a health professional to understand what makes patients' breathing relatively easy, so that these conditions may be reproduced in the future.

As one aspect of treatment, the patient is reminded to do or to avoid doing various things in order to minimize the possibility of another asthmatic episode. When an episode has occurred, even the most considerate and pleasant style of interacting with patients may not conceal the implicit message that the patient did something wrong and that something needs to be changed. This is especially the case since the vast majority of health professionals who deal with asthmatic patients believe that it is important to communicate the message that "You can manage your asthma."

Accordingly, when a problem occurs, the expert attempts to specify the reasons for the asthmatic episode. The questions posed by the professional may convey the message to the patient that she has departed from what "should" have been done. With this focus on problem solving, it is not clear how many health care professionals communicate that there is also an inherent variability to the disease process of asthma. Perhaps the aforementioned message "You can manage your asthma" is in need of a modifier. That way, patients may come to understand that while they are expected to comply with the appropriate treatment, there is a possibility that certain factors leading to an asthmatic episode may present themselves in an unexpected manner. A complicated balance is needed here, given that the health professional does not want to detract from the central message that asthma is manageable.

Question four serves the purpose of allowing the health professional to learn from the patient, contrary to the typical path of knowledge exchange, that goes from clinician to patient. This information might even be generalizable in some way to the health care professional's future dealings with other patients.

Another factor that makes these types of questions "patient centered" is the fact that they specifically seek the patient's input on a number of occasions. Question five, for example, asks the patient to reflect on what s/he typically does in response to breathing difficulty and how well these effects work. In most traditional interactions, the health professional determines what techniques work best to treat the child's asthma. In contrast, by posing a question such as number five, the clinician communicates the message to the patient before the visit even begins that she, although an expert, does not always know what works best for this particular patient. This message is intrinsic to one of the major premises of a partnership, namely that no one, not even a health professional, is a mind reader.

These six questions hopefully allow the child to reflect on what makes breathing easy and difficult and to provide a detailed description of these factors. Bodily self-awareness, an important component to asthma maintenance, is thereby heightened in these children. Awareness of one's bodily sensations has been found to facilitate the early detection of an asthmatic episode. Participants in a focus group of seven adult asthmatics, conducted by Snadden and Brown (1992), advocated the recognition of "signals from your body" as an important component of asthma treatment. One participant elaborated upon this idea:

> I am always conscious of what's going on with myself. I am always listening to my own breathing to see if I am whistling or wheezing or whatever. I guess it's subconscious but I know I do it a lot. (p. 1356)

Health care professionals may benefit in a number of ways through the use of these types of questions. The first benefit, mentioned in summary point two, is that these questions are a time saving procedure. Since the parties involved have already taken the time to reflect on the child's breathing experiences, they will be more likely to arrive at the physician's office prepared to engage in a discussion about the child's asthma. Accordingly, the clinician should require less time during the actual interview to elicit relevant information. Also, through the use of these questions, the physician is provided with a more complete set of data on the patient's experiences, rather than merely the parent's evaluations, which often consist mainly of negative experiences.

The second phase of the medical visit focuses on the *actual interaction* between the clinician and the patient. The health care professional evaluates the patient's medical condition and, calling on her normative knowledge of pediatric asthma, makes diagnoses and treatment recommendations. Many health care professionals often repeat similar explanations or descriptions of illness and treatment to patients.

Byrne and Long (1976) point out that when explaining illnesses and treatment "most doctors use the same form of words for most of their patients" (p. 21).

Pantell (1996) articulates this sameness of presentation, specifically in the domain of pediatrics.

> Remarkably, there was very little difference between 5- and 15-year olds. In other words, physicians treated all children as a generic child. . . . physicians tend to overestimate the understanding of younger children, and underestimate the understanding of older children: everybody is 9 years old in the minds of physicians, even pediatricians. (p. 15)

Those in psycholinguistics typically refer to these similarities of explanation as "scripts." Nelson (1986) defines a script as:

> An ordered sequence of actions appropriate to a particular spatial-temporal context and organized around a goal. Scripts specify the actors, actions and props used to carry out those goals within specified circumstances. . . . For example, in a restaurant script a waiter or waitress is assumed, as are a menu, food, a bill, and a tip. (p. 15)

In the world of medicine, the counterpart of the script is the "protocol." A protocol for a cold would lead a health professional to offer an explanation to a patient about what may have caused the cold and how it can be treated. Primarily words and possibly a model or picture of the chest or head may be used in this explanation, which in all probability, varies little from case to case. The interaction would end with advice from the health professional, together with a prescription, if needed.

An important, positive aspect of a reliance on the use of protocols is the assurance that information is provided to patients as accurately and consistently as possible. However, the limitations of standardized explanations have been brought out earlier in the chapter in message one and two, namely that patients differ widely in terms of their cognitive ability to assimilate information. The recognition that all people, including patients and medical experts, demonstrate considerable intraindividual variability requires flexibility on the part of health professionals.

The advice offered by a physician through a protocol often takes the form of orders, rather than what they truly are: recommendations. While it is crucial for a physician to share biomedical knowledge of the disease, this must be done in an empathic way in order to increase the likelihood of successful treatment. These points indicate the need to ask, not assume. This policy benefits not only the patient, but the medical expert as well. By espousing this type of open attitude, a health professional has the opportunity to learn things about patients that most likely would not automatically occur to the physician.

After the visit, the child and parent can be invited to provide two different types of feedback. The first kind of evaluation, discussed in summary point three, deals with the child's and the parent's feelings regarding the visit. This type of feedback involves their opinions as to what they got out of the visit, whether or not all of their questions were answered, and their beliefs about the feasibility and usefulness of the health professional's recommendations.

The second type of feedback, addressed in summary point four, relates to the degree to which the child and parent have understood and assimilated the information that the professional has provided. This is an opportune time to assess the child's and the parent's understanding of what the health professional said earlier regarding both diagnosis and treatment. Follow-up by the health professional can correct any misunderstandings by the child or parent. As discussed earlier, the use of another mode of communication, such as a drawing or an analogous activity, might be even more beneficial. The purpose of this task is to ensure that the parent and patient have a clear understanding of the health care professional's recommendations. The use of these two types of feedback again delivers the message that physician, patient, and parent are all partners, in a medical interaction, each with a different, but important, contribution to make. As a result, children will most likely provide health professionals with more honest responses, rather than simply a repetition of the expert's own words.

It is further suggested in summary point five that keeping on file the written responses of the parent and child allows the health care professional to obtain a longitudinal record of the child's experiences with asthma. This type of subjective information complements the long-term, objective, biomedical records routinely obtained for every patient.

By having access to this information, health care professionals can assess the intraindividual variability experienced by each child and parent, thereby avoiding the overuse of scripts discussed by Byrne and Long (1976). Again, variability is an unavoidable aspect of the disease for most asthmatics, requiring continuity of care, thus making this type of longitudinal data extremely useful to health care professionals. As suggested in summary point six, sharing longitudinal data with child and parent enables reflection. Children and parents are able to compare and contrast the circumstances that facilitate or hinder breathing, across a longer period of time.

CONCLUSION

By applying features of the partnership model to the treatment of pediatric asthma, health care professionals make a commitment to accounting for "where the patient and parent are coming from" by negating the myth of physician omnipotence and avoiding the use of the apostolic function. Thus, the degree of complementarity in the relationship among health professionals, parents, and children is actualized. The results benefit children in that they receive continuous care, which is crucial given the variability inherent in the disease and a reduced likelihood of future asthmatic episodes. Benefits to health care professionals include optimal use of the limited time available for most medical interactions, more honest feedback from patients and parents, and a greater likelihood that their partners will follow through with the most appropriate treatment.

REFERENCES

Baron, R. J. (1981). Bridging clinical distance: An empathic rediscovery of the known. *The Journal of Medicine and Philosophy, 6,* 5–23.

del Barrio, C. (1988). The development of biological process explanations: How children understand illness and cure. *Infancia y Appendizaia, 42,* 81–95.

Bibace, R., Sagarin, J., & Dyl, J. (1998). The heuristic value of Werner's co-existence concept of development. *Journal of Applied Developmental Psychology, 19,* 153–163.

Bibace, R., Schmidt, L., & Walsh, M. E. (1994). Children's perceptions of illness. In G. N. Penny, P. Bennett, & M. Hebert (Eds.) *Health psychology: A life-span perspective.* London: Harwood.

Bibace, R., & Walsh, M. E. (1980). The development of children's concepts of illness. *Pediatrics, 66,* 912–917.

Bibace, R., & Walsh, M. E. (Eds.) (1981). *Children's conceptions of health, illness and bodily functions.* San Francisco: Jossey-Bass.

Bibace, R., & Walsh, M. E. (1982). Conflict of roles: On the difficulties of being both scientist and practitioner in one life. *Professional Psychology, 13,* 389–396.

Budwig, N. (1991). The conduit metaphor: Language and informed consent. *Family Systems Medicine, 9,* 313–327.

Burke, K. (1945). *A grammar of motives.* New York: Prentice-Hall.

Byrne, P. S., & Long, B. E. L. (1976). *Doctors talking to patients: A study of the verbal behaviour of general practicioners consulting in their surgeries.* Exeter, England: The Royal College of General Practitioners.

Cazden, C. (1988). *Classroom discourse.* Portsmouth, NH: Heinemann.

Cole, M., & Cole, S. R. (1993). *The development of children.* New York: W. H. Freeman.

Cowley, G., & Underwood, A. (1997, May 26). Why Ebonie can't breathe. *Newsweek, 129,* 58–64.

Crider, C. (1981). Children's conceptions of the body interior. In R. Bibace & M. E. Walsh (Eds.), *Children's conceptions of health, illness and bodily functions* (pp. 49–65). San Francisco: Jossey-Bass.

Epstein, N. B., Bishop, D. S., & Baldwin, L. M. (1982). McMaster model of family functioning: A view of the normal family. In F. Walsh et al. (Eds.), *Normal family processes* (pp. 115–141). New York: Guilford Press.

Flavell, J. H. (1996). Piaget's legacy. *Psychological Science, 7,* 200–203.

Flavell, J. H., & Markman, E. M. (1983). Preface. In P.H. Mussen (Series Ed.) & J. H. Flavell, & E. M. Markman (Vol. Eds.), *Handbook of child psychology: Vol. 3. Cognitive development,* (pp. viii–x). New York: Wiley.

Hadamard, J. (1949). *An essay on the psychology of invention in the mathematical field.* Princeton, NJ: Princeton University Press.

Hilton, S., Sibbald, B., Anderson, H. R., & Freeling, P. (1986). Controlled evaluation of the effects of patient education on asthma morbidity in general practice. *Lancet, 1,* 26–29.

Hogshead, N. (1998, May 2–3). Asthma and exercise. *Pediatric asthma: Promoting best practice.* Meeting sponsored jointly by the American Academy of Allergy, Asthma and Immunology and the National Heart, Lung and Blood Institute, Washington, DC.

Hogshead, N., & Couzens, G. S. (1989). *Asthma and exercise.* New York: Henry Holt.

Jenkins, D., Davison, J., Jones, S., & Hawtin, P. (1988). Comparison of effects of a self-management booklet and audio cassette for patients with asthma. *British Medical Journal, 297,* 267–270.

Keil, F. C. (1998). Commentary: Words, moms and things: Language as a roadmap to reality. In S. A. Gelman, J. D. Coley, K. S. Rosengren, E. Hartman, & A. Pappas (Eds.) *Beyond Labeling: The role of maternal input in the acquisition of richly structured categories* (pp. 149–157). Chicago: Monographs of the Society for Research in Child Development Vol. 63.

Larsen, G. L. (1992). Asthma in children. *The New England Journal of Medicine, 326,* 1540–1545.

Mehan, H. (1979). *Learning lessons.* Cambridge, MA: Harvard University Press.

Munro, J. F., Haire-Joshu, D., Fisher, E. B., & Wedner, N. J. (1996). Articulation of asthma and its care among low-income emergency care recipients. *Journal of Asthma, 33,* 313–326.

National Institutes of Health. (1997). Guidelines for the diagnosis and management of asthma. *Expert Panel Report II.* Bethesda, MD: author.

Nelson, K. (Ed.) (1986). Event knowledge and cognitive development. *Event knowledge: Structure and function in development* (pp. 1–20). Hillsdale, NJ: Lawrence Erlbaum.

O'Connor, M. C., & Michaels, S. (1993). Aligning academic task and participation status through revoicing: Analysis of a classroom discourse strategy. *Anthropology and Education Quarterly, 24,* 318–335.

Pantell, R. (1996, September 29–October 1). Improving the process and outcomes of medical care for children: How effective communication impacts children taking medicine. *Children and medicines: Information isn't just for grownups.* United States Pharmacopeia Conference, Reston, VA.

Piaget, J. (1952). *The origins of intelligence in children.* New York: International Universities Press.

Piaget, J. (1978). Development and learning. In J. K. Gardner (Ed.), Readings in developmental psychology (pp. 228–237). Boston: Little, Brown.

Platts-Mills, T. A. E., & Carter, M. C. (1997). Asthma and indoor exposure to allergens. *The New England Journal of Medicine, 336,* 1382–1384.

Reddy, M. (1979). The conduit metaphor—A case of frame conflict in our language about language. In A. Ortony (Ed.), *Metaphor and thought.* Cambridge: Cambridge University Press.

Roter, D. L., & Hall, J. A. (1997). Gender differences in patient–physician communication. In S. J. Gallant, G. Puryear-Keita, & P. Rotak-Schaler. *Health care for women: Psychological, social and behavioral influences* (pp. 57–71). Washington, DC: American Psychological Association.

Schilder, P., & Wechsler, D. (1935). What do children want to know about the interior of the body? *International Journal of Psycho-Analysis, 16,* 355–360.

Shure, M. B., & Spivack, G. (1979). Interpersonal cognitive problem solving and primary prevention: Programming for preschool and kindergarten children. *Journal of Child Psychology, 8,* 89–94.

Siegler, R. S. (1994). Cognitive variability: A key to understanding cognitive development. *Current Directions in Psychological Science, 3,* 1–5.

Siegler, R. S., & Crowley, K. (1991). The microgenetic method: A direct means for studying cognitive development. *American Psychologist, 46,* 606–620.

Sigel, I. E. (1979). On becoming a thinker: A psycho-educational model. *Educational Psychologist, 14,* 70–78.

Sigel, I. E. (1993). The centrality of a distancing model for the development of representational competence. In R. R. Cocking & E. Renninger (Eds.), *The development and meaning of psychological distance* (pp. 141–158). Hillsdale, NJ: Lawrence Erlbaum.

Sinclair, J. M., & Coulthard, R. M. (1976). *Toward an analysis of discourse: The English used by teachers and pupils.* London: Oxford University Press.

Snadden, D., & Brown, J. B. (1992). The experience of asthma. *Social Science and Medicine, 34,* 1351–1361.

Susman, E. J., Dorn, L. D., & Fletcher, J. C. (1987). Reasoning about illness in ill and healthy children and adolescents: Cognitive and emotional developmental aspects. *Developmental and Behavioral Pediatrics, 8,* 266–273.

United States Pharmacopeia. (1998). *Ten guiding principles for teaching children and adolescents about medicines: A position statement of the United States Pharmacopeia.* Rockville, MD.

Werner, H. (1948). *Comparative psychology of mental development.* New York: International Universities Press.

Werner, H. (1957). The concept of development from a comparative and organismic point of view. In D. B. Harris (Ed.), *The concept of development: An issue in the study of human behavior.* Minneapolis: University of Minnesota Press.

Werner, H., & Kaplan, B. (1963). *Symbol formation: An organismic-developmental approach to language and the expression of thought.* New York: Wiley.

18

FACULTY PHYSICIAN GROUPS

Roger Bibace
Clark University and
University of Massachusetts Medical School

ABSTRACT

This chapter is a retrospective of two faculty physician groups in the Worcester, Massachusetts, area that have been meeting regularly for a number of years. These groups allow faculty physicians a much higher degree of openness and honesty than the classical Balint group. Given that the leader in the Worcester groups alternate from week to week, this format is also much more egalitarian than the Balint, single-leader approach. Most importantly, members of these faculty physician groups have been given the opportunity to admit that they sometimes do not know what to do, with regard to a particular patient or personal/familial situation. This high degree of openness has enabled group members to benefit from one another's experience without the pressure of evaluation.

This description of faculty physician groups focuses primarily on two different faculty physician groups from a partnership perspective. The two faculty physician groups are composed of faculty family physicians and of faculty obstetricians. The groups are quite different in size, though similar in overall orientation. The historical roots for both group meetings draw on the practices and traditions of Michael Balint's (1964) work with "general practitioners" in England, dating back to the 1950s. Balint was a psychoanalyst who argued that the "doctor was the drug" and that a very important therapeutic aspect of the doctor–patient relationship was the doctor's personality. The aim of such groups was to help the doctor to cope more adaptively with "difficult patients," through an awareness of his unconscious apostolic function.

In a Balint group, a psychoanalyst, familiar with the mind's unconscious defenses, would act as the group leader. While the doctor takes the role of healer in his or her everyday practice, the physician, by his or her very presence, recognizes that s/he is a "wounded healer." Specifying the nature of the wounds and the best means of healing them were aspects of the leader's role. It was also sometimes assumed that a physician was required to have undergone psychoanalysis or intensive psychotherapy in order to become a group leader. There are striking differences between a classical Balint group and the faculty physician groups that have evolved in Worcester, Massachusetts, over the past quarter century.

The University of Massachusetts Faculty Family Physician group began in September of 1974. It has been meeting weekly since then, every Thursday morning. The name "Thursday Morning Group" was adopted because the group did not limit its discussions as in traditional Balint-type groups. Membership in the group is open to any faculty family physician except the chairperson. The evaluative role of the chair can inhibit optimal participation among group members. For instance, it can be difficult to have some topics discussed when the chair, who is involved in matters related to merit raises, is present. However, this is not always the case. The personality of the chair and the relationship between him/herself and the faculty determines whether the chair's presence can be a comfortable actuality. Currently, for instance, the chair is a member of the Thursday Morning Group.

Partnerships encourage debate and discussion of alternatives in a nonhierarchic way. A complete antithesis can be appreciated with respect to attempts at establishing a group of faculty physicians in the military. The ranking officer had ordered a group to be formed! Some officers were puzzled as to why this group ever got started. It is important that the group dynamics be person, not authority, focused. The academic rank or administrative position of individuals in the group should be subordinated to the group processes, that are organized to be nonhierarchical.

Another major and important difference between a classical Balint group and the Thursday Morning Group is that the role of group moderator rotates among group members. In a Balint group, there is one, predetermined leader. Further, the leader is often an "expert" who is not a family physician. Typically, it is a psychoanalyst or psychiatrist in England or a behavioral scientist in this country. The leader of a Balint group could also be an "expert" family physician who has undergone special training.

In the Thursday Morning Group, there is no pre-set leader. Rather, the "moderator" is the person who is "presenting" on that given day. It is also entirely congruent with partnership ideals to note how this practice of rotating the leadership came about. This practice actually was not initiated within the faculty group. It began with the third-year resident group and was later adopted by the faculty. This offers a striking example of more symmetrical learning, wherein faculty family physicians learn from residents in family medicine.

In keeping with this "role rotation," the behavioral scientists, over the years, were afforded an opportunity to present their own personal problems and professional perspectives. In contrast, the "expert" in a classical Balint group would never present his own difficulties to a patient. The Balint group leader, as expert, also never discussed his personal/familial difficulties. This of course is highly consistent with Balint's framework, in which the analyst was supposed to remain an "ambiguous" figure, who does not reveal his own personal conflicts to patients. The current practices of the Thursday Morning Group serve to mitigate any illusions entertained by group members regarding the personal or professional abilities of any "expert." Furthermore, such continuous, weekly experiences among group members help to make clear to everyone that any "expert" also has an "agenda." Classical Balint groups typically have a limited life span, usually one or two years. When a group lasts as long as the Thursday Morning Group has, it becomes much easier to appreciate that all of our relationships, not just the doctor–patient relationship, bear the stamp of an "apostolic" mission.

The continuity of the Thursday Morning Group over the years has also made clear (to many of us) the truth of the following aphorism attributed to Will Rogers: "There is nothing so stupid as an educated man, if you get off the thing that he was educated in" (Stevenson, 1934, p. 529). Conversely, the group appreciates the special expertise of each of the group members, in areas as diverse as gender issues, family dynamics, religion, hand surgery, geriatrics, and so on. "I must ask 'X' about 'Y'" is a common refrain. The members have all learned that there is great value in consulting with a peer colleague.

Above all, the Thursday Morning Group permits an expert to begin by acknowledging what is so difficult for most experts to say: "I don't know. Please help me." It is even more difficult for a faculty physician, who is supposed to know how to address any problem that may arise, to say "I don't know how to deal with this patient." This is not an instance of a professor of family medicine acknowledging a general issue: "We don't know what causes this disease." In the Thursday Morning Group, the presenter deals with a personal problem, not an impersonal issue. The contrast with other traditions in academia is clear. In a Grand Rounds, the speaker sometimes "grandly" informs others of how wonderful s/he is, what marvelous results were obtained either clinically or through a study, and so on. In the Thursday Morning Group, the opposite is most frequently the case. The difficulties, failures, frustrations, and anxieties, related not only to patient relationships, but also to teaching a resident, or to relationships with colleagues in other departments, are the frequent foci. Even more difficult are the discussions about a group member's own difficulties as a patient, as a spouse, or as a family member.

Most striking to me is the difference between conversation in this group and professional interactions in academic psychology departments. I have visited numerous psychology departments, as a representative of the American Psychological Association. Unfortunately, psychology, like many other departments in academia, puts a very high premium on two features of interpersonal interactions:

cleverness and criticality. Often, the criticality and cleverness occur at the expense of the other person!

In the Thursday Morning Group, the moderators' acknowledgement that they "don't know" and the request for help from other group members have eliminated the kind of critical comments that denigrate the presenter. Allowing time at the end of most group meetings for the presenter's feedback to the group—regarding what was and was not particularly helpful—enhances this aspect of the group process. This way, the presenter is both the one who is asking for help and the evaluator of what was "helpful." Often, a group member will, toward the end of the meeting, ask the presenter if the group has "answered" or dealt with "your questions" properly.

Different specialties in medicine have diverse properties. Differences between the faculty family physician group and the faculty obstetrician group include a major disparity in size. The former is a much larger group (some 10 to 15 members on a particular day) compared to the latter group (with a maximum of 4 and often only 2 faculty present). The informality of the smaller group makes taking turns to present unnecessary. There are more similarities than differences between the two groups with respect to issues in doctor–patient relationships. However, it is much more frequently the case that a psychologist will not understand the technical, biomedical issues in obstetrics, compared with the psychosocial focus in family medicine groups. Another difference between my experiences in the two groups is the priority assigned to "knowledge creation" or research. The emphasis on research is much greater with the group of obstetricians. Faculty in obstetrics participate or think they should be involved in empirical research.

In retrospect, my experiences as a member in both groups ranks as one of the best learning opportunities of my life. It is quite a relief not to have to be clever, not to be evaluated, or act as the evaluator (I have always disliked grading as a teacher!). I have enjoyed the opportunity to admit "I don't know" at times.

Lastly, I want to tell the reader why the group came to be called the Thursday Morning Group. Over the years, the group has covered many areas beyond the scope of a classical Balint group. For instance, we had many sessions devoted to what is usually labeled "faculty development" in areas such as teaching or even research. Initially, there was one area that was considered to be taboo: administrative issues. However, even that barrier has been breached in recent years. These foci transcend, by far, the classic Balint group, which is specifically aimed at "difficult doctor–patient relationships."

Given the success of the Thursday Morning Group, a number of other departments in medical schools throughout the country have asked for advice regarding how to start a faculty group. A summary of the suggestions we have made is given in the Appendix.

APPENDIX: SO YOU WANT TO START A FACULTY GROUP?

Suggestions from the Thursday Morning Group, UMASS Worcester, Family Practice

1. Keep it open to any faculty family physicians who want to join![1]
2. Let people discuss anything they want to.
3. Meet regularly (once a week is ideal) to maintain continuity.
4. Allow 1½ hours for the meeting.
5. Keep a record of your meetings. Rotate the role of recorder.
6. For presenting, write down what you and the patient said and did; or provide audiotape or videotape of the interaction.
7. Provide for coffee (our group provided breakfasts for those who want it).
8. Select a time that most members find suitable.
9. Select a suitable meeting place—acceptable to all.
10. Rotate the role of the group moderator.
11. Allow time for the person presenting to give the group feedback—what was and wasn't helpful to the presenter.
12. Employ a behavioral scientist knowledgeable about family medicine. Make sure there is science in your behavioral science.

REFERENCES

Balint, M. (1964). *The doctor, the patient and the illness* (2nd ed.). New York: International Universities Press.

Stevenson, B. (1934). *The home book of quotations.* New York: Dodd, Mead.

[1] The one exception is the departmental chairperson. Evaluative role of chair may inhibit optimal participation among group members.

19

PHYSICIAN PARTNERSHIPS WITH PATIENTS THROUGH TEMPORAL AND INTERPERSONAL SEQUENCES

Roger Bibace
Clark University and
University of Massachusetts Medical School

ABSTRACT

This chapter focuses on the sequence of behaviors occurring in a doctor–patient relationship from a partnership perspective. Important activities are believed to occur *before* and *after*, as well as *during*, the actual doctor–patient interaction itself. This three-step process is a key difference between a partnership approach and past frameworks for the doctor–patient relationship. Thus, in a partnership perspective, the doctor–patient relationship extends beyond the limits of traditional medical interaction. Given that complementarity and reciprocity are accentuated in this approach, each doctor–patient interaction provides opportunities for questions, answers, and feedback between doctors and patients, both of whom have the opportunity to benefit from this more symmetrical interaction.

This chapter focuses on the sequence of behaviors occurring in a doctor–patient relationship from a partnership perspective. The key difference between this approach and past frameworks for the doctor–patient relationship is that in a partnership approach, important activities are considered to occur *before* and *after*, as well as *during,* the actual doctor–patient interaction itself. Thus, in a partnership perspective, the doctor–patient relationship extends beyond the limits of the traditional medical interaction. The idea put forth in this chapter is that each doctor–patient interaction provides opportunities for questions, answers, and feedback between doctors and patients, both of whom have the opportunity to benefit from this more symmetrical interaction.

Temporally, this symmetrical relationship allows for both macro- and micro-*sequences* of questions, answers, and feedback between doctor and patient. The macro-sequences include activities on the part of both patients and doctors, taking place before and after the actual interaction. The micro-sequences refer to the questions, answers, and feedback that occur specifically *during* the doctor–patient interaction. The activities occurring at these times are centered around providing the patient with the opportunity to voice relevant questions and concerns, while the physician benefits by gaining greater assurance that the patient has understood any necessary treatment recommendations.

Byrne and Long (1976) were among the first researchers to break down the specific sequence of exchanges between patients and physicians taking place during medical interactions. They posited that six sequentially organized activities should occur during a medical interaction (See the Appendix for an overview of four models of doctor–patient interactions). The work of Byrne and Long differed from past research, that centered around pointing out desirable personality characteristics for physicians. However, Byrne and Long's research, like most of the literature on medical interviewing, focuses almost entirely on the role of the doctor in the medical interaction.

This approach to doctor–patient interactions has been elaborated thoroughly by British and Canadian family physicians. For instance, the Calgary/Cambridge Observation Guide to the Consultation (Kurtz & Silverman, 1996) divides the doctor–patient interaction into five main parts, all of which should be completed during a successful medical visit. The first step is initiating the session, which involves establishing initial rapport and identifying the patient's reasons for making the appointment. Second, the physician must gather the necessary information in order to make treatment recommendations. This step is comprised of exploring the patient's problems, from the patient's own perspective, while attempting to provide structure to the interaction. Third, the physician makes an effort to develop rapport with the patient and involve him or her in the process of deciding on what would be best for his/her health. In the fourth part, explanation and planning, the physician provides information to the patient, while incorporating his/her perspective and opinions in the decision-making process. The physician closes the session in the fifth and final portion of the interaction by summarizing treatment recommendations.

The medical model closest to the partnership perspective is the "Disease/Illness Model" formulated by McWhinney (1984). This model sharply differentiates between the medical "disease" viewpoint of a physician and the "illness" perspective of a patient. The "disease" viewpoint of the physician centers around biomedical information related to symptoms, signs, syndromes, and the course of a disease.

However, according to McWhinney's Disease/Illness Model, physicians must also come to "understand the patient's unique experience of illness." It is in this respect that the Disease/Illness Model, corresponds closely with the main assumption of a partnership ideal, which is that *no one is a mind reader.* The physician must *ask* and *not assume* that they are aware of all of the features that comprise a particular patient's "illness framework." According to McWhinney, an understanding of the "patient's unique experience of illness" requires an appreciation of the "patient's agenda." This agenda is comprised of the individual's own ideas, concerns, expectations, thoughts, and feelings.

The partnership approach, however, is more specific with respect to the relationship between the physician and the patient. In conceptual terms, the objective is to seek ways in which *both* the physician's "disease" framework and the "illness" framework of the patient can be concretely implemented so as to result in the integration of the two perspectives.

The questions, answers, and feedback sequence advocated in a partnership approach provides the specific means to achieve a negotiated understanding between doctor and patient. The symmetrical sequences posited as ideal according to a partnership perspective focus on the concrete activities in which doctors and patients are to engage. The partnership approach is considered preferable in that it is more specific than McWhinney's "parallel search of two frameworks" (1984, p. 3), in regard to these activities.

In addition to the *interpersonal sequences* between doctor and patient, characterized by symmetrical questions, answers, and feedback, the partnership approach to the doctor–patient interaction is also examined with respect to *temporal sequences.* A visit to the doctor involves three temporal phases, comprising patient activities:

1. before the actual doctor–patient interaction,
2. during the actual doctor–patient interaction itself, and
3. those activities occurring after the completion of the doctor–patient interaction.

ACTIVITIES TAKING PLACE BEFORE THE DOCTOR–PATIENT INTERACTION BEGINS

In the patient activities taking place before the visit with the doctor, the emphasis is on the patient's beliefs, questions, and concerns. The patient is also asked to complete a number of questionnaries, which should allow the doctor to better know the patient as a person.

Similar to Byrne and Long (1976) and Kurtz and Silverman (1996), a partnership perspective emphasizes a patient's reasons for scheduling an office visit. The "call" made by a patient to schedule an appointment is the psychological end point of a sequence of events. These events may include "public" (behavioral) or "private" (intrapsychic) events in that person's life (bodily, psychological, family events). There may be numerous variations in these events (behavioral and/or psychological) taking place before the patient calls to make an appointment, involving attitudes, behaviors, memories of past doctor–patient interactions, or anticipated hopes or fears regarding what the doctor might "say" or "find out." All of these events may be "concealed" or "marginalized" during patient visits. So from this perspective, it is assumed that the events occurring in the patient's life between visits, in terms of family, friends, and occupation, may play a role in determining why a patient called for an appointment at a particular time. This is a well-known and accepted aspect of doctor–patient interactions in family medicine. The patient may not have been feeling well for a number of days. But what led her to seek an appointment today?

Health professionals can acknowledge the importance of a patient's concerns and questions by setting aside a distinct place to serve this purpose. Such a place might be called the "patient activities room." In practical terms, such a room would be designated by a portable sign so that any empty room could be temporarily designated as a "patient activities room."

Ideally, it is desirable to have both a "waiting room" and a "patient activity room." The waiting room area is "traditional" in that many individuals including mothers and children, parents, and relatives would be present. The noise often associated with a waiting room should be absent from the patient activity room, where patients are asked to complete two sets of materials. The first set centers around patient beliefs, questions, symptoms, and concerns. These responses should be read by the health professional or doctor so that a patient's questions or concerns can be answered and addressed. Clinicians are made aware that patients are asked, as part of their evaluations completed after the visit, whether the doctor answered the patient's questions and whether the answers were satisfactory to the patient.

The rationale for such "patient activities" occurring prior to the doctor–patient interaction is explained to the patient, either in written form (in various languages) or conveyed by a volunteer who is trained to differentiate between merely "providing information to a patient" as opposed to "assessing whether the patient has understood." (For further discussion of the difference between providing information and promoting understanding, refer to Chapter 17. Instructions to the patient should include time that is "set aside" for articulating such patient-centered questions and concerns prior to each clinic visit. Typically, about 30 to 40 minutes would be required on the first visit with approximately 10 to 15 minutes required thereafter. Such time estimates can be individually tailored by the doctors and patients themselves.

The following points could be included for both patients and health professionals as part of the rationale for the patient activity room. First, it is a place where the patient can, without any time pressure, write down (or have a volunteer write down) any questions and concerns they might have. These may include questions that patients believe to be too "difficult" to say to the doctor directly. The patient activity room also provides patients with a context where they can ask for further clarification, confirmation, and modifications of interactions based on "previous" visits. In other words, the patient can question the doctor in a less direct manner. Questions could refer to both diagnosis and treatment, such as: "What did you mean when you told me I had to . . . or should. . . ."

The second set of materials to be completed prior to the doctor–patient interactions includes items such as the following:

1. Questions regarding the patient's own health beliefs, both generally and specifically related to this visit:
   a. What are your symptoms?
   b. When did they start?
   c. What do you think made you sick (i.e., what is the cause of your illness)?
   d. What do you think will make you better?
2. Questionnaires related to the psychology of the patient.
   a. Such questionnaires vary depending on the preferences of the health professionals in a group practice. For instance, self efficacy measures are favored by the OPD of the obstetrical services at UMass/Memorial Healthcare.
   b. Another suggestion is to include the following two topics, which pertain to a patient's general outlook and experiences
      i. The most important thing that my doctor should know about me as a person is . . .
      ii. If I had three wishes I would wish for:
3. Relevant family-oriented information. This should be a family genogram with specific information regarding parents, grandparents (maternal and paternal), and so on of which the doctor should be aware in order to make treatment recommendations for the patient.
4. Information on past medical history that currently is most frequently asked at the beginning of actual doctor–patient interactions.

Some of the above aspects of the patient's activities occurring prior to the doctor–patient interaction are of a "first-time-only"variety, while others should be repeated during each visit to the clinic. Such questionnaires are changed periodically. Data collected is analyzed and the analysis reviewed by doctors as well as other allied health professionals. Feedback from patients is also sought. This feedback should be part of an ongoing process, thus allowing for systematic, comprehensive changes to be made in the information sought prior to the visit.

Such aspects of a patient's background contribute to his or her "agenda" for making the visit to the clinic. The term "patient's agenda" has often been conflated or condensed as something "latent" or "hidden" within the patient. Unfortunately, some physicians believe it is their "apostolic function" (Balint, 1964) to determine what is the "real" reason for the patient's visit. At best, a physician should "ask and not assume" they know the "real" reason why a patient has decided to visit the clinic.

Physician competence in the biomedical domain justifiably allows doctors to diagnose and treat a patient's body. However, psychoanalytic frameworks have encouraged some physicians to take this a step further and interpret the patient's "unconscious" motives. Some physicians and behavioral scientists, working within psychoanalytic frameworks, believe that they are capable of determining a patient's "real" reasons for making office visits. The patient's stated reasons (the manifest content) may then be viewed as secondary or dismissed entirely by professionals who adhere to such a theoretical framework. In sharpest contrast, according to a partnership approach, the patient is assumed to be capable of clarifying her own agenda both to herself as well as to the doctor.

THE ACTUAL DOCTOR–PATIENT INTERACTION

This intermediate phase of a medical visit has been best articulated in the literature on medical interviewing (refer to Lipkin, Putnam, & Lazare, 1995, for a recent comprehensive review). For our present purposes, we focus on only those aspects of the actual doctor–patient interaction that are directly related to this partnership perspective. Many of the features considered to be desirable, such as silence, reflecting, and clarifying are also viewed favorably from a partnership perspective. Such patient-centered activities are also complementary to a number of essential, physician-centered activities such as gathering information and "probing."

The patient activities taking place prior to the visit should minimize the time required for the traditional physician-centered activities. The time that is saved can then be used by physicians to address the patient's questions and concerns. As a result, the actual doctor–patient interaction becomes more patient-centered. In the literature, the emphasis is overwhelmingly on the doctor's behavior, regarding what the doctor should say and how s/he should say it. This over-emphasis has minimized the importance of the patient's role in the interaction.

From a partnership perspective, the objective is to move away from an exclusive reliance on asymmetrical interactions in which doctors initiate questions, patients respond, and doctors evaluate (IRE sequences) (Cazden, 1988; Mehan, 1979; O'Connor & Michaels, 1993; Sinclair & Coulthard, 1976), toward more symmetrical question–answer–feedback (QAF) interactions. A more symmetrical QAF interaction can be fostered in two ways: first, through the patient activities *before* and *after* the doctor–patient interaction and second, with the focus on more symmetrical QAF *during* the doctor–patient interaction. The sequence taking place during the doctor–patient visit could, from this perspective, begin with an acknowledgement of the patient's questions and concerns.

The second step optimally results in a doctor's attempts to determine whether their answers to the patient's questions make sense. It is during this second phase when the physician can point out what sort of information should be obtained, through physical examinations and clinical tests, so that the patient's questions and concerns may be clarified. The patient's agenda is acknowledged, and her questions and concerns are now concretized with respect to the means that the physician, as expert, believes are necessary. Modifications can then be negotiated between doctor and patient. These modifications may be based on matters as practical as time ("Well, we can do this today. But we will have to schedule another visit for that other test") or as psychologically central as values, related to the physician's professional integrity as well as the patient's own value orientations and preferences. In a partnership approach, the idea of patient as consumer and doctor as provider is rejected. When the patient is considered to be a consumer, the provider is under pressure to accept patient preferences. However, some patient requests can be rejected when they violate a physician's professional integrity or personal values.

The third step in the doctor–patient interaction focuses on

a. the doctor's agenda, comprised of any issues the physician wants to address, that were not included in the patient's agenda,
b. the rationale for the physician's agenda, and
c. the relationship between the patient and the physician's agenda.

During the course of the visit, the physician may need to focus on the patient's preferences regarding alternative approaches to diagnosis and treatment. Emphasizing the importance of patient preferences, Clancy and Eisenberg (1998) point out that "traditional measurements of health . . . offer few insights about the meaning of health states to an individual's daily life" (p. 245).

An example of a physician oversight of patient preferences occurs when the physician "orders" the patient to adhere to "complete bed rest" disregarding the fact that the patient's family relies on this individual for manifold activities. The realistic demands on the patient in his/her everyday activities should be addressed and negotiated between doctor and patient. Indeed, some physicians are unaware of the incongruities in their prescribed treatments. For instance, a doctor warned his patient to stay in bed and to use a bedpan in order to avoid walking to the bathroom. Yet this physician was unaware of the incongruity between the prescribed emphasis on bed rest and asking the patient to return to his office next week!

A focus on patient's preferences during the actual doctor–patient interaction can be complemented by measures (Clancy & Eisenberg, 1998) that the patient is asked by the doctor to complete *after* the interaction is completed. Similarly, through such "functional measures," physicians can assess the implications of their diagnostic and treatment suggestions with respect to their impact on the "ability of individuals to carry out daily activities that are important to them, ranging from general activities of daily life to functions specific to a particular organ or body part" (Clancy & Eisenberg, 1998, p. 245).

The next steps in the actual doctor–patient interaction are "traditional," with regard to obtaining or completing the medical history, the conduct of the physical examination, and prescribing further diagnostic tests and treatment.

In summary, from a partnership perspective, physicians should attempt to determine whether:

1. the patient has understood what was said regarding diagnosis and treatment;
2. the physician understands the patient's questions; and
3. the physician has answered the patient's questions to the patient's satisfaction.

During this last phase of the doctor–patient interaction, the doctor emphasizes the importance, for both parties, of the patient activities occurring after the interaction ends and before the patient leaves the clinic.

PATIENT ACTIVITIES AFTER THE DOCTOR–PATIENT VISIT

Patient activities occurring after the doctor–patient interaction recognize that the visit does not end when the actual interaction with the doctor is over. The feedback provided by the patient after the visit focuses on a) the patient's satisfaction with the visit and b) the patient's understanding of the physician's statements including, but not limited to, medical diagnosis and treatment. Both of these foci constitute feedback for the physician. These types of activities would be considered feedback, according to Briggs, in that they serve to keep "things in check" (1992, p. 116).

The "personal satisfaction" evaluation provides the physician with feedback regarding how the patient "feels" about the interaction. It also addresses the issue of the patient's satisfaction with answers the doctor gave to the patient's questions. Specifically, patients should evaluate a physician's answers with respect to their comprehensiveness, appropriateness, and clarity.

The patient's satisfaction with the visit is important because "interpersonal aspects have been shown to influence adherence to recommended treatments and advice, as well as individuals' ability to manage their own condition" (Clancy & Eisenberg, 1998, p. 245). The questionnaires utilized to determine patient satisfaction are usually generated by experts (e.g., Greenfield, Kaplan & Ware, 1985). In contrast, a partnership perspective would favor questionnaires generated by groups of patients themselves. The patient-generated set of questions, utilized in the OPD Obstetrical Department of Umass/Memorial Health Care, begins with a personal issue: Does the doctor greet the patient by name *or* does the doctor refer immediately to the medical condition? Patients want to be recognized as *individuals,* not as a "case." As one patient explained, "when a doctor uses my name it reassures me that it is *me* who is being treated, not someone else!!!" Such patient satisfaction evaluations have been summarized and used in order to provide periodic feedback to physicians. Indeed, there are currently examples of HMOs where "patient satisfaction" has been relied on as *one* aspect of gauging physician performance and eligibility for "merit" pay raises.

Whereas these activities are considered to be patient-centered, the second set of activities taking place *after* the completion of the doctor–patient interaction are more doctor-centered. The first aim is to address the patient's "understanding" of what the physician has stated regarding diagnosis and treatment. Repeatedly, I have observed misunderstandings and misconceptions by patients of what their physicians have just told them. Having the patient write down (or tell a volunteer) what the doctor said, according to his or her "understanding," is a necessary precaution against the fallacy of assuming that the information provided by the physician is automatically transformed into understanding by the patient. This procedure allows physicians and allied health professionals to determine the "fit" or agreement between statements made by doctors and a patient's understanding. Any misunderstanding can then be followed up, by phone for instance, in order to clarify and correct the physician's original statements. Such clarifications and corrections should obviously not convey "negative" evaluations of the patient by the doctor. Rather, they should be understood as part of the dialogicality between two people attempting to reach an "understanding" of complicated and important issues, namely the patient's health.

It is important that this assessment of the patient's understanding take place immediately *after* the doctor–patient interaction. Studies have shown that patient recollection of what the doctor said is clearly correlated with "recency." In other words, memory is at its best immediately following the visit. Kaplan (1995) explains

> That the storage capacity of long-term memory is essentially unlimited and that the relatively small information capacity of working memory is the limiting factor in man's ability to process information. As such working memory has been the subject of much scrutiny. (p. 24)

Encouraging patients to *write down* what they understand should facilitate recall. The patient is a *recipient* of the verbal message from the doctor. Now the patient is an *active* agent, through writing, conveying what they have selectively remembered. The rationale here is that the *repetition* of doctor statements facilitates recall because the patient is using a different *mode* (writing) as a psychological activity. The reliance on a different mode makes it less likely that the patient will "merely repeat" what the doctor said.

The "cumulative" record of a patient's understanding over time and across visits can be extremely useful for physicians and allied health professionals. Such longitudinal information enables health professionals to assess the patient's understanding of her illness over time, both in terms of variability and consistencies. Given this information, health professionals would then be able to determine what type of progress the patient has made in her understanding over time. It is important to highlight both what improvement the patient has made, as well as what still needs to be changed. Similarly, the patients can review the same information themselves and comment on whether they believe that they have changed with respect to understanding of the illness and health-related behaviors. Patients and physicians are then able to use this information in order to learn more about what facilitates or hinders changes in adherence behaviors over time.

The "medical record" contains the physician's notes at the time of the visit. Similarly, getting the patient's written understanding for each visit also has medical-legal advantages for both patient and doctor. The recollection of "past events" weeks, months, and even years after an event are not as accurate as immediate recall. When the events in a particular instance of a doctor–patient interaction are at issue, as in cases of malpractice, the "memory" of the events is mediated by the lawyers for the plaintiff and the defense. Lawyers construe their aim as providing the best case for their client, irrespective of whether they are pleading for the plaintiff or the defense. For this reason, the story that the doctor or patient tells will have been "smoothed out" by their lawyers. It is assumed that the clearest evidence would be the written statements made by the doctor in the medical record at the time of the visit *and* the written statements completed by the patient immediately following the visit.

The macro-sequence of patient activities before and after the doctor–patient interaction are a practical requirement in the contemporary health care system. The current system in place in the United States actually penalizes physicians for time spent with patients that does not contribute to reimbursement for "clinical services rendered." Therefore, time spent by physicians empathically eliciting the patients' own ideas regarding their concepts of illness, concerns, feelings, and expectations is not recognized by the health care system as an activity worthy of "reimbursement." Having a patient write down these aspects of their "illness framework" *prior* to meeting with the physician represents not only a necessary adaptation to current realities but also an attempt on the part of a physician to learn more about the patient's "illness agenda."

Similarly, the activities taking place *after* the conclusion of the interaction allow the physician to determine whether the objective of "explanation and placing medical recommendations in terms the patient can understand and accept" (McWhinney, 1984) has been accomplished from the patient's perspective. This cognitive aspect of feedback should be complemented by an affective component in which the patient is asked to convey her satisfaction with the visit.

APPENDIX: A SUMMARY OF FOUR MODELS OF DOCTOR–PATIENT INTERACTIONS

Doctors Talking to Patients (Byrne & Long, 1976)

Six phases of activity on the part of doctors, that form a logical structure to the consultation:

Phase I: The doctor establishes a relationship with the patient
Phase II: The doctor either attempts to discover or actually discovers the reason for the patient's attendance
Phase III: The doctor conducts a verbal or physical examination or both
Phase IV: The doctor, the doctor and the patient, or the patient (in that order of probability) consider the condition
Phase V: The doctor, and occasionally the patient, detail further treatment or further investigation
Phase VI: The consultation is terminated usually by the doctor

The Calgary–Cambridge Approach to Communication Skills Teaching (Kurtz & Silverman, 1996)

A set of skills found to aid doctor–patient interactions. The following is the structure of the consultation they propose:

1. Initiating the session
   a. establishing initial rapport
   b. identifying the reason(s) for the patient's attendance
2. Gathering information
   a. exploration of problems
   b. understanding the patient's perspective
   c. providing structure to the consultation
3. Building the relationship
   a. developing rapport
   b. involving the patient
4. Explanation and Planning
   a. providing the correct amount and type of information
   b. aiding accurate recall and understanding
   c. achieving a shared understanding: incorporating the patient's perspective
   d. planning: shared decision making
5. Closing the session

The Disease/Illness Model (McWhinney, 1984)

A "transformed clinical method."

A. Patient presents problem

Gathering information

Parallel search of two frameworks

Illness framework	Disease framework
Patient's agenda	Doctor's agenda
Ideas	Symptoms
Concerns	Signs
Expectations	Investigations
Feelings	Underlying Pathology
Thoughts	
Effects	
Understanding the experience of illness	Differential Diagnosis

B. Integration

Explanation and planning in terms the patient can understand and accept

The Partnership Approach

A partnership between patients and physicians requires communication from patients to doctors and vice versa. Each partner asks and receives answers to his/her questions and provides the other with feedback. A patient's partnership with a physician includes three activities, taking place during each visit. Patients should plan to allow time for these activities:

1. Activities occurring *before* the interaction with the doctor
   a. Think of (preferably write down) any questions for the doctor
   b. Assess the patient's health perceptions*
   c. Answer questions that help your doctor to know you as a person
2. Activities taking place *during* the interaction with the doctor
   a. Doctor collects necessary information verbally and through a physical examination
   b. Patient brings to doctor's attention relevant information from step 1
   c. State patient preferences and functional measures*
3. Activities *after* meeting with the doctor
   a. Determine level of patient satisfaction*
   b. Patient notes any remaining, unanswered questions
   c. Patient writes down what the doctor said regarding medical recommendations and what should be done in response to these recommendations
   d. Read any educational materials and view videotapes suggested by the doctor

*From Clancy and Eisenberg (1998)

REFERENCES

Balint, M. (1964). *The doctor, the patient and the illness* (2nd ed.). New York: International Universities Press.

Briggs, J. (1992). *Fractals: The patterns of chaos*. New York: Simon and Schuster.

Byrne, P. S., & Long, B. E. L. (1976). *Doctors talking to patients: A study of the verbal behavior of general practitioners consulting in their surgeries*. Exeter, England: The Royal College of General Practitioners.

Cazden, C. (1988). *Classroom discourse*. Portsmouth, NH: Heinemann.

Clancy, C. M., & Eisenberg, J. M. (1998). Outcomes research: Measuring the end results of health care. *Science, 282*, 245–246.

Greenfield, S., Kaplan, S., & Ware, Jr., J. E. (1985). Expanding patient involvement in care. *Annals of Internal Medicine, 102,* 520–528.

Kaplan, C. (1995). Hypothesis testing. In M. Lipkin, Jr., S. M. Putnam, & A. Lazare (Eds.), *The medical interview: Clinical care, education and research* (pp. 20–31). New York: Springer-Verlag.

Kurtz, S. M., & Silverman, J. D. (1996). The Calgary-Cambridge referenced observation guides: An aid to defining the curriculum and organising the teaching in communication training programmes. *Medical Education, 30,* 83–89.

Lipkin, Jr., M., Putnam, S. M., & Lazare, A. (1995) (Eds.) *The medical interview: Clinical care, education and research*. New York: Springer-Verlag.

McWhinney, I. R. (1984). Changing models: The impact of Kuhn's theory on medicine. *Journal of Family Practice, 1,* 3–8.

Mehan, H. (1979). *Learning lessons.* Cambridge, MA: Harvard University Press.

O'Connor, M. C., & Michaels, S. (1993). Aligning academic task and participation status through revoicing: Analysis of a classroom discourse strategy. *Anthropology and Education Quarterly, 24*, 318–335.

Sinclair, J. M., & Coulthard, R. M. (1976). *Toward an analysis of discourse: The English used by teachers and pupils.* London: Oxford University Press.

part IV

Partnerships in Interprofessional Collaboration

20

UNIVERSITY–COMMUNITY–SCHOOL PARTNERSHIP*

Mary E. Walsh
Boston College

Dita G. Andersson
Boston College

ABSTRACT

Partnerships between institutions constitute an important domain in the intersection of science and practice. Recently, universities have become active participants in interinstitutional partnerships. In the last decade, universities have become more cognizant of the changing societal issues and problems faced by their local communities and schools. Realizing that the application of traditional research findings to issues confronting youth and families is not sufficient to meet the contemporary needs of children and families, universities are beginning to shift toward a new model of research, working "with" rather than "in" communities. With this shift comes a multitude of changes in the way communities and universities work together. In this chapter, we describe various aspects of creating a partnership between an urban public school, the local community, and a university.

* The preparation of this manuscript was supported in part by grants from the DeWitt Wallace Reader's Digest Fund and the U.S. Department of Education (Fund for the Improvement of Post Secondary Education).

America's youth and families face a historically unprecedented set of problems. The number of children and adolescents living in poverty, experiencing educational and school failure, and engaging in high-risk behaviors such as drug and alcohol abuse, unsafe sex, and delinquency, is higher than ever before in this country's history (Lerner, 1995). In response to these problems, universities are increasingly making interdisciplinary and collaborative efforts to bring their knowledge to bear more directly on the needs of the community. Boyer (1994) signaled this change in direction when he called for a "New American College" that would be less fragmented, focusing less attention on specific specialties and more attention on the university's connections to the greater community. At local and national levels, growing numbers of university faculty have begun to develop collaboration across professions as well as university–community partnerships (Fitzgerald, Abrams, Church, Votruba, & Imig, 1996; Harkavy, 1997; Lerner & Simon, 1998; McHale et al., 1996; Small, 1996; Weinberg & Erikson, 1996).

Relationships between universities and communities are not a new phenomenon. Historically, university researchers have always recognized that their applied scholarship had significant potential for addressing the social and economic problems that communities faced. Many of the difficult problems encountered by practitioners across a variety of professions have been ameliorated through the application of university-based research. However, the application of research findings to community problems most often occurred at an abstract level and did not directly engage the university and the community in ongoing relationships. The research findings were "available" to local communities to apply as they were able.

Furthermore, in the cases where the university–community relationships were more direct and immediate, the focus was almost exclusively on the needs of the universities. The research needs of university faculty led them to seek out individuals and groups in the community who could serve as research subjects. For example, it has come to be common practice for researchers to enter local schools in order to study particular aspects of children's psychological development (i.e., cognitive or socioemotional processes). Relationships between universities and communities also emerged from the university's need for field sites in which to train students. For decades, community schools, hospitals, clinics, and social service centers served as practicum placements for the various professions. The bulk of university–community relationships were limited to one-way arrangements in which the university sought to meet the needs of its research or teaching functions.

In the last decade, universities have become more cognizant of the societal issues and problems that local communities face. They have come to recognize that, as universities, they have multiple resources that may help to address some of these important issues. They have realized that the application of research findings to general problems and issues is important, but insufficient, in connecting the university and the community in collaborative problem solving. Universities are beginning to acknowledge the significant distance, described by Schon (1987), between the "application" of research findings and on-the-ground problem solving.

> In the varied topography of professional practice, there is a high, hard ground overlooking a swamp. On the high ground, manageable problems lend themselves to solution through the application of research-based theory and technique. In the swampy lowland, messy, confusing problems defy technical solution. The irony of this situation is that the problems of the high ground tend to be relatively unimportant to individuals or society at large, however great their technical interest may be, while in the swamp lie the problems of the greatest human concern. (Schon, 1987, p. 3)

In many universities, there is now a notable shift of concern from "the hard high ground" to the "messy lowland." In the process of shifting, the university has recognized the need to work with the community in a different type of relationship. In contrast to the typical arrangements in which the university has more power than the community in terms of knowledge, resources, and student "workforce," some newly emerging collaborations have embraced a more bilateral relationship. In these relationships, the community brings a set of resources and knowledge that is different from and necessary to the university. Universities are beginning to recognize that community and university are more effective when the power of the collaborative is balanced.

In this chapter, we describe a university–community collaboration in which a group of our university faculty and students are engaged in a partnership with our local community to address the needs of children, youth, and families. More specifically, we have engaged in a process of negotiation with the community and schools not only to work on "solutions," but also first to codefine "the problem." Through this process, we have learned from one another by engaging in dialogue that was open to the unique contribution and perspective of each other. In short, our aim has been to achieve a more ideal model of partnership in which the gains for each member, while different in content, are equal in significance and in which the exchange of ideas between members is both symmetrical and reciprocal.

Our work with a local elementary school is the most developed example of our partnership efforts to date. Over the past five years, our goal in working with this traditional, urban school is to be stable, contributing partners as the school staff intensify and broaden their own efforts to develop curricula and programs that promote the positive development of the children and families of their school community. In this chapter, we describe the origins and development of our unique partnership, our conceptual assumptions, the short-term outcomes of our work, and the difficulties we have faced in our efforts to engage in a partnership that is distinct from our previous relationships with the community. It should be noted that in contrast to other chapters of this book that have applied the partnership ideal to various kinds of interpersonal contexts, our efforts have been directed toward applying the partnership ideal to collaboration between institutions.

THE ORIGINS OF OUR RELATIONSHIP WITH THE SCHOOL

Located in a Boston neighborhood about four miles from the Boston College campus, the Gardner Elementary School faces the complex issues typical of urban schools across the country (Wang & Kovach, 1996). Of the population of 500 students, 80 percent are students of color and 80 percent meet the federal poverty guidelines. For 78 percent of these children, English is a second language, with more than 31 different languages spoken among their families.

As psychologists, we first became involved with the Gardner School in a manner typical of academics, that is, collecting data for a research study. At the conclusion of the data collection, as we said our usual "thanks and farewell," the Gardner teachers and administrators interrupted our leave-taking with a request for assistance from the university in solving problems that were important to the school. They believed that issues related to students' health, safety, psychological well-being, economic circumstances, immigration status, and family problems were interfering with the academic success of their students. They expressed a hope that university professionals would provide them with "answers" and "solutions." While we viewed the school as a useful avenue for the accumulation of knowledge relevant to the university's purposes, the school wanted our work to generate a knowledge base useful for them in their efforts to improve the lives of their students.

Initially, we turned away from their requests for assistance. "Partnering" with the school around their concerns had not been our intent, and we felt unable to commit our time to efforts that might distract us from what we viewed as our primary responsibility to produce and publish "new knowledge." However, conversations that had begun to take place among the faculty within the university led us to change our minds. That is, our eventual decision to respond to the school's request was reflective of a shift in the way that many university faculty and administrators had begun to think about academic knowledge and its applicability to larger community issues.

THE DEVELOPMENT OF THE PARTNERSHIP

Shifts Within the University

At the same time that the local school requested our assistance, university faculty members were beginning to address the relevance of knowledge for addressing complex social issues. Within the Boston College community, a small group of faculty and administrators from across various professional preparation programs (law, social work, nursing, education, psychology, management, pastoral ministry) and arts and sciences departments had become increasingly interested in conducting research that was responsive to the human issues of its local community. More specifically, they had begun meeting informally to address a common set of concerns about the condition of America's children and families, particularly those living in poverty (Brabeck, Walsh, Kenny, & Comilang, 1997). A continuing series of conversations among these faculty highlighted the isolated character of each profession's approach to working with what they variously referred to as "clients," "patients," or "students." Consistent with what many policy experts had been pointing out, these conversations made clear that community problems could not be defined in discipline-shaped boxes, and that an individual seeking assistance from one or more of these professions would most likely experience fragmented and uncoordinated care (Lerner & Simon, 1998; Peterson, 1995; Schorr, 1997). To be effective, "outreach scholarship" that "generated, transmitted, and applied knowledge for the purpose of addressing societal problems as defined in concert with the community" (Lerner & Simon, 1998, p. 4) would require collaboration both across professions and with the local community.

Creating partnerships with the community that would involve collaboration across professions, as well as colearning with the community, was new to the university (Walsh, Howard, & Brabeck, 1997). Consequently, faculty recognized the need to develop structures within the university to shift the effort from an ad hoc activity to a more permanent part of the work of the university. In order to create such a structure at Boston College, faculty and administrators committed themselves and substantial resources to the development of the Center for Child, Family, and Community Partnerships. The center's purpose was to promote interprofessional collaboration in the university as well as outreach scholarship in the community. The center brings together faculty and graduate students from across professional specialties to collaborate in research and practice that might lead to more effective practice with children and families.

While collaboration across professions and disciplines was indeed an asset to the work of the university, the faculty did not view it as sufficient to meeting the new goals we had set. As academics, we had limited firsthand experience in the community. As researchers, we focused on universal processes such as "cognition" and "affect," rather than on persons. We engaged people as "research subjects," rather than as members of the human community. For example, as developmental psychologists, we often did not hear the life stories of children living in seriously stressful conditions because we relied almost exclusively on standardized measures of their feelings or cognitive processes. As lawyers, we addressed issues in larger systems, such as the juvenile justice system, while often overlooking the individual adolescents in youth services detention. While a focus on abstract processes has long been the norm for research by a wide range of academic professionals, we quickly realized that our efforts would remain ungrounded unless our work was informed and shaped by community-based professionals who had experience "in the trenches."

After two years of dialogue within the university, we realized what a unique and valuable opportunity had been presented to us by the Gardner School's request for assistance. It was the kind of opportunity that would allow us to match the needs and interests of the university with issues confronting the community. It would simultaneously serve as a site for integrating the realities of practice with the theory of interprofessional collaboration.

Our first collaborative effort with the Gardner School focused on developing educational experiences for future teachers, social workers, and counselors that might better prepare them for working with the wide range of student's needs such as those faced by children at Gardner. The school and university staffs recognized that the barriers to learning experienced by schoolchildren were not merely psychological, but were also economic, legal, and health related. For this reason, new features of the curriculum were designed to prepare future teachers, counselors, and social workers to work collaboratively, not only with families and mental health service providers, but also with legal and health professionals. The influx of professionals-in-training significantly assisted the Gardner staff to meet the needs of children better. The success of this collaboration encouraged us to continue working with the Gardner School in order to address their concerns in a more immediate manner. Preparing future teachers and counselors was important, but the Gardner School faced immediate difficulties that could not wait for the next generation of professionals to be addressed.

SHARED ASSUMPTIONS

In the years that followed, university and school professionals engaged in a dialogue that would attempt to codetermine not only the answers and solutions that the school staff were looking to find, but more fundamentally, the very definition of "the problem" (Walsh, Buckley & Howard, 1998). Our ability to identify the problem and develop common goals was aided in no small part by our shared beliefs about the nature of human development. All of the partners—both university and community—had a fundamentally similar view about how people develop into productive and healthy adults. We briefly describe the shared assumptions that have been articulated by developmental psychologists and that laid the groundwork for our work together.

Development in Context

University and public school faculty were firmly committed to the notion that all aspects of a child's environment are connected and relevant to his or her development, that is, it was agreed that development occurs in context. By focusing on underlying processes, traditional psychological approaches have tended to view the individual abstractly and in isolation from his or her context. New understandings suggest that youths develop in relationship to the various contexts in which they are embedded. That is, their development occurs in families who have particular cultural orientations and who live in particular neighborhoods or communities. As a result, collaboration between schools and families has come to be seen as vital to develop intervention strategies that are context specific, culturally relevant, and grounded in family and community. This orientation is supported by the considerable evidence that suggests that intervention programs that exclusively service individuals in isolation from their social contexts are especially vulnerable to failures in long-term maintenance (Peterson, 1995; Schorr, 1997). In her review of programs aimed at preventing negative developmental outcomes in youth, Schorr (1997) points to the limits of a-contextual interventions and argues that "one of the most difficult lessons for policymakers to learn is that most successful interventions cannot be imposed from without and that there is no simple model that can just be parachuted in" (p. 7). Similarly, the Council of State Policy and Planning Agencies which conducted field research into "best practices" in anti-poverty programs found that very little held true when context is disregarded and that "the successful programs are the ones which respond to the needs of the community and reflect the character of its people" (Schorr, 1997, p. 8). For these reasons, all partners in the university–school collaboration were committed to devising interventions that considered the child's familial and community context.

Multiple Levels of Organization

The range of professions represented in the initial conversations in the university exemplified the fact that no one believed that fostering the education and development of youth was the province of a single profession. Because of their understanding of the complexity of children's lives, the faculty could only conclude that multiple professions needed to be involved in developing effective solutions. In parallel, school staff realized that it had to respond not only to the educational, but also to the psychological, social, and health needs of its students. Together, university and community shared a vision for schooling grounded in the belief that development occurs at multiple levels (e.g., biological, psychological, social, and cultural) and that these levels are continually impacting one another (Lerner, 1996). With our commitment to this assumption, we recognized that it was necessary to include people from a number of different professions working with the children and families, and that it was not enough for these professionals to simply work "side by side." To the contrary, professionals would necessarily interact and coordinate their efforts with one another. They would share in a negotiation process to define questions, design interventions, and evaluate outcomes. In short, given the understanding that development occurs at multiple levels, it was clear that prevention and intervention would have to address the many aspects of each individual child rather than focus exclusively upon cognitive capacities.

Life Span Perspective

Another shared assumption emerging from our discussions was the belief that any intervention program designed to enhance the development of the Gardner School children should also address the issues confronting their respective families. Because adults are continually developing, particularly in regard to their familial roles, the influence of parents on their children depends, to some extent, on the parents' developmental level (Lerner & Fisher, 1994). Recognizing the variation in the developmental pathways not only of children, but also of adults, prevention and intervention activities would need to support both children and parents in their development (Lerner, Walsh, & Howard, 1998).

Resilience

A final assumption shared by all members involved the recognition that developmental outcomes were not fixed, and children had individual strengths that enabled them to overcome significant developmental obstacles. This shared belief in resilience led us to move away from a deficit model of youth development that would have focused on addressing and blocking negative developmental outcomes. Instead, we moved toward a model that bolstered the particular strengths of each individual child. While such a program certainly involved interventions to address existing developmental difficulties, it balanced such efforts with preventive activities to provide each child with services and conditions likely to promote positive development. Consistent with the positions of Lerner, Ostrom, and Freel (1995) and Eccles (1996), our efforts have attempted to move beyond "band-aid" interventions to focus on factors that are believed to promote positive youth development.

NEGOTIATING DIFFERENCES: DEFINING "THE PROBLEM" AND DESIGNING AN INTERVENTION

While the partnership between the school and the university was grounded in many shared conceptual assumptions about human development, there were also important differences between the partners that would require negotiation. These differences were particularly evident around the definition of the "problem." At the level of theory, university faculty were committed to the principle that the barriers to learning experienced by each of these children were ultimately the product of numerous external social, political, and economic forces. However, at the level of practice, we assumed that the problem could be addressed by developing interventions at the level of the individual child. We assumed that the changes that would benefit the children and families of the Gardner School could be brought about by delivering individual services to children within the context of the school building. The problem, as we defined it, was to determine how to improve each child's level of academic achievement; that is, we hoped to "fix" the child within the context of the school.

The school principal, however, quickly challenged this definition. "The problem is not located in the child," she said, "nor is it restricted to the context of the school." The problem, as the principal viewed it, was "in the many worlds that the child must traverse." She clearly saw the child as embedded in many contexts and she located the "problem" in the relationship between the child and those contexts. She viewed the school's difficulties as part of the problems of the larger community and suggested that the school should play a vital role in helping to build stronger families and communities that, in turn, would better support the development of their children. She pointed to particular stressors that interfered with parents' ability to support their child's education (e.g., inadequate after-school care, limited English proficiency, lack of access to necessary health care, immigration-related legal difficulties). The principal argued that the school had a responsibility to work to alleviate some of these difficulties rather than to continue to view such problems as irrelevant to its objectives. For university professionals, these identified issues did not fit within the parameters of what they had ordinarily viewed from a clinical perspective as "the problem" (Bibace, Dillon, & Dowds, in this volume). "Fixing the child" within the school was a far cry from actually intervening in the systems that encompassed the child outside the school walls (Lerner, Walsh, & Howard, 1998).

What emerged from these discussions was a decision by all members that the partnership should be expanded from a school–university partnership to a school–community–university partnership. Incorporating the community into the partnership brought community members, agencies, businesses, and public services into the conversation to develop a concrete intervention strategy. Comprised of parents, community members and agencies, and university faculty, the partnership met weekly for two years to plan a response to the school and community's concerns about their children.

With funding from the DeWitt Wallace Readers' Digest Foundation, the intervention, which seemed to the partners to flow logically from the needs of the children and families as well as from the capabilities and resources of the partners, was the transformation of the Gardner school into an Extended Services School. An Extended Services School would not only extend the school day into after-school, weekend, and summer hours, but it would also focus specifically on integrating academic instruction with opportunities for enrichment, career exploration, youth development, and family support services. It would provide adults with health care, legal assistance, mental health services, job counseling, ESL courses, and computer training. As Dryfoos (1994) has described, community schools combine education with the supports needed for the healthy development of children and families, and it does so in one place.

THE ROLE OF THE EXPERT

University faculty from various professions and disciplines began interacting around specific issues confronting the school. Working as partners forced them to redefine the role of "expert" vis a vis one another. Similarly, if the public school and community were to participate equally in the identification of research questions and in the design and implementation of interventions, university faculty would need to relinquish their stance as "the" experts so that responsibility and authority for the project could be shared. In essence, a "co-learning" model, that is, a model involving a synthesis of expertise in schools, communities, and universities, needed to be developed (Lerner & Simon, 1998). By adhering to such a model and by no longer setting priorities independently of the school and community's key issues, we, as academics, could take on the role of the "learner." It was no longer assumed that we "knew best" or that we alone were responsible for the project's leadership. As Eccles (1996) has stated, the time had come for us to move the study of youth development "out of the laboratory and into the full complexity of real world problems" and to begin to "listen to the wisdom of practitioners" (p. 81).

While useful knowledge was gained in our movement toward a "partnership," potential difficulties also emerged. Since the responsibility for the project no longer lay exclusively with either the university or the school, but rather with the partnership, the sense of structure and order that exists when there is a designated "expert" was lacking. Unable to call upon a single external "expert" for solutions, teachers and administrators were overwhelmed by the diversity of issues and problems presented by students, by the range of ethnic and cultural differences, and by the varying levels of cognitive and emotional maturity manifested by the students. What emerged from their frustration was the incipient belief that there may be no way to support adequately the development of these children. What was particularly potent was their increasing skepticism about the ability of the partners, previously considered "experts" (i.e., the university professionals) to come up with "answers." They reported growing despair about the usefulness of the university's contributions.

At the same time, the university was experiencing similar angst. Academics from different professions and disciplines began to realize that no single profession or discipline had the "answer"; they had been unable to establish universally applicable and effective interventions even through their interdisciplinary efforts. In effect, the deemphasis on the role of the "expert" had not immediately solved the problem, but rather appeared to contribute significantly to the problem. Both the university and the school needed the expertise of the other for certain problems and issues. It became clear that the role of the expert should not be eliminated, but rather should be shared as a function of the task. There were issues about which the school simply knew more, just as there were some issues about which the university knew more. Negating this was as problematic as assuming that one partner, the university, had all the answers. What was needed was the dissolution of a permanent hierarchy among members and the creation of flexible hierarchies which could respond differently to the needs of the moment. For example, while the university may well be the "expert" in quantitative aspects of program evaluation, the public school's expertise would most likely be required to design mechanisms that integrate health and human services in the school. Thus, for those working within a university partnership, it is assumed that universities have as much to learn about the schools and communities with which they partner as they have knowledge to offer. Their "expertise" is viewed as a contribution to the partnership's ongoing dialogue, rather than as a "proclamation from the mountain top."

We view the history of this partnership as an evolution. We began with a rather traditional approach to knowledge that assumed that specialized individuals working in isolation would generate the most useful research; we ultimately came to assume what Prilleltensky (1997) has referred to as a "communitarian stance." This perspective deemphasizes self-determination and, instead, stresses reciprocal or mutual determination. It shows a concern and responsibility not only for the individual, but also for the disempowered communities within which the individual exists.

As part of this shared communitarian world view, all partners agree that a good society is one in which members operate as a collective to ensure that its children are safe, well-educated, and have access to those services that are most likely to facilitate their healthy development. Furthermore, they agree that to achieve this end all members must share equal authority and responsibility and that they be able to participate in a democratic and collaborative manner. In this way, communitarianism is not only concretized through partnership, but is also fundamental for its success.

OUR MODEL OF PARTNERSHIP

In the literature on collaboration, "partnership" has been defined in a number of different ways. Following the work of Bibace, Dillon, and Dowds (in this volume), we describe ideal partnerships as being characterized by "complementarity, symmetry, and reciprocity" between members. Successful partnerships are those in which each member is able to "share learning" by contributing knowledge to and receiving information from other members. Both the Interprofessional Collaboration Project at the university and the Gardner Extended Services School in the community reflect this understanding of "partnership."

Inherent in this view of partnership is the notion that the problem definition and the solution will be negotiated. In describing their model for university–community partnerships, Ostrom, Lerner, and Freel (1995) point out that university faculty working within a partnership should not "enter the community with the goal of making a pre-established set of content recommendations or with pre-planned research agendas to implement" (p. 491). To do so would be to "superimpose the university's belief system on the community and to fail to listen to and learn from the community about its needs" (p. 491).

A successful partnership, in contrast, is a partnership that is continuously self-evaluating. Members question their own understanding of each member's perspectives, values, and experiences, and they question whether each member's position has been acted upon (Schorr, 1997; Thorkildsen & Stein, 1996). This involves an ongoing dynamic process that ensures that what one "heard" from another member was indeed what that member meant. The members work from extremely varied positions, languages, and professional cultures, and this necessitates continuous feedback about intentions and interpretations. As Bibace and colleagues have argued, it is precisely this complementarity between members that distinguishes the partnership model from other collaborative models: "the aim of a partnership approach to research is to move toward symmetry regarding the opportunity to ask questions, to have one's questions answered, and to provide feedback to one's partner" (Bibace, Dillon, & Dowds, in this volume).

As a result of engaging in this university–community partnership, a fundamental shift has begun to occur in our university faculty's self-perception. In contrast to their earlier stance that the university is "in, but not of" the community, the faculty have now begun to see themselves and the university as part of the community. The community has also perceived this change. Describing her experience in the Gardner School project, and the shift in the university's approach to such work, the director of the community-based coalition with which we have collaborated reported, "For the first time, we are dealing with the real guts of the university—professors and students—not just the Community Affairs Office."

While this shift in approach with respect to the university's role is clearly beneficial to the local community, it also offers important benefits to the university. As Lynton (1996) has suggested:

> New knowledge is created in the course of the application of outreach, and as a source of new insights, it is of great pedagogical value for faculty to have had direct involvement in such projects, to have worked collaboratively with practitioners, and to have acquired first hand knowledge of the field in this way. (p. 16)

The most critical shift in the university, however, has occurred in the faculty's approach to scholarship. In a traditional approach to research, the researchers frame the questions, which constitute the core of the research process. The researchers have typically initiated the sequence of asking and answering and discussing questions. Academics have framed and asked the questions, the community members have responded. Discussion and/or negotiation may or may not follow. Contrary to this traditional sequence, in the partnership model as we have engaged it, the community initiated the questions and the university responded. The discussions that led to co-defining of the problem and identifying tentative solutions have reflected a process of continuing negotiation. The relationship between the university and the community is more symmetrical than the researchers involved in the project previously experienced. This model of partnership follows the model that has been articulated by Bibace and colleagues (in this volume) in clinical and research contexts. While it involves a relationship between institutions rather than individuals, it is built on the same core assumptions about the differences between symmetrical and asymmetrical relationships.

SYSTEMIC CHALLENGES

This partnership has not been without challenges. There are numerous systemic obstacles that make this particular kind of relationship between schools, universities, and communities difficult to implement (Lerner & Simon, 1998; McHale et al., 1996; Weinberg & Erikson, 1996). These challenges involve the community's perceptions of the university, the university reward system, and the traditional way in which distinct disciplines interact within the university.

Schools and communities have grown distrustful of universities in recent years (Boyer, 1994; Eccles, 1996; Weinberg & Erikson, 1996). Universities have come to be seen as self-interested, unresponsive to the needs of the community, and exploitative. As Carl Bell, professor of psychiatry and public health at University of Illinois at Chicago has pointed out:

> When you consider what's on the researcher's plate, you see that they're getting Ph.D.'s, careers, funding, sabbaticals and publications while the community is getting "the project" but then the funding is over and everybody leaves, and what do they have then? (Clay, 1997)

Our partnership was able to begin to address this substantial issue through a shift in the usual arrangements for funding. In contrast to the typical school–community–university collaborations in which the university serves as the recipient of and fiscal agent for the funding, our partnership made the decision to locate the largest of its grants not with the university but with the community partner, the local YMCA. This represented a fundamental shift in the orientation of the university. Ordinarily, in grant production and management, the university receives the "overhead" from faculty-authored grants. As a Jesuit university, whose mission statement explicitly calls for the generation of knowledge that can lead to real difference in human lives, Boston College recognized the central importance of partnering with the community in the practice of meaningful scholarship, of engaging in "outreach scholarship" with the community. For this reason, Boston College was willing to relinquish control of the funds involved in this community partnership.

The university reward system presents another set of challenges that must be confronted by university faculty as they attempt to participate in a "partnership" with the local schools and community. In the present organization of universities, reward systems promote independent scholarly contributions; little or no collaborative or community engagement is required or encouraged. Consequently, untenured faculty members have little incentive to invest the time required for outreach scholarship (Lerner & McHale, 1996; Harkavy & Puckett, 1991).

"Turfdom among the disciplines" presents another impediment to community–university collaborations (Weinberg & Erikson, 1996). Unfortunately, such "academic territorialism" can become particularly entrenched in departments with overlapping missions. Education, psychology, and social work are then at particular risk for territorialism as each works in the domain of child and youth development (Lerner & Fisher, 1994). The Gardner School partners found that maintaining an emphasis on the children and families that the project served helped the partners to shift the attention away from the battle lines of turf wars.

While these systemic obstacles make partnership difficult, studies of successful intervention programs suggest that partnership, while difficult to accomplish, is the approach that is most effective in promoting the healthy development of America's disadvantaged youth (Foley, 1997; Schorr, 1997; Thorkildsen & Stein, 1996). In her review of successful interventions, Schorr (1997) found that the most effective programs were those that were comprehensive, flexible, and responsive to the needs of the local community. They were the programs that viewed children in the context of their families and communities and that had evolved in response to the changing needs of its members.

Similarly, in a review of various nationwide efforts aimed at university–school collaboration, Thorkildsen and Stein (1996) found that successful interventions were derived from partnerships that had worked to cooperatively identify goals and questions, that had shared decision making among all members, and that had an ongoing and dynamic process of evaluation through which changes in goals, objectives, and activities could be initiated. Outcomes of these partnership studies have not supported the claim made by Peterson (1995) which stated that university partnerships that are directed at intervention should focus less upon the needs of particular communities and more upon identifying a universally applicable model of prevention and intervention. In fact, Schorr (1997) suggests the opposite. Schorr found that America has not been successful in replicating "what works" in particular communities onto a larger scale because doing so has eliminated many of the critical contextual details that made the initial, smaller-scale intervention effective in the first place. That is, such larger-scale efforts have consistently eliminated important components of the smaller-scale intervention despite the fact that evaluators of the original models had indicated that it was precisely the interaction of its multiple components that had made the smaller programs successful.

Partnership offers universities a framework for conducting research and designing interventions in a way that is appreciative of the interacting influences of family, school, and community in the lives of children. In sharing responsibility and authority, and in alternating the role of the expert between members according to particular problems and contexts, our partnership has been able to move forward in response to the complex problems presented by the students, parents, and families of the Gardner School. By requiring that all members be open to the distinct contributions of the "other," our partnership has attempted to demonstrate the flexibility that Schorr (1997) deemed essential in responding to human problems.

As children in America today continue to face unprecedented levels of poverty and its accompanying problems, the public is growing ever more weary of universities that separate themselves from society and remain aloof from real-world problems (Eccles, 1996; Harkavy & Puckett, 1991; Weinberg & Erikson, 1996). As

Harkavy and Puckett (1991) have noted that while communities have "problems," universities have "departments." If we are to strengthen the role of higher education, it is essential that we work together with schools and communities to devote our intellectual resources toward humane applications of scientific knowledge. We, as academics and as universities, can no longer afford to insulate ourselves within specialized departments, nor can we afford to conduct research that ignores the questions that the community considers to be important. As our work with the Gardner School has revealed, the university's questions and the university's solutions are simply not as useful as the questions and solutions that the university and community co-construct in ongoing partnership with one another.

REFERENCES

Brabeck, M., Walsh, M., Kenny, M., & Comilang, K. (1997). Interprofessional collaboration for children and families: Opportunities for counseling psychology in the 21st century. *The Counseling Psychologist, 25* (4), 615–636.

Boyer, E. L. (1994, March 9). Creating the new American college. *Chronicle of Higher Education,* p. A43.

Clay, R. (1997, November). Psychologists seek closer ties with communities they study.*APA Monitor,* pp. 30–31.

Dryfoos, J. G. (1994). *Full service schools: A revolution in health and social services of children, youth, and families.* San Francisco: Jossey-Bass.

Eccles, J. (1996). The power and difficulty of university–community collaboration.*Journal of Research on Adolescence, 6* (1), 81–86.

Fitzgerald, H., Abrams, A., Church, R., Votruba, J., & Imig, G. (1996). Applied developmental science at Michigan State University: Connecting university and community via programs for children, youth, and families. *Journal of Research on Adolescence, 6,* 55–69.

Foley, E. (1997). *Lessons from a three-year project to advance interprofessional education in nine universities.* New York: National Center for Schools and Communities.

Harkavy, I. (1997). Organizational innovation and the creation of the new American university. In R. M. Lerner and L. A. K. Simon (Eds.), *University–community collaboration for the 21st century: Outreach scholarship for youth and families* (pp. 275–289). New York: Garland.

Harkavy, I., & Puckett, J. (1991). Toward effective university–public school partnerships: An analysis of a contemporary model. *Teacher College Record, 92* (4), 557–577.

Lerner, R. (1995). *America's youth in crisis.* Thousand Oaks, CA: Sage.

Lerner, R. (1996). Relative plasticity, integration, temporality, and diversity in human development: A developmental contextual perspective about theory, process, and method. *Developmental Psychology, 32* (4), 781–786.

Lerner, R., & Fisher, C. (1994). *Applied developmental psychology.* New York: McGraw-Hill.

Lerner, R., & McHale, S. (1996). University–community collaborations on behalf of youth. *Journal of Research on Adolescence, 6* (1), 1–7.

Lerner, R., Ostrom, C., & Freel, M. (1995). Promoting positive youth and community development through outreach scholarship. *Journal of Adolescent Research, 10,* 486–502.

Lerner, R., & Simon, L. (Eds.). (1998). *University–community collaboration for the 21st Century: Outreach scholarship for youth and families.* New York: Garland.

Lerner, R., Walsh, M., & Howard, K. (1998). Developmental-contextual considerations: Person-context relations as the bases for risk and resiliency in child and adolescent development. In T. Ollendick (Ed.), *Comprehensive Clinical Psychology: Vol. 4* (pp. 1–24). New York: Elsevier Science.

Lynton, E. (1996). Ensuring the quality of outreach: The critical role of evaluating individual and collective initiatives and performance. *Journal of Public Service and Outreach, 1* (2), 16–22.

McHale, S., Crouter, A., Fennelly, K., Tomascik, C., Updegraff, K., Graham, J., Baker, A., Dreisbach, L., Ferry, N., Manlove, E., McGroder, S., Mulkeen, P., & Obeidallah, D. (1996). Community-based interventions for young adolescents: The Penn State PRIDE Project. *Journal of Research on Adolescence, 6* (1), 23–36.

Ostrom, C., Lerner, R., & Freel, M. (1995). Building the capacity of youth and families through university–community collaborations: The development-in-context evaluation (DICE) model. *Journal of Adolescent Research, 10* (4), 427–448.

Peterson, G. (1995). The need for common principles in prevention programs for children, adolescents, and families. *Journal of Adolescent Research, 10* (4), 470–485.

Prilleltensky, I. (1997). Values, assumptions, and practices: Assessing the moral implications of psychological discourse and action. *American Psychologist, 52* (5), 517–535.

Schon, D. (1987). *Educating the reflective practitioner.* San Francisco: Jossey-Bass.

Schorr, L. (1997). *Common purpose: Strengthening families and neighborhoods to rebuild America.* New York: Anchor Books.

Small, S. (1996). Collaborative, community-based research on adolescents: Using research for community change. *Journal of Research on Adolescence, 6* (1), 9–22.

Thorkildsen, R., & Stein, M. (1996). Fundamental characteristics of successful university–school partnerships. *The School Community Journal, 6* (2), 79–92.

Walsh, M., Howard, K., & Brabeck, M. (1997, August). A theoretical framework for engaging in interprofessional collaboration. In *Opportunities for counseling psychology: Interprofessional collaboration for children and families.* Symposium conducted at the annual meeting of the American Psychological Association, Chicago.

Walsh, M., Buckley, M., & Howard, K. (1998). Critical collaborations: School, family and community. In R. Haney & J. O'Keefe (Eds.), *Conversations in Excellence: Providing for the diverse needs of youth and their families* (pp. 63–84). Washington, DC: NCEA.

Wang, M., & Kovach, J. (1996). Bridging the achievement gap in urban schools: Reducing educational segregation and advancing resilience-promoting strategies. In B. Williams (Ed.), *Closing the achievement gap: A vision for changing beliefs and practices* (pp.10–36). Alexandria, VA: Association for Supervision and Curriculum Development.

Weinberg, R., & Erikson, M. (1996). Minnesota's children, youth, and family consortium: A university–community collaboration. *Journal of Research on Adolescence, 6*(1), 37–53.

part V

A Partnership Ideal

21

A PARTNERSHIP IDEAL

Roger Bibace
Clark University and
University of Massachusetts Medical School

ABSTRACT

Traditional, asymmetrical relationships in education, medicine, and research are characterized by asymmetry in that an "expert" typically controls the sequence and goals of the interaction. In contrast, partner relationships are typified by complementarity and reciprocity, but not equality, between both parties. Whereas in a traditional interaction, professionals initiate questions and then evaluate the counterpart's responses, partner relationships rely on reciprocal interactions, in which nonexperts are encouraged to ask their own questions and provide feedback to the expert. The primary assumption of a partnership approach is a commitment to a differentiation between self and other. Sigel's Psychological Distancing Activities offer a means by which behaviors of both partners may be changed in order to meet this assumption. In addition, an understanding of the coexistence concept of development may help to bring about a higher level of empathy between partners, which is a critical element in partnerships.

OVERVIEW

The previous chapters have illustrated various aspects of a partnership approach in three domains: medicine, education, and research. However, none of the previous chapters attempted to articulate partnerships as an *ideal*, though they were all animated by the ideal. Ideals are posited as alternatives to perceived realities or actualities. The issues that prompted these proposals for a partnership ideal were the *practices*, the concrete everyday behaviors of professionals in the aforementioned areas. The partnership ideal has evolved over the past five years and the various chapters in this book reflect the diverse aspects of partnerships relied on by the contributors. Now I synthesize these various experiences in this chapter, which outlines the concept of partnerships as an ideal.

My central assumptions related to a partnership ideal draw on my citizenship as an American. It is the wisdom inherent in the American Constitution that I admire most generally. The constitutional guarantees put forth in the Bill of Rights, allowing Americans "the right to be left alone," according to Justice Louis Brandeis, (Wriston, 1960, p. 37) are most appealing and worthy of support. The Constitution, of course, recognizes that the state requires order. This degree of order legally constrains the freedom of individuals. But it is this ubiquitous, ongoing, irresolvable tension between individuals and groups that I take to be the main premise that human sciences should address. The nature of this tension requires constant reinterpretations.

For instance, many psychological theories do not clearly deal with the *complexities* implicit in this tension between individuals (the one) and the state (the many). Indeed psychology is polarized into two "cultures" (Kimble, 1984). The first of these "cultures" favors the many, the study of groups, the understanding of impersonal psychological processes as their goal. These psychologists, cutting across content areas such as social, developmental, personality, or even clinical psychology, favor experimental, "objective" methods for arriving at truth. In contrast, there are groups of psychologists who consider themselves to be humanists. Such groups insist on exploring and understanding individual "subjectivity."

This polarization has been institutionalized by universities that prefer and promote the "science" of psychology. That is, science as understood from the perspective of those psychologists who seek to uncover significant differences between groups. In contrast, clinicians, long derogated by academia, have argued for a shift away from an exclusive focus on such nomothetic aims, toward an increased emphasis on ideographic pursuits. It would take us too far afield to pursue the omnipresent conflicts between these two "cultures." Suffice it to say that the irresolvable disagreements, quarrels, and name calling between the two groups led to the creation of a new national association, the American Psychological Society (APS), which places emphasis on the "scientific" side. The APS now rivals the American Psychological Association (APA).

I am calling attention to this longstanding division within psychology because I take it to be indicative of a lack of wisdom. Of course, both national associations (the APA and the APS) promote the values of "diversity." We should all respect differences in ethnicity, religion, and so on. However, it is quite clear to me that psychology and psychologists have been so "busy" exporting their "insights" to the larger society that we have not learned to tolerate individual differences *within* the discipline. What is true at the national level is also true in many departments of psychology, or between departments of psychology and other departments in education and in the social and behavioral sciences. Indeed, the *respect* for differences between individuals, discussed by Dillon in Chapter 10, is often lacking in many departments of psychology.

Before pursuing some further implications of these conflicts for psychology, I want to return to the tensions between individuals and the state in the United States Constitution. I follow Sowell's (1987) lead in construing these irresolvable, ubiquitous tensions as due to "conflicts of visions," that can be schematically portrayed as "constrained" versus "unconstrained" visions. In the realm of everyday life, these visions are debated by feuding political parties, that *tend* to favor one or the other vision. I say "tend" because both Democrats and Republicans reenact and subscribe to both constrained and unconstrained visions depending on the issue. It is not simply that there are differences between Democrats and Republicans. There are intraindividual differences with respect to the composition of many individuals' visions. The conflicts in our outlooks are not consistent across various issues.

The intent of this chapter is not to "resolve" this longstanding conflict between visions. Rather, the intent is to discuss partnerships as a framework, which may help professionals and their counterparts to work together in complementary and reciprocal relationships.

The types of professional interactions to be addressed in this chapter are limited in at least two ways. First, there are "boundary issues" between professionals and their partners. Violations of the boundaries established by society as a whole and by specific professions may result in disciplinary action against professionals. These violations may entail moral, as well as legal, consequences for both participants.

Secondly, partnerships constrain the relationships between professionals and their partners through the practical issues of time. Professionals such as physicians, teachers and researchers interact with a particular patient, student, or research participant on a time-limited basis. Indeed, if a professional spends too much time with any one person, s/he may be accused of a boundary violation by members of that profession. This time limitation is frequently invoked by professionals as an example of how the actualities of everyday practice deviate from the ideal. Further, some professionals blame the social system for imposing such temporal constraints on their practices as physicians or as teachers.

Researchers often operate under strict time constraints as well. In the effort to maximize the statistical power of their studies, researchers typically impose limits on the amount of time they can spend with each individual, so that they might be able to include as many as possible. In addition, many researchers believe that scientific "objectivity" is enhanced when clear-cut answers are sought from research participants. These short, pointed responses also tend to decrease the amount of time needed for each subject.

This chapter consists of two main sections. The initial section begins with an overview of traditional, asymmetrical relationships in the domains of education, medicine, and research. In addition to providing descriptions of traditional relationships, the reasons behind their widespread acceptance are explored, as well. The alternative, partnership approach is then explained, with emphasis on the "complementarity" and "reciprocity" required in such relationships. After providing the basic framework for each, the two types of interactions are then compared and contrasted.

The partnership ideal is examined more thoroughly in the next section. The basic assumption of a partnership ideal, namely the differentiation between the self and other, is discussed. The idea of differentiation was previously articulated by Werner (1948, 1957), as part of his orthogenetic principle of development. Sigel's (1978, 1993) psychological distancing strategies and the coexistence concept of development (Bibace, Sagarin, & Dyl, 1998; Bibace, Dillon, & Sagarin, in this volume) is offered as means of advancing toward a partnership ideal. This section concludes with an examination of the value orientations inherent in a partnership ideal.

TRADITIONAL AND PARTNER RELATIONSHIPS

This section provides a description of both traditional, asymmetrical interactions as well as the alternative, partnership ideal. The focus of the first part of this section is on traditional, asymmetrical relationships. Observations of these traditional relationships in education, medicine, and research led to the conception of a partnership ideal. In short, my colleagues and I observed that professionals, as persons in authority, almost always either occupied or sought positions of control in their professional interactions. The everyday activities of these professionals rely on practices that, historically, have been most clearly acknowledged and criticized in the educational domain. These practices are characterized as an Initiation-Response-Evaluation (IRE) sequence of behaviors by a number of researchers (e.g., Cazden, 1988; Mehan, 1979; O'Connor & Michaels, 1993; Sinclair & Coulthard, 1976).

The educational IRE is a bottoms-up generalization that is characterized here as an asymmetrical, interpersonal interaction. This is the case because the professional's counterpart is not usually in the position of initiating questions and evaluating a professional's answers. In this book, the various authors have illustrated that IRE sequences often occur in the interactions between medical professionals and patients and psychological researchers and research participants, as well. Given the degree of consistency with which professionals initiate questions and evaluate responses, the IRE is specified as leading to "asymmetrical relationships" between professionals and their counterparts in all three domains. A partnership ideal provides a clear alternative to such traditional, asymmetrical relationships between professionals and patients, students, and research participants.

The second part of this section examines some of the initial, defining terms in a partnership. In order to foster greater symmetry between professionals and their counterparts, complementarity and reciprocity in the sequence of questions, answers, and feedback (QAF) are necessary features in interpersonal interactions. For complementarities to exist, professionals must recognize, encourage, and appreciate the distinctive contributions that patients, students, and research participants bring to the relationship.

It is important to stress that while partnerships require complementarity and reciprocity, equality between participants is not assumed. In addition, complete agreement between partners is not predicated as a necessary component of partnerships. Indeed, the primary assumption is that individuals are different, and that no one is a "mind reader."

So, partnerships are especially valuable *because of*, not in spite of, the fact that professionals and counterparts have distinctly different contributions to make to the relationship. Given this emphasis on differentiation between the self and other, disagreement is bound to occur between partners, at least on occasion. But, if the participants have similar objectives and can come to some degree of concurrence as to the proper means of achieving these goals, partnerships are still feasible.

The greater degree of symmetry between partners is manifest in the reciprocal back-and-forth pattern of QAF taking place between them. Such reciprocity, also recognized as a dialogue between people, is the interpersonal process that may lead to a negotiated understanding between partners. It should be clear that symmetry in QAF is not a mechanical set of activities that inevitably lead to partnerships. Psychologically, partnerships are distinct from the legal or business meanings attached to the term. Partnerships are fragile. If one partner fails to respect the viewpoint of the other, the partnership could be permanently jeopardized. On the other hand, partnerships between professionals and their counterparts are bound by the parameters of their professional relationships. Partnerships need not address ideological or political differences between partners.

After providing overviews of the traditional, asymmetrical interaction and the alternative, partnership model, these two perspectives are compared and contrasted. These types of relationships can be most usefully contrasted according to the ways in which the professional approaches the following three aspects of the interaction: 1) the rigidity or flexibility with which questions are asked and responses are provided, 2) the goals of the relationship, and 3) the treatment of nomothetic versus ideographic issues.

In a partnership, a recognition is needed, on the part of professionals, that the questions posed by patients, students, and research participants must be attended to and answered in a manner that is satisfactory to the partner. These concerns expressed by patients, students, and research participants complement the traditional questions and evaluations generated by professionals. Bilateral feedback from professionals to their partners and vice-versa is thus an integral component of any successful partnership. The term "feedback" is meant to include both "formative" and "summative" evaluations on the part of patients, research participants, and students. The concrete goals of the partnership are made possible by the complementarity, the reciprocities of QAF between partners. The more flexible dialogue between partners is compared to traditional relationships, that typically rely on invariant IRE sequences.

Traditional, asymmetrical presentation precludes optimal accommodation by professionals to their partners. In other words, professionals in these types of interactions often do not take into account "where their partners are coming from." Rather, they are socialized to assimilate and accommodate to the relevant knowledge and skills of their professions. But such "norms," or "generalizations" that are currently favored by a given profession should be utilized in ways that take into account the "particularities" of *this* patient, *this* research participant, or *this* student. An overemphasis on group norms may result in the appearance of *negative* stereotypes, on the part of both professionals and their counterparts.

Often a particular individual is automatically assimilated and homogenized to a class of "patients," "students," or "research participants." This "amalgamation" of the individual to a group represents a violation of the primary assumption that partners must differentiate themselves from one another. Similarly, significant individual differences within groups of physicians, teachers, and researchers are often marginalized by patients, students, and research participants who "stereotype" the professionals with whom they interact.

The goals of professionals in traditional and partner relationships vary as well. In many cases, the goal of an asymmetrical interaction is to solve problems. By implication, problems have solutions and such problem solving constitutes a substantial aspect of a professional's socialization. A partnership ideal requires a recognition that the enduring aspect of the interaction must address *issues* as well as problems. In contrast to problems, issues do not have solutions. Rather, proposed solutions for issues often generate new problems. Recognizing the enduring presence of issues requires partners to take steps to assure that they will continue to work together over time. Problem-solving approaches often lead to the assignment of "blame," when a solution is not reached. When a patient does not get "cured," or a student does not "learn," the physician or teacher is usually viewed as blameworthy.

There are several reasons why such asymmetrical relationships between professionals and their counterparts are so widespread and deeply rooted. These include:

1. the accepted discrepancy in power and knowledge between the professional and the layperson,
2. the apostolic function of the professional who attempts to convert patients and students to his/her perspective, as an example of professional self-centeredness, and
3. the link between "sequence" and "cause," present in everyday life and in most domains, including medicine, the humanities and psychology.

After engaging in an asymmetrical interaction with a professional, a counterpart still may not have a clear understanding of the information that has been presented.

Many patients, students, and research participants accept the expert's position of privilege with respect to knowledge and power, so they will frequently avoid questioning the professional regarding any information they do not understand. The acceptance of a disparity in status is one of the main reasons for the perpetuation of asymmetrical relationships.

The "apostolic function," articulated by Balint (1964), is an attitude frequently displayed by professionals in asymmetrical interactions. Some professionals enter an interaction with the attitude that since the other individual came to see him or her, this person needs to receive the pertinent information, without consideration for where s/he is coming from. In the medical field, an example would be a physician with the opinion that "my job is to diagnose and treat and your job is to do what I say." This traditional, authoritarian outlook is now widely rejected in medical schools, but is still present in medical practice. Such an attitude violates the assumption that the patient's "subjectivity" must be valued. It is important to distinguish between the physician's expertise in the biomedical domain and the patient's own knowledge, with respect to her psychological self, familial relationships, and sociocultural context.

The intrapersonal basis for acceptance of asymmetrical interactions is rooted in the correlation between cause and sequence in the psychology of both professionals and their counterparts in our society. The term "intrapersonal" refers to the philosophical assumptions being made in the relationships between cause and sequence. It is the intuitive assumption that associates cause and sequence, that regulates the interpersonal activities of both professionals and their counterparts.

Traditional Asymmetrical Relationships in Education, Medicine, and Research

Traditional relationships in education are characterized by what has been called an Initiation-Response-Evaluation (IRE) sequence. This sequence begins with the professional initiating the question, followed by the patient, student, or research participant briefly responding, and then the professional evaluating the response. Relationships between doctors and patients, teachers and students, researchers and research participants illustrate such traditional, asymmetrical relationships.

O'Connor and Michaels (1993) explain that much of the research on classroom discourse "has been on classroom language use within the traditional lesson format, featuring the initiation-response-evaluation (IRE) sequence" (p. 319). They define the traditional IRE as an interaction in which the teacher aims to:

> coordinate the sequencing of the academic task. . . . In that type of sequence, the teacher reserves the right to evaluate the student's response, and the turn structure provides no opportunity for the student to negotiate the meaning of his or her contribution. (pp. 319–323)

This type of asymmetrical sequence in education has been discussed by a number of researchers (e.g., Mehan, 1979; Cazden, 1988), including Lemke (1990), who referred to it as the "triadic dialogue." As these and other researchers have discussed, this sequence consists of a high rate of initiation moves by the teacher, usually involving questions with known answers. This is followed up by a response from the student, often a simple response to the question. The third move in the sequence is prototypically the teacher's evaluation statement (or elaboration, follow-up, or feedback) in reference to the student's response (1. "What's the capital of Arkansas?" 2. "Little Rock." 3."Good.").

In this book, the contributors and I have argued that the traditional IRE, which itself is a generalization in education, may be further applied to the domains of medical care and psychological research. Table 21.1 demonstrates the diversity with which the traditional IRE has been generalized.

This generalization *transcends* the kinds of professionals and counterparts involved, the contexts in which such professionals and their counterparts work, along with the goals and means typically relied on by such professionals as they interact with their counterparts. The content of the generalization has three referents: questions, answers, and evaluations. That is, all three groups of professionals rely on questions, answers, and evaluations in their interactions. But the generalization has a specific *formal* character. The form of organization is the *sequence* in which questions, answers, and evaluations occur. In addition, this generalization refers to the consistency, across the three domains, regarding *who* initiates the questions and evaluates the responses, in contrast to the person who provides the answers.

Such generalizations are widely applicable because of their abstract quality. These abstractions are possible through "analogies" from one domain to another. The generalization is a triple analogy, or a formal parallel, in Werner's (1948, 1957) terms: the doctor is to the patient; as the teacher is to the student; as the researcher is to the research participant.

In *Comparative Psychology of Mental Development* (1948), Werner relies on *analogies* as the basis for comparing diverse sequences of development. Drawing on microgenesis, ontogenesis, phylogenesis, and psychopathology, Werner argued

TABLE 21.1
The IRE Sequence in Diverse Contexts

Agents	Context	Ends	Means	Individual/Group
Professional physicians/patients	Medical settings	Curing & caring	Diverse medical assessments/ procedures	Mostly individuals
Teachers/students	Schools, colleges	Teaching/ learning	Lectures, seminars, tutorial	Mostly groups
Researcher/ research participants	University laboratories	Knowledge creation	Diverse methods, experiments, interviews	Individuals & groups

for "formal parallels" or analogies among such developmental sequences. In this case, the analogy is the formal organization of an asymmetrical sequence of questions, answers, and evaluations asked by a professional of the other person. The professional *constrains the parameters of the answers* that are permissible. The "form of organization" that is analogized is the asymmetrical sequence, as a means relied on by professionals in all three domains.

The same type of asymmetrical IRE sequence previously noted in education is also the "hallmark" of many medical interviews. In the following example, the physician's questions restrict a patient's responses to monosyllabic "no's" after only two conversational moves.

D Have there any cases of tuberculosis diabetes (acantees) suicide among your relatives.
P (h)......(h) My father had tuberculosis oh:h ....tst twenty ohgee twenty five thirty years ago he was in the hospital......... he was there two years.
D Twenty five years ago herng:h? ....
P ....Oh maybe longer than that. (h) I was a little boy. Twenty five— Yeah I'd say twenty five years ago.
D Have you (within) the last ten years been intimately associated with anyone having tuberculosis?
P .... No.
D Have you ever consulted a doctor suffered from any illnesses or diseases of the brain or the nervous system?
P No.
D Heart, blood vessels or lungs?
P No.
D Stomach or intestines.
P No.
D Skin glands (nurr) your eyes?
P No.
D Have you ever had rheumatism bone disease or syphilis.
P No.
D Have you ever seen a doctor suffered from any illness or disease not included in the above questions other than for routine colds?
P No.

(Mishler, 1986, p. 56. Transcription according to psycholinguistic criteria for conversational analysis: each period is equivalent to a one-second pause.)

Such traditional medical interviews are still very common, particularly in subspecialty areas in medicine. In these cases especially, physicians have been socialized to elicit, as quickly as possible, the "information" that they, as experts, consider relevant. However, by limiting the patient's responses in this way, the physician may be preventing him- or herself from obtaining the proper information. In answering "No" to the physician's question "Have you ever had rheumatism, bone disease, or syphilis?" the patient in the above example may be implying one of two things. One, the patient truly has not had any of these ailments; or two, the patient does not know what these illnesses are and therefore negates the possibility of ever having them. Without an attitude of openness and reciprocity in the interaction, a patient may not feel comfortable in asking a physician about a particular illness of which s/he has none or little knowledge.

Adherence to a "protocol" is even more frequently the case in researcher/research participant interactions. This strict adherence is sustained by a belief that such practices ensure "objectivity." In psychological researcher–research participant interactions, the short-term, episodic nature of the relationship highlights the researcher's initiative in making clear *what* the study is about, the objectives of the study, and the demands to be placed on the research participant. As a voluntary contributor to a study, a research participant is viewed as unlikely to "know," or to care about, the researcher's aims. A major concern for the research participant is that the requirements of the researcher not be too onerous or time-consuming. The dual aims of the researcher—objectivity and brevity—coincide with the goals of the research participant. Single-word answers (yes or no) also fulfill these aims. The popularity of "narratives," of "discourse analysis" or of "conversational analysis" in recent years provide an exception, but such approaches still run counter to mainstream methods in psychology.

The Definition of a Partnership Model as a Movement Toward Reciprocal Relationships

The definition of an ideal partnership can be constructed by emphasizing some of the ordinary, everyday meanings of four key words: complementarity, reciprocity, symmetry, and equality. (The meanings of these words are taken from *The Compact Edition of the Oxford English Dictionary*, 1971.) Partnerships as an ideal certainly draw on the notion of "complementarity," meaning "to make complete . . . to supply what is wanting."

"Reciprocity" adds the meaning of "an alternate backward and forward motion." Since sequences are a part of the formal analysis of partnerships, the notion of alternating the motion of questions and answers backward and forward is important. The contributions of professionals to the dialogue should, ideally, be complemented by the questions, answers, and evaluations of their partners in order to "supply what is wanting."

The term "symmetry" is introduced in order to compare traditional relationships between professionals and their counterparts with our ideal. Again, in the traditional, asymmetrical relationship, professionals initiate questions. Patients, students, or research participants subsequently answer the questions, with the professionals then evaluating the responses. The ideal in a partnership is the *movement toward* "symmetry" in the sense that the relevant parts and the sequence (that is questions, answers, evaluations) are "balanced" and therefore, more harmoniously arranged.

The repetition of these symmetrical sequences constitutes a dialog. This interpersonal "give and take" between partners relies on broad psychological processes, as outlined by Piaget. In Piaget's terms, the process of "adaptation," comprised of assimilation and accommodation, is here constructed as "negotiated understanding" (Piaget & Inhelder, 1969). The *assimilation* by each partner of the other person's statement may require major or minor accommodations of each individual's beliefs or assumptions to those of their partners.

These repeated, more symmetrical sequences should ideally demonstrate the oscillations, the variabilities of statements by each of the partners when viewed separately. But together, such variabilities now can be characterized as demonstrative of empathic sensitivity of one to the other. These sequences contribute to what we designate as a "dialogue," or as dialogicality, referring to the repetitions of more symmetrical mutualities between partners.

In turn, it is from dialogicality as a process that negotiated understanding comes about. Such negotiated understanding yields more stable and meaningful agreements because they are based on a partnership, with respect to mutually agreed-upon decision-making processes, as well as the content or outcomes of such dialogical processes and negotiations.

Lastly, by way of contrast, I should address the word "equality." Partnerships in the sense being used here, do not imply "equality." One cannot assume that a professional's relationship to their partners is of "the same level . . . of power, or the ability, of achievement" or of "having the same rights and privileges," as is stated in the definition of the word "equal." Indeed, the status of the professional is here equated with different rights and privileges. Simply put, patients cannot write prescriptions, students do not assign grades to their instructors, and research participants do not publish papers on the studies in which they have been involved.

In a partnership, a health care professional's medical knowledge should complement a patient's understanding of his/her own thoughts and feelings. To draw a parallel, a university professor's "learning how to learn" approach complements a student's choice of topic. Conversely, the professor gains a greater understanding of topics about which s/he may have little or no previous knowledge. In terms of the research domain, a researcher may learn from questions generated by participants. Such questions may not have occurred to the researcher on his/her own, without the input of the partner.

A Comparison Between Traditional Asymmetrical and Symmetrical Partner Relationships

In order to clarify the differences between asymmetrical and symmetrical (traditional) partnership interactions, these two types of relationships are compared and contrasted in three ways. First, the invariant sequencing of questions, that typifies an asymmetrical interaction, is contrasted with a focus group method, that exemplifies an attempt at a more symmetrical approach. Secondly, the goals of professionals in each of the three domains (medical, education, and research) are examined. Thirdly, the divergent manner in which conflicts between the nomothetic and the ideographic are treated in the two types of interactions is discussed.

Sequence and cause in traditional and partnership interactions

Traditional and partner relationships differ as to the manner in which three psychological activities (questions, answers, and evaluations) are addressed. In traditional relationships, the authority of the professional is made manifest through his/her control over the *sequence* in which questions are posed. These questions are answered by the counterpart and are then evaluated by the professional. The formal, determinative feature of a question has been clearly articulated by Levy (1943):

> an ordinary question intends its answer. It calls for it, requires it. In itself it (i.e., the question) is incomplete and establishes a vector towards completion. Once a proper answer is given, question and answer form a complete closed whole. (p. 61)

The *whole* to which I am calling attention is the totality of the three activities: questions, answers, and evaluations. The initiator of a question and the evaluator of the answers, in effect, sets the parameters of the "whole."

The appropriateness, the correctness, and the features of the answer deemed relevant are all aspects of both the vector intended in the question and the evaluation. This evaluation by the professional is meant to assess the comprehensiveness, completeness, and accuracy of the answer provided by the counterpart. The dynamics of these formal features among questions, answers, and evaluations occur both intrapsychically and interpersonally.

In sum, a partnership ideal requires a movement toward more symmetrical sequences characterized by reciprocities and complementarities between individuals. What must be clarified further is the manner in which sequence and cause are connected. The claim is that sequence and cause are fused in traditional relationships. As a result of such fusion, what is associated in time or contiguous in space is also construed as causally related. The concept of fusion is explored further in a later discussion of the relevance of Werner's orthogenetic principle (1948) to a partnership model.

The traditional, asymmetrical IRE sets limitations on who initiates the questions in a one-on-one relationship between a professional and counterpart. In such contexts, there is considerable pressure to conform to IREs. The use of focus groups provides a contrast in that the child or the adult can discuss, argue, disagree, or contradict one another as peers. In a focus group, time is the only limitation, because there is no one particular response that ends the dialogue (see Chapter 5).

Piaget and Werner have favored the so-called "clinical method" in order to address the psychological processes underlying a response given by a research participant. However, a one-on-one relationship in a "process-directed inquiry" ends when the researcher receives what s/he considers to be a satisfactory response or when the research participant stops answering due to a lack of energy. Repeated questions by the researcher in a one-on-one relationship may convey to the research participant the message that the answers s/he has previously given were unsatisfactory. Since the researcher eventually stops asking questions at a certain point, the research participant may infer that the answers given at that point in sequence were the correct or approved ones.

Questioning often ceases when the researcher thinks that s/he has obtained a set of classifiable responses from a research participant. These responses typically accord with the category system employed by the researcher. In this case then, what the researcher considers to be a satisfactory explanation, in relation to his/her predetermined categories of analysis, determines the objective of the inquiry.

The goals of professionals

The goals of professionals are different in traditional, asymmetrical interactions, as opposed to the more symmetrical relationships required in a partnership model. In turn, these differences have to do with general attitudes that regulate the behavior of the professional toward the counterpart. This general attitude entails the contrast between problem-solving versus issue-centered interactions. The problem-solving approach is dominant in medicine, education, and research. Once adopted, this approach favors the traditional IRE because it is primarily the professional's task to formulate the problem, to rely on accepted methods and procedures to solve it, and to evaluate the results. A problem-solving approach imposes major constraints on such answers.

In contrast, issue-centered interactions between professionals and partners involve very different assumptions. These assumptions clearly make the professional aware that every so-called "solution" gives rise to new problems. The realization that issues transcend all solutions is one of the defining characteristics of the dialogue that typifies a symmetrical, partnership interaction. Family medicine in the 1970s proposed and implemented this distinction. While accepting that the traditional medical goal of "curing" is applicable to one set of problems, namely episodic illness, advocates of family medicine also claimed that by far the largest number of doctor–patient interactions should be focused on "caring" for the patient. Caring for the patient as a goal is necessary because there are no "cures," or "solutions" for chronic disease, nor for many of the risky behaviors in which people engage that contribute greatly to morbidity and mortality.

Similarly, in education there is a sharp division between educators who are committed to learning and communicating the particular contents to be taught, and those who are directed toward assisting students in "learning how to learn." The former can be assessed much more easily than the latter. The educational issues and psychological processes implicit in "learning how to learn" are much more complicated and variable, because the issues involved transcend content. What remains unanswered is the generality of the learning over time, in different contexts and with varying tasks. Clearly, from this perspective there is no definitive solution or simple answer that can be considered valid and generalizable. However, the potential benefits of a "learning how to learn strategy" are great enough to warrant its exploration.

In research contexts in psychology, there is one tradition that has partially accommodated to the constraints imposed by the researcher's questions. This accommodation involves beginning with relatively open or unstructured questions and only later introducing more specific, structured questions. Often researchers adhering to such an approach may, at the end of a set of questions, ask the research participant for their reactions to the study. This is sometimes analyzed as "qualitative data" and utilized to generate further studies, together with the implications from the quantitative results.

Such accommodations are desirable, though there are limitations to such procedures. Asking the person what s/he thinks or feels at the end of the study, may well be more of a reflection of the contents covered by the questions, rather than the initial opinion of the research participant, based on her personal background. This sequence also sets constraints on what the research participant assumes is relevant to the area being studied.

In a traditional sequence, it is often the case that the goal and the context are taken as "obvious," so that the remaining questions focus on the means, processes, or procedures required to attain the goal. It is often presumed that the goal of a student is to learn from the teacher, that a patient is there to be cured by a doctor, or that a research participant cooperates with the researcher. Such assumptions cannot be taken for granted in more symmetrical sequences. In doctor–patient interactions in which caring as well as curing are deemed relevant and important, there is considerable indeterminacy for the professional, because what constitutes caring may vary from patient to patient. The professional is thus required to accommodate to the patient's subjectivity as an individual. These types of individual idiosyncrasies go beyond biomedical knowledge. Only the individual herself is aware of her own thoughts and feelings. It is this type of subjective information with which a professional must be concerned, in order for reciprocity to be maintained.

Similarly, in education a traditional teacher's focus on the lesson to be learned is different from the teacher who is concerned about the learner. Educationists have recognized this distinction between "formative" and "summative" evaluations. The former constitutes feedback that is intended to help the learner overcome difficulties. The latter is synonymous with a more objective final evaluation, as in the assignment of a grade.

The emphasis placed on the nomothetic versus the ideographic

The dynamics and tensions between a focus on the citizen versus the state during the time of our nation's founding serves as an analogy to the divisiveness and difficulties inherent in attending to both individuals and groups, an issue perennially faced by professionals and their counterparts. Epistemologically and ethically, this is the tension between a nomothetic and ideographic focus.

All three groups of professionals (physicians, teachers, and researchers) voice similar complaints. The ideal espoused here is derided or ridiculed as being unrealistic because society, through the health care system, the educational system, or the institutions that require and support research, does not encourage, endorse, or even permit the realization of such goals. Contemporaneously, there is considerable evidence, from the perspective of professionals, to support the view that institutions constrain professionals with respect to time, the number of students in a class, the number of patients to be treated, or the number of studies that have to be published.

Professionals in a particular occupation internalize the normative values and practices of their respective professions. These conventions may include a commonly accepted manner of dealing with groups of people categorized as patients, as students, or as research participants. For example, psychologists in the 1950s (and even later) were socialized into the assumption that, conceptually, the discipline's cornerstone was the "individual." One agent with one personality, in all its vicissitudes and development, would engage in "interactions" with others. When theories became more comprehensive and moved away from "unilateral" effects of the individual on the environment or vice-versa, the favored term became "transactions." The effects were bilateral. But the general conceptual assumption remained: the unit of analysis was *one*, not two.

The normative values and practices of a given profession, in effect, act as constraints on the ways in which professionals can accommodate to the individuals with whom they traditionally interact. Each of these professional groups are constrained in particular "worlds of action" in their everyday practices and by similar "reality" pressures. The theme in all three domains may be summarized as: "Too much to do, for too many people, too few resources, and too many constraints on my professional freedom." These complaints are more concretely expressed through too many patients, students, or publications required to survive. In addition, there is too little time, fewer resources, less freedom, and less remuneration for many of these professionals.

What is remarkable is the number of professionals who, despite these barriers, remain committed to the ideals congruent with partnerships. One consequence of such commitment is the frustration voiced by professionals who know and want to do what they think should be done, but who are frustrated by the organizational characteristics of the medical, educational, or research institutions to which they belong. For an ideal to remain viable, it is important that one recognize such systemic issues, which will now be briefly addressed.

In medicine, the health care system imposes continuous, pervasive limits on the quality of care offered to patients by requiring doctors to treat a specified number of patients in a particular time period. Physicians are given monthly computer printouts, which gauge productivity as "average" or "below average." In some health care systems, the average time allowed or considered desirable for an interaction with a patient is 8 to 10 minutes! What is even worse is that the permitted treatments (medication, procedures, clinical tests) are monitored by outside parties who are not directly involved with the individual patient. This reaction is an outgrowth of societal cynicism directed at physicians who were judged to be helping themselves unduly.

Though this might be true in some cases, there has been an overreaction. This overreaction is only now becoming the source of national political debates, as "scandals" regarding such inappropriate constraints by health care systems become a source of congressional investigations. What should be clear, from a partnership perspective, is that there will *not* be a "solution" to this "issue." But nonetheless, partnerships in particular doctor–patient interactions are currently possible and realistic occurrences. This is the case because a number of doctors and patients have negotiated an understanding that enables both partners to be reasonably satisfied with each other, despite such unavoidable constraints such as time.

In education there are quite similar pressures. The resources, financial and otherwise, are too limited. The students are too numerous! Expectations of the teacher now go beyond the classroom and the material to be learned. As Walsh's chapter, entitled "University–Community–School Partnerships," illustrates, some principals consider the community context in which the school is located as a central consideration to be taken into account. Many teachers report that they have to provide needed educational materials for teaching at their own personal expense!

Time is again an issue and some school systems (e.g., charter schools) are extending both the school year and the school day, mainly due to the demanding lifestyles of adults in our society. When both parents work, the school has been enlisted to provide "services" both before and after the regular school day. And again, societal rewards for teachers reflect the relatively low priority assigned to education. Adversarial sentiments on the part of many individuals are a major factor: resentment at the money earned by physicians and at the vacation time that teachers enjoy.

Researchers in psychology face major pressures from the institutions that require such activities. Clearly, the pressure to "publish or perish" has increased enormously. It used to be the case that a good teacher who was scholarly but did not publish a great deal could not only survive, but be a valued member of his/her college or university. This is rarely the case nowadays. The American Association of University Professors guidelines are such that the pressure to publish now has very specific temporal markers. Such time constraints clearly limit what can realistically be undertaken as research. For instance, it would be unrealistic for an untenured assistant professor to embark on long-term longitudinal studies! More subtly, the methods and procedures foster what in the jargon of researchers are referred to as "quick and dirty" studies. These types of studies are safely within traditional paradigms, utilize traditional methods and preferably objective procedures, typically yielding some minor contribution to knowledge.

The reliance on statistical analyses in studies such as these entails a focus on significant group differences, that has contributed to the subordination of individual differences within groups. Indeed, such individual differences are sometimes consigned to the category of "error variance"—not only unexplained variance, but variabilities not worthy of an explanation.

The tensions among the members of *all* three groups (physicians, teachers and researchers) are exacerbated by a specialization of function created and maintained by administrative personnel. Administrators oversee groups of professionals, in contrast to the professionals themselves who deal with individual patients, students, and research participants. These administrators wield a considerable degree of power and control over the behaviors of professionals.

Some administrators who "manage" groups of professionals, "negotiate" with other administrators. The values and daily practices of professionals who previously worked in the "trenches"—in clinics, classrooms, or research settings—are often transformed when one becomes an administrator. Such administrators, who once worked on a hands-on basis are, in many cases, now isolated and protected from daily encounters with patients, students, or research participants.

This isolation often breeds further conflicts between values and practices for groups of professionals and the exigencies of a particular professional's attempts to accommodate to *this* patient, *this* student, or *this* research participant. The particulars of an individual are more likely to be dismissed as "outliers" by an administrator who does not actually experience the frustrations of having to deal with such a person directly. The subordination of the individual to the group, of the ideographic to the nomothetic, is fostered by values and practices, that are dictated by what is considered "administratively convenient." Ideals are sometimes dismissed in a condescending manner or grudgingly acknowledged as "unrealistic." The justification is based on utilitarian values of "efficiency" and "cost/benefit" analyses for "groups" or "categories," but not of individuals.

Why Are Asymmetrical Relationships Accepted?

The linkage between causality and sequence refers to two distinct realms of psychological activities. First are the intERpersonal, psychological activities that facilitate the linkage between cause and sequence. Second, is the conceptual, or intRApersonal, linkage between causality and sequence, or the assumptions made by an interpreter regarding causal claims. Here, these activities focus on the asymmetrical or symmetrical sequences of questions, answers and feedback between professionals and their counterparts.

The interpersonal level

There are several reasons why asymmetrical relationships between professionals and their counterparts are so widespread and deeply rooted. These reasons include: 1) the accepted discrepancy in power and knowledge between professionals and laypeople; and 2) the apostolic function of professionals attempting to convert patients and students to their perspectives, as an example of professional self-centeredness.

Differences in knowledge are also recognized as differences in power. This sort of power makes itself evident in similar practices, espoused by quite different professional groups. These practices privilege professionals in a variety of ways. For instance, the task of defining the ends and the means of attaining the goal at hand are taken, by both parties involved, to be part of the privileges and responsibilities of the professional. Certainly, such rights and privileges are circumscribed for "professionals," and the boundaries between professional and personal relationships are articulated for the professional groups themselves, by societal mores and laws. The very fact that patients show up to the doctors office; that research participants agree to participate in a study; that students are enrolled in school is indicative of the implicit agreement regarding the respective roles of the professional and her counterparts. Thus, the context, as well as the ends, serve to buttress the power of the professional in relationships with his/her counterparts.

Traditionally, the professional's power is also manifest through the context in which s/he functions and is concretely implemented by the professional's questions, that determine *what* is relevant to the goals to be achieved in that encounter. Further, the questions are also assumed to be essential in determining the changes that need to be brought about—changes regarded as treatment in medicine, as learning in an educational setting, and as an intervention, assessment, or evaluation required by a particular research study.

The professional's control over these two activities—questions and evaluations—imply control of the third aspect; that is, what answers are to be considered relevant, appropriate, or satisfactory. In a traditional relationship, the professional does not have to systematically include, consider, and respond to the questions, answers, and input of the counterpart. In contrast, the consideration of this type of feedback is considered necessary to the implementation of the values required by a partnership ideal. These activities by the partner are precisely the reciprocal of those three activities (questions, answers, and evaluations) enacted by professionals and constitute a necessary degree of complementarity to the activities of the authority figure. It is only when both the professionals and their partners (either single individuals or groups) have fostered such reciprocity that the values inherent in "mutualities" can be fostered.

Many professionals exhibit behavior that typifies an "apostolic function." Egocentricity or self-centeredness is a ubiquitous and pervasive issue both epistemologically and with reference to values. In the humanities as well as the human sciences, there is a general recognition that the tendency toward "privileging oneself" is a major issue. Privileging oneself occurs at every level of analysis and of practice. Foucault (1973), for instance, has argued that all professionals within a particular "historical era" privilege themselves with respect to what constitutes "progress" in their respective fields. By progress, Foucault means a comparison between the knowledge and practices employed currently to those of previous historical eras. A corollary of Foucault's idea is that all professionals and scientists are circumscribed by the "episteme" that dominates a historical era. The very few exceptions are those creative scientists who contribute to the structure of scientific revolutions by altering the very terms of what is taken for granted. It is this change that has been described as a "paradigm shift" by Kuhn (1970).

How are such abstract assumptions regarding "self-centeredness" in the humanities and sciences expressed in the daily lives of physicians, teachers, and researchers? The link between values, theory, and practice for the professional is what Balint referred to as the "apostolic function" of the professional. Balint (1964), referring to physicians, stated:

> Apostolic mission or function means in the first place that every doctor has a vague, but almost unshakably firm, idea of how a patient ought to behave when ill. Although this idea is anything but explicit and concrete, it is immensely powerful, and influences, practically every detail of the doctor's work with his patients. It was almost as if every doctor had revealed knowledge of what was right and what was wrong for patients to expect and to endure, and further, as if he had a sacred duty to convert to his faith all the ignorant and unbelieving among his patients It was this which suggested the name of "apostolic function." (p. 216)

It has taken me many more years to recognize that a similar apostolic function occurs among experts in psychology, in both research and teaching. Many psychologists behave as if it were their sacred duty to convert to their "faith," to their brand of psychology, all of the ignorant and unbelieving among patients, students, and colleagues, both in their departments and in other disciplines. This is the case because such folks are, from that psychologist's perspective, "unenlightened" or "misguided."

The intrapersonal level

On the intrapersonal level, the concepts of "cause," "sequence," and "power" are related in meaningful ways. It may be helpful to clarify the term "cause" as used here, through Aristotle's four types of causes: "final," "formal," "material," and "efficient" (Irwin, 1998, p. 419). Here the connection between sequence and cause focuses on "cause" as form. The forms can be referred to as asymmetrical when compared to more symmetrical sequences in partner relationships. But it is also "cause" as "final," as "telos," as implying *the* answer to the questions asked by professionals that underlies the power and control exercised by professionals in their traditional reliance on IRE interactions. Attitudinally, the IRE sequence is based on the implicit and very general question: "Do you know what I know?" Or in another variant of the same assumption by the professional, "Since you don't know and can't know what I know, just answer my questions and I will decide what you should do and evaluate what you say."

Like Aristotle, Handlon differentiated between "final" and "formal" causes. In addition, Handlon articulated "causes" as "enduring" (Handlon, 1960, p. 56). The repetitive, formal aspects of "enduring," with respect to the "sequences" of the three activities, (questions, answers, and evaluations) have been acknowledged in generating what is referred to as the IRE. Earlier, the applicability of the IRE to traditional sequences in doctor–patient and researcher–research participant relationships was discussed. Lastly, Handlon articulated "cause" as "radical." Focusing on the formal features of sequence, one can point to radical, abrupt shifts in the traditional sequence of the three activities (questions, answers, and responses). As when a student said to a professor: "That's the first question I've heard you ask where you don't know the answer!" Surely a professional involved in such an encounter with a patient or a student would be surprised!

Cause and effect logically can be stated as a sequence of antecedent and consequent, meaning that the "cause" precedes the "effect." In the realm of concrete everyday activities, children and adults have many opportunities to experience this sequence. A mechanical cause, for instance, pushes an object from here to there as an effect. Such intuitive, concrete experiences become internalized by individuals. This abstraction is no longer dependent on "cause" as concrete, material, and efficient. Rather, cause and affect are abstracted as *forms of organization,* that are inherent in any sequence. What comes "before" is interpretable formally as influencing what comes "after."

Our adherence to "material," concrete, mechanical cause-and-effect sequences has obscured the "formal" and more abstract meaning of cause being espoused here. And yet such sequential forms of organization appear to constitute one basis for the authority of any person who is societally sanctioned to "ask questions." From this perspective then, it is a gross violation of "common sense" to reverse the sequence. One cannot bring about a "cause" by manipulating the "effect." True, one may hypothesize what the "cause" might have been in order to account for such an "effect," but the sequence of a cause leading to an effect remains intact. Mill's canons dictate that one must progress from the general to the particular and from what is known, to what is unknown. In other words, the "antecedent" *precedes* the "consequent"(Cohen & Nagel, 1934). In a given series of experimental trials, a hypothetical *cause* is tested to determine if there is an invariant *effect*. Our logic requires this transformation. It is this sequence that is persuasive.

Conversational analysts have focused on "turn taking" in conversations to assess interpersonal dominance. "Turn taking" is, of course, an index of interpersonal sequence. Here, it is important to stress another aspect of "sequences," namely questions, answers, and evaluations.

Thus, in widely different areas, cause and effect are understood through sequence as a form of organization. In the domain of research, counterbalancing is required in order to control for sequence. This process of counterbalancing acts as a control in the experimental design for the purpose of preventing potential confounds regarding inferences, with respect to the specification of whatever one variable or factor was the cause of or, conversely, the effect of, the same factor.

In the medical domain, algorithms and flow charts indicate "sequences" of events. That is, sequences ostensibly refer to "causes," depending on how strongly the reader is persuaded of the "processes," through which event A precedes event B. Thus, both algorithms and flow charts are forms of organization, that communicate the idea of "cause through sequence."

Similarly, models are forms of organization, used with concepts and theories in psychology, that may convey multiple causes in their sequential orders, including complicated "feedback" and recursive processes. In all of these abstractions, cause is equivalent to sequence in the events that are being explained. Formal sequences, not concrete, mechanical forms, are the representations of cause.

Many individuals and professionals, in their everyday lives, adhere quite unconsciously, to Hume's concept of causality. In Hume's view,

> every representation of causality should ultimately be derived from the representation of *mere coexistence*. Two contents which have appeared together in consciousness with sufficient frequency are ultimately transposed, through the mediating psychological function of "imagination," from a relationship of *mere contiguity, of mere spatial coexistence or temporal succession, into a causal relation. Mere local or temporal contiguity is transformed into causal by a simple mechanism of "association."* (Cassirer, 1955, p. 44, emphasis added)

I am in agreement with Cassirer, in his critique of Hume and also in his endorsement of Kant:

> According to Kant the principle of causality is a synthetic principle which enables us to spell out phenomena and so read them as experience. But this (i.e. Kant's) causal synthesis, like the synthesis which takes place in the concept of the object, involves a very specific analysis. Here again synthesis and analysis are necessary complements to each other. The fundamental flaw in Hume's psychology and his psychological critique of the concept of causality is that he does not sufficiently recognize this *analytical* function. (1955, pp. 43–44)

The generality of this form of causal reasoning based on "mere contiguity, of mere spatial co-existence" is emphasized by Cassirer, "we must come to the astonishing conclusion that Hume, in attempting to analyze the causal judgement of science, rather revealed a *source of all mythical explanations of the world*" (1955, pp. 44–45, emphasis added). The application of this generalization to both professionals and their counterparts draws on two cornerstones of Werner's (1948) comparative psychology of mental development.

First, Werner's concept of *formal parallels* underlies *analogous psychological processes* in widely differing populations and contexts. Here, the analogous psychological processes refer to the linkage, intrapsychically and interpersonally, between causality and sequence for both professionals and their counterparts.

Second, the heuristic value of Werner's concept of development reasserts that the magical (or mystical) forms of causal reasoning in which "mere coexistence or mere spatial contiguity" is relied on as sufficient for causal claims, coexist in the same individual with more mature forms of reasoning. These less mature forms of cognition coexist with levels of reasoning that require analysis (or differentiation in Wernerian terms) and the construction of a synthetic principle that *integrates* the sequences of events into the coherent causal explanations required in science, law, or the humanities.

The development of individuals in our society facilitates the linkage between cause and sequence in interpersonal interactions. In childhood, the authority of the parents is often misinterpreted as parental omnipotence and omniscience. The overly sharp distinction between "experts" and "novices" in many aspects of life favors the persistence of the misattribution of omnipotence and omniscience to professionals. Both omnipotence and omniscience are violations of one of our fundamental assumptions: the differentiation between self and others. Such an assumption leads to necessary constraints, resulting from a professional's realization that another person's life is distinct from one's own.

In addition to such intrapsychic assumptions that spuriously link cause and sequence are the traditional asymmetrical sequences between professionals and their counterparts. A major reason for the persistence of traditional, asymmetrical interactions is the assumption, commonly made by all parties involved, that the nonexperts *do not know* and are therefore not in a position to inquire about, or to contradict the questions asked by the professional. The latter is assumed to be addressing the important, valid, and relevant topics at hand, even when such questions do not make sense to the patient, student, or research participant. They may shrug (mentally), but in most instances counterparts feel that they are required to answer the professional's questions in the manner in which they were asked.

FEATURES OF A PARTNERSHIP IDEAL

The previous section focused on comparing traditional and partner relationships. In the following section, four features of a partnership model are addressed. These are:

1. differentiation between self and other as a basic assumption,
2. changing both partners' behaviors through Sigel's Psychological Distancing Activities (PDAs),
3. a coexistence concept of development as facilitating empathy between partners, and
4. the value orientations regulating partnerships—namely reciprocal altruism and by-product mutualism.

No One Is a "Mind Reader": Differentiation Between the Self and Other as a Basic Assumption

Because no one is a "mind reader," the first main feature of a partnership ideal to be addressed is the importance of differentiation between one's own beliefs, assumptions, and needs and those of others. This theoretical premise is an aspect of a developmental orientation, as a very general implication of the orthogenetic principle, outlined by Werner (1948, 1957). Here the differentiation principle requires the professional to determine "where the other person is coming from." Professionals may attain a greater understanding of what the other person knows through a reliance on the other person's questions and feedback regarding the professional's initiatives. These activities are prerequisites to a negotiated agreement between partners.

Differentiation between partners in an interaction is necessary in order to acknowledge not only the fact that professionals and counterparts are different from one another, but also that patients, students, and research participants have their own distinctive contributions to make to a partnership. This differentiation between the contributions of professionals and counterparts must be recognized as part of the sequence leading to a negotiated understanding between partners.

From this perspective, the traditional, asymmetrical IRE is interpreted as resulting in fusion between the self as professional and others as patients, students, or research participants. Concrete exemplars of "fusion" attitudinally may include conversations that center around the assumption that "since you don't know what I know, I will tell you." This attitude equates "difference" between self and others with the notion that the professional "knows" and the "other" (patient, student, research participant) does not know what the professional knows. In terms of such knowledge, professionals erroneously assume that ignorance is not knowing versus knowing things that may or may not be congruent with the professional's own belief system.

Such professionals erroneously subscribe to the "conduit metaphor" (Reddy, 1979). In doing so, they assume that information can be directly "transferred" from themselves to their counterparts; rather than positing that communication, entails the transformation of *messages* by the recipient of the message from the sender (the professional), and conversely from the patient to the professional.

There are two other formal possibilities that deviate from the ideal of differentiation as articulated in Werner's principle of orthogenesis (1948): 1) differentiation and isolation between partners; and 2) differentiation and conflict between partners. In the case of differentiation and isolation, there is recognition of the differentiation between professional and counterpart but no *explicit* attempt is made by the professional to bridge the distance between him/herself and their counterparts. Attitudinally, this is manifest in a "take it or leave it" approach. The professional's attitude is one of "doing their job, period," which entails the traditional assumptions of the IRE.

The difference between "lack of differentiation" and "differentiation and isolation" is that in the former case, the professional assumes that the "transfer" of information will occur. In the latter case, the professional makes no such assumption. Rather, there is a clear acknowledgment that their counterpart is "different" and might not immediately and completely comprehend the messages they have sent. But professionals, through their evaluations, distance themselves from their counterparts. Under this assumption, it is the patient's, the student's, or the research participant's "responsibility" to "hear" what is being told to her. They are evaluated, either positively or negatively, with respect to this stance by the professional. There are articulate concepts and vocabularies relied on by professionals that "justify" the negative evaluations by professionals of their counterparts.

The literatures on noncompliance in medicine, unmotivated and disinterested students in educational contexts, and uncooperative participants in research demonstrate that professionals need go no further than to "affix" such a label in order to be "understood" within their community. The reasons for noncompliance, however, are not sought. "Where the other person is coming from" need not be a legitimate question. Consequently, these professionals feel that it is not their responsibility to work to overcome the isolation between the professional and their counterpart. Such labels could be interpreted as low-level distancing acts according to Sigel's model of psychological distance (1978, 1993).

A "formal" description of differentiation and conflict between professionals and their counterparts subsumes two kinds of conflict: 1) conflicts between professionals and their counterparts with respect to the concrete goals which are *implicit* in the relationship; or 2) acceptance of the concrete goals between professionals and their counterparts *but* the existence of conflict (implicit or explicit) regarding the means to attain the agreed on ends.

Conflicts regarding *ends* between professionals and their counterparts are often revealed, in all three domains, when the "vague, overall ends" that have been agreed to by patients, students, or research participants *are* concretized and made specific. A patient may tell their doctor "fine, I understand that we both want me to be cured of X, but I was not clear that becoming cured of X would *also* mean that I subscribe to this *other goal* with which I disagree."

In research interactions, the ends of the researcher in a particular study may not be clear to the research participant. Thus, the research participant may initially agree to be involved in a study. However, when the study gets under way and the goals of the researcher become clearer to the research participant the latter may no longer agree to participate. It is precisely for this reason that institutional review boards require that the researcher make clear to the research participant that the latter may, for any reason, refuse to continue participating at any time during the course of the study.

Similarly, in educational contexts, the initial goals of a course may entail subordinate or auxiliary goals that, as they become clear, constitute the basis for a conflict between teacher and student. This formal distinction of differentiation and conflict is important to the overall partnership approach. Unless this distinction is thoroughly recognized as a *possibility*, there is the danger that the "partnership" ideal becomes "pollyannish." Partnerships require *differentiation* and recognize that various conflicts may impede or indeed disrupt the partnership. It may well be the case that no partnerships can be envisaged because of pervasive and conflicting goals between potential partners. There is the further assumption that conflicts with regards to "means," where the ends are shared, are more negotiable, when compared to explicit conflicts between ends as principled and central values.

In contrast with these deviations, the ideal of differentiation and integration is an essential component of a partnership ideal. The formal concept of integration in Wernerian psychology is grounded here in the particulars of the criteria for a partnership ideal. The movement toward *more* symmetrical sequences between partners regarding questions, answers, and feedback is required of both partners. According to the principle of orthogenesis, the formal ideal is integration. In a partnership ideal, the principle of orthogenesis is actualized through *microgenetic changes* (in contrast with lifelong ontogenetic change) in the interactions between partners. These microgenetic changes may lead to a negotiated agreement between partners.

Changing Both Partners Through Sigel's Psychological Distancing Activities

The partnership ideal relies on Sigel's (1978, 1993) Psychological Distancing Activities (PDAs) as the psychological processes most conducive to positive change. Sigel's seminal, programmatic studies have shown the comparative value of high-level, versus low-level, psychological distancing activities. Interactions based on low-level distancing strategies (e.g., labels, descriptions, demonstrations) are consistently less effective than high-level distancing acts (e.g., comparisons, contrasts, and evaluations).

The partnership ideal relies on a speculative extension of Sigel's PDAs. This speculation goes beyond the teacher–student and child–parent interactions Sigel studied, by applying PDAs to the domains of medicine and research as well. For instance, when a patient or research participant is required to "produce information" or to "describe and define" as an answer to the professional's question, this serves as an example of the type of low-level distancing strategies typified in traditional interactions (for a further discussion of PDAs, please refer to Chapter 10).

In partnerships, there is pleasure and joy for the professional or expert who learns from a so-called novice, be it a patient, a student, or a research participant. The story of a 36-year-old man with Down's Syndrome, who was diagnosed with cancer, provides an illustration of an instance when an expert could learn a great deal from a patient. Rather than calling his affliction "cancer," as normal adults would, this man referred to it as a "boo boo." A traditional reaction to such a label by physicians and research psychologists would be to simply say that the patient is "wrong." Or to put it in a more derogatory fashion, a person who refers to cancer as a "boo boo" would be called "weird."

In contrast, a partnership approach would *require* the professional to explore this person's world. This exploration would lead the professional to a better understanding of how this patient's interpretation of cancer as a "boo boo" correlates with the ways in which the man, more generally, makes sense of his everyday life. The student who told me this story had an interesting question regarding cancer as a "boo boo": Did this *interpretation*, on the part of the patient, lessen his experience of the fears, pain, and anxiety ordinarily suffered by cancer patients? This type of question, which indicates an arousal of curiosity, would be an ideal reaction, on the part of a professional, when encountering a patient with radically different conceptions of illness.

A Coexistence Concept of Development Facilitates Empathy Between Partners

The difference in knowledge between professionals and their potential partners might be large, in some cases. Nonetheless, in partnerships professionals should be able to *empathize* with their respective partners. In developmental psychology, a coexistence concept of development (Bibace, Sagarin, & Dyl, 1998; Bibace, Dillon, & Sagarin, in this volume) offers a means through which this degree of empathy may be achieved by professionals. A coexistence concept of development accounts for the presence of both mature and immature concepts and irrational beliefs and feelings in all people. These immaturities coexist in professionals as well as in children and laypersons. A competent professional has presumably transcended these less mature conceptions, with respect to the parameters of professional interactions with their partners. But the coexistence of such immaturities in the person's concepts of illness can still be observed, as sometimes occurs when a physician becomes a patient!

A coexistence concept of development subscribes, epistemologically, to Will Rogers's aphorism "There is nothing so stupid as an educated man, if you get off the thing that he was educated in" (Stevenson, 1934, p. 529). In the domain of morality, the coexistence of good and evil is a cornerstone of Judeo-Christian tradition. Both epistemologically and morally, the coexistence concept focuses on variabilities *within* each and every person, not merely on differences *between* people. These variabilities posit a broad range of psychological processes, present within each person.

The coexistence concept of development is offered as a necessary modifier and counterbalance to the numerous concepts that are used to validate consistencies between individuals. In developmental psychology, the search for order has resulted in concepts such as stages, phases, and so on. Nomothetic order is necessary for science. But competency as a professional *requires* flexible accommodation to the variabilities within one's self and one's partner, as well. Empathic accommodations must be based on an understanding by the professional of his/her own limitations, variabilities, and lack of knowledge and understanding.

Most importantly, it is helpful for professionals to appreciate their own microgenesis, an awareness of progressions from their own past ignorance to their present level of understanding. The opportunity for a professional to *learn from* his/her partner presents a great challenge.

Some readers may think that such "ideals" are unrealistic, that such bridges cannot be forged between professionals (with their highly advanced knowledge), and patients, students, or research participants. Yet evidence suggests that such "bridges" are not only possibilities, but are an *acknowledged* aspect of the way in which professionals experience their lives. The "acknowledgement" section of many books written by physicians and teachers often explicitly states how much they have learned from their patients or students, though this is much less frequently the case for researchers in psychology. Seldom will an experimental psychologist thank his/her research participants in a similar fashion. My unsubstantiated guess is that this widespread lack of recognition on the part of researchers stems from the fact that many behavioral scientists still believe that it is their task to "run subjects," rather than interact with persons in their studies.

The biblical "golden rule," that we should "do to others as we would have them do to us," has many contemporary counterparts in psychology. One such counterpart favored by developmental psychologists is "taking the role of the other." Even more widespread is the importance attributed to "empathy" by many human service professionals.

From a partnership perspective, empathy is valuable in many cases. According to Zahn-Waxler and Radke-Yarrow (1990), "empathy refers, in various ways to the experiencing of another's affective or psychological state and has both affective and cognitive components" (p. 108). When a professional acts with empathy and sensitivity toward the discrepancy in power between themselves and their partners, the likelihood is greater that the partner will choose to ask questions and provide clear and direct feedback to the professional.

But while empathy is a significant component to a partnership ideal, this value must be subordinated to differentiation. It is expected that empathy would consist of "A's" personal thoughts and feelings regarding how "B" thinks and feels. But problems arise when empathy is relied on as justification for "A's" actions with respect to "B."

At times, "A's" empathy for "B" may not be limited to his/her sensitive thoughts and feelings about "B." Rather, "A's" thoughts and feelings are translated into action, with empathy as justification. "A's" empathy has therefore moved beyond the intrapsychic realm and into her interpersonal relationship with "B."

Conversely, when differentiation between self and other is taken as the primary assumption, empathy is relegated to a subordinate role. While empathy is considered to be a desirable trait, it is neither necessary nor sufficient, in many cases. Empathy is not necessary in many partner relationships because "A" should first ask "B" what s/he wants. Or, "A" should verify with "B" whether the assumptions s/he has made are correct. Empathy is not sufficient in that such a basis for action is, from this perspective, interpreted as a lack of differentiation between one's self and others.

The sequence required in a partnership is to assign priority to the questions "A" should ask of "B." "A" should avoid making unwarranted assumptions that the answer s/he prefers is also favored by "B." Even such questions and answers between "A" and "B" prior to an act constitute only two aspects of the ideal, symmetrical partnership. Ideally both "A" and "B" should provide each other feedback after the activity agreed on in the question/answer sequences, that took place prior to the act.

The persistent reliance by some professionals on "empathy" as "justification" for actions is here interpreted as another example of "self-centeredness." The reliance on "personal associations," labeled as empathy, as a rationale for actions is rejected in a partnership ideal. The analytical principle, required by Kant, in contrast to Hume's associations, applies here. In this case, the relevant, analytical principle is the symmetrical sequence. As noted repeatedly above, the behavioral referents, in symmetrical, partner relationships, in comparison with traditional, asymmetrical relationships, are questions, answers, and feedback.

Value Orientations Regulating Partnerships

The value orientations regulating such partnerships draw on many sources, focusing on the bilateral, symmetrical mutualities between partners. Partnerships are distinctive in that they ground such values and mutualities in the everyday activities required of professionals and their partners. Questions and answers are intrinsic to traditional interactions.

Questions, answers, and feedback are the concrete means, the psychological processes behind the implementation of partnerships. In a partnership, a recognition of the importance of both "giving" and "getting" is needed. Such values transcend the traditional dichotomy, that dictates that the professional be the "giver" of knowledge. Some of the numerous fields that have contributed to these value orientations include religion, sociology, and more recently, evolutionary psychology (e.g., Mesterton-Gibbons & Dugatkin, 1997). The latter field differentiates between reciprocal altruism and by-product mutualism. I have interpreted the former as related to "give and take," the reciprocities that occur in the present between both partners. In contrast, by-product mutualism addresses that which is beneficial to both the group and society, along with the immediate participants in the partnership.

There is little originality in the abstract goals, or the telos of partnerships as an ideal. Such goals have been reiterated by professionals in many different fields. This interpretation of partnerships is most compatible with the "mutualities" advocated by Erik Erikson (1963). The mutualities between mother and infant as a nursing couple espouse "complementarity" and "reciprocity," but not equality. The behavioral activities of the mother as "giver" and the baby as "getter" are specified as the complementarity and reciprocity involved in this relationship.

At a sociocultural level, the French sociologist Mauss has argued that "socialization" depends on the "gift." When an individual "gives" to another, such an activity is conducive to the reciprocal activity of "getting." Certainly, anthropologists have described such relationships. The "potlatch" among Kwakinbl Indians depends on reciprocal "giving" and "getting" of blankets between members of the tribe. Interestingly, "giving" results in higher social status in this tribe. The person who "gives" the greatest number of blankets is the most highly regarded among his/her peers.

This interpretation of partnerships relies on Werner's "world of action," the practical, everyday activities as the analogous processes, that constitute the basis for abstractions. These abstractions include values or principles that are intrinsic to the identity of a professional.

CONCLUSION

The inherent tensions between individuals and groups, that I began discussing at the opening of this chapter, are also present within a partnership ideal, as illustrated in the juxtaposition of two significant assumptions in partner relationships. On the one hand, it has been argued that through a coexistence concept of development, similarities between partners constitute a basis for bridging the knowledge gaps between them. On the other hand, the *differentiation* assumption posits that the differences between self and other are primary. In balancing coexistence and differentiation, I favor the primacy of the differentiation assumption. The general implication is to subordinate empathy and assumptions regarding the benevolent intentions of professionals, to the value of differentiation.

From a partnership perspective, the biblical "golden rule" gives primacy to what is referred to here as coexistence, the empathic basis for similarities between self and other. Certainly, that aspect of the "golden rule" is endorsed by a partnership ideal. But partnerships, first and foremost, require an attitude of differentiation between the actions, the activities we would want others to "do" for us, or with us, compared to what *we assume* others want us to "do" for them or with them. The primacy of differentiating between the self and other in this version of partnerships requires the "doer" to "ask and not assume" that the partner thinks and feels the same way as one's self.

Benevolent intentions based on one's own thoughts and feelings are insufficient. Such thoughts and feelings are often important ingredients in the *sequence* of activities between partners. It is the questions and answers that *precede* the actions that are considered primary in partnerships. Further, the tentativeness, the fragility of the partnership, is underscored if one assumes that questions and answers by both partners are sufficient. The consequences of the actions, agreed on by both partners, must also be assimilated by both individuals. This "back and forth" between partners leads to modifications or adjustments, which themselves are aspects of the interpersonal processes that lead to an agreement "understood" in both thought and action by the members of a partnership.

The concept of conflict has positive connotations in the Piagetian sense of "disequilibrium" or "tension" between partners. This type of tension constitutes the telos, or *drive* toward "dialogicality," the reciprocal moves backward and forward in which partners are engaged as they work toward a negotiated understanding. There is pleasure inherent in the *complementarity* of a partnership, since one partner "supplies what is wanting" to the other.

Without initial diversity there would be no need for reciprocity and complementarity. Again the concept of "differentiation" between the self and other is a guarantor that the differences between individuals should be taken into account and valued by each of the partners. Further, even partners who have known each other over long periods of time, for example, a family physician who has known a patient for decades, should subscribe to the differentiation assumption. This assumption recognizes not only "individual differences," but also the importance of intraindividual variability, that may emerge as discontinuity; behaviors that neither the patient themselves, nor the doctor are able to explain. For instance, some patients who have been very clear with "advanced directives" in the doctor–patient relationships may radically change their wishes at some later time.

The *ideal* of differentiation and integration between partners has been expressed by Kahilil Gibran (1923) in a poem. This poem has been frequently used by ministers performing marriage ceremonies:

> Give your hearts, but not into each other's keeping.
> For only the hand of Life can contain your hearts.
> *And stand together yet not too near together:*
> *For the pillars of the temple stand apart.*
> And the oak tree and the cypress grow root in each
> other's shadow. (p. 20, emphasis added)

The differentiation idea is clearly expressed in the italicized couplet and the image of the shared end of the pillars of the temple is also clear. The negative consequences of lack of differentiation (growth does not occur in each other's shadow) is also explicit.

REFERENCES

Balint, M. (1964). *The doctor, the patient and the illness* (2nd ed.) New York: International Universities Press.

Bibace, R. Sagarin, J., & Dyl, J. (1998). The heuristic value of Werner's co-existence concept of development. *Journal of Applied Developmental Psychology, 19,* 153–163.

Cassirer, E. (1955). *The philosophy of symbolic forms: Vol. 2. Mythical thought.* New Haven: Yale University Press.

Cazden, C. (1988). *Classroom discourse.* Portsmouth, NH: Heinemann.

Cohen, M. R., & Nagel, E. (1934). An introduction to science and logic. New York: Harcourt Brace.

The compact edition of the Oxford English dictionary. (1971). Oxford, England: Oxford University Press.

Erikson, E. (1963). *Childhood and society.* New York: W. W. Norton.

Foucault, M. (1973). *The birth of the clinic: An archaeology of medical perception.* New York: Random House.

Gibran, K. (1923). *The prophet.* New York: Alfred A. Knopf.

Handlon, J. H. (1960). A metatheoretical view of assumptions regarding the etiology of schizophrenia: Implications for research. *Archives of General Psychiatry, 2*, 53–70.

Irwin, T. H. (1998). Aristotle. In E. Craig (Ed.), *Routledge encyclopedia of philosophy.* (Vol. 1) (pp. 414–435). London: Routledge.

Kimble, G. A. (1984). Psychology's two cultures. *American Psychologist, 39,* 833–839.

Kuhn, T. S. (1970). *The Structure of Scientific Revolutions.* Chicago: University of Chicago Press.

Lemke, J. L. (1990). *Talking science: Language, learning, and values.* Norwood, NJ: Ablex Publishing Co.

Levy, E. (1943). Some aspects of the schizophrenic formal disturbance of thought. *Psychiatry (Journal of the Biology and Pathology of Interpersonal Relations), 6,* 55–70.

Mehan, H. (1979). *Learning lessons.* Cambridge: Harvard University Press.

Mesterson-Gibbons, M., & Dugatikin, L. A. (1997). Cooperation and the prisoner's dilemma: Towards testable models of mutualism versus reciprocity. *Animal Behavior, 54,* 551–557.

Mishler, E. G. (1986). *Research interviewing: Context and narrative.* Cambridge: Harvard University Press.

O'Connor, M. C., & Michaels, S. (1993). Aligning academic task and participation status through revoicing: Analysis of a classroom discourse strategy. *Anthropology and Education Quarterly, 24,* 318–335.

Piaget, J., & Inhelder, B. (1969). *The psychology of the child.* New York: Basic Books.

Reddy, M. (1979). The conduit metaphor—A case of frame conflict in our language about language. In A. Ortony (Ed.), *Metaphor and thought.* Cambridge: Cambridge University Press.

Sigel, I. E. (1978). The development of pictorial comprehension. In B. S. Randhawa & W. E. Coffman (Eds.), *Visual learning, thinking, and communication* (pp. 93–111). New York: Academic Press.

Sigel, I. E. (1993). The centrality of a distancing model for the development of representational competence. In R. R. Cocking & E. Renninger (Eds.), *The development and meaning of psychological distance.* Hillsdale, NJ: Lawrence Erlbaum.

Sinclair, J. M., & Coulthard, R. M. (1976). *Toward an analysis of discourse: The English used by teachers and pupils.* London: Oxford University Press.

Sowell, T. (1987). *A conflict of visions.* New York: William Morrow.

Stevenson, B. (1934). *The home book of quotations.* New York: Dodd, Mead.

Werner, H. (1948). *Comparative psychology of mental development.* New York: International Universities Press.

Werner, H. (1957). The concept of development from a comparative and organismic point of view. In D.B. Harris (Ed.), *The concept of development: An issue in the study of human behavior*. Minneapolis: University of Minnesota Press.

Wriston, H. M. (1960). The individual in the American assembly. In *Goals for Americans.* New York: Prentice-Hall, Inc.

Zahn-Waxler, C., & Radke-Yarrow, M. (1990). The origins of empathetic concern. *Motivation and Emotion, 14,* 107–130.

AUTHOR INDEX

SUBJECT INDEX

www.ingramcontent.com/pod-product-compliance
Ingram Content Group UK Ltd.
Pitfield, Milton Keynes, MK11 3LW, UK
UKHW041131071026
15587UKWH00009B/411

9 781567 504545